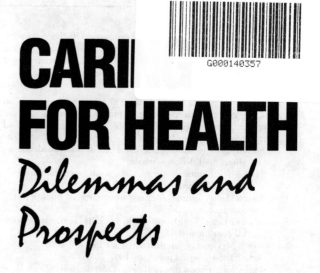

CARING FOR HEALTH
Dilemmas and Prospects

prepared by the U205 Course Team

THE OPEN UNIVERSITY
Health and Disease   U205   Book VIII
A Second Level Course

THE OPEN UNIVERSITY PRESS

The U205 Course Team

U205 is a course whose writing and production has been the joint effort of many hands: a 'core course team', colleagues who have written on specific aspects of the course but have not been involved throughout, editors, designers, and the BBC team.

Core Course Team

The following people have written or commented extensively on the whole course, been involved in all phases of its production and accept collective responsibility for its overall academic and teaching content.

Steven Rose (neurobiologist; course team chair; academic editor; Book VI coordinator)

Nick Black (community physician; Book IV coordinator; Book VIII coordinator)

Basiro Davey (immunologist; course manager; Book V coordinator)

Alastair Gray (health economist; Book III coordinator; Book VII coordinator)

Kevin McConway (statistician; Book I coordinator)

Jennie Popay (social policy analyst)

Phil Strong (medical sociologist; academic editor; Book II coordinator)

Other authors

The following authors have contributed to the overall development of the course and have taken responsibility for writing specific sections of it.

Lynda Birke (ethologist; author, Book V)

Eric Bowers (parasitologist; staff tutor)

David Boswell (sociologist; author, Book II)

Eva Chapman (psychotherapist; author, Book V)

Andrew Learmonth (geographer; course team chair 1983; author, Book III)

Rosemary Lennard (medical practitioner; author, Books IV and V)

Jim Moore (historian of science; author, Book II)

Sean Murphy (neurobiologist; author, Book VI)

Rob Ransom (developmental biologist; author, Book IV)

George Watts (historian; author, Book II)

The following people have assisted with particular aspects or parts of the course.

Steve Best (illustrator)

Sheila Constantinou (BBC production assistant)

Gerald Copp (editor)

Ann Hall (indexer)

Debbie Crouch (designer)

Mark Kesby (illustrator)

Liz Lane (editor)

Vic Lockwood (BBC producer)

Laurie Melton (librarian)

Peggy Stevens (course secretary)

Jacqueline Stewart (managing editor until January 1985)

Sue Walker (editor)

Peter Wright (editor)

External consultant

Gerry Stimson (medical sociologist) Department of Sociology, Goldsmiths College, University of London.

Book VIII Assessors

Michael Clarke Professor of Epidemiology, Department of Community Health, University of Leicester.

Howard Glennerster Professor of Social Administration, Department of Social Science and Administration, The London School of Economics and Political Science.

Gordon Horobin Deputy Director, MRC Medical Sociology Unit, University of Aberdeen.

Acknowledgements

The course team wishes to thank the following for their advice and contributions:

Sheila Adam (community physician) North West Thames Regional Health Authority.

John Ashton (community physician) Department of Community Health, University of Liverpool.

Robert Dingwall (medical sociologist) Centre for Socio-Legal Studies, Wolfson College, Oxford.

Alex Gatherer (community physician) District Medical Officer, Oxfordshire Health Authority.

Lyn Jones (operational researcher) Department of Community Medicine, University of Edinburgh.

Anne Murcott (sociologist) Department of Sociology, University of Cardiff; Department of Psychological Medicine, Welsh National School of Medicine.

Chris Pond Low Pay Unit, London.

Adrian Sinfield (social policy analyst) Department of Social Administration, University of Edinburgh.

Barbara Stocking (health policy analyst) Kings Fund College, London.

Malcolm Walker (medical practitioner) Department of Cardiology, University of Oxford.

About this book

A note for the general reader

Caring for Health: Dilemmas and Prospects is the eighth of a series of books on the subject of health and disease. The book is designed so that it can be read on its own, like any other textbook, or studied as part of U205 *Health and Disease*, a second level course for Open University students. As well as the eight textbooks and a Course Reader, *Health and Disease: A Reader*,* the course consists of eleven TV programmes and five audiocassettes plus various supplementary materials.

Open University students will receive an *Introduction and Guide* to the course, which sets out a study plan for the year's work. This is supplemented where appropriate in the text by more detailed directions for OU students; these study comments at the beginning of chapters are boxed for ease of reference. Also, in the text you will find instructions to refer to the Course Reader. It is quite possible to follow the argument without reading the articles referred to, although your understanding will be enriched if you do so. Major learning objectives are listed at the end of each chapter along with questions that allow students to assess how well they are achieving those objectives. The index includes key words (in bold type) which can be looked up easily as an aid to revision as the course proceeds. There is also a further reading list for those who wish to pursue certain aspects of study beyond the limits of this book.

*Black, Nick *et al.* (1984) *Health and Disease: A Reader*, Open University Press.

A guide for OU students

In this book we examine the dilemmas that confront those involved in caring for health and consider the prospects for the solutions that are currently being proposed. The book has two major themes. The first is that the dilemmas we face will only be resolved by adopting a broad strategy that combines and integrates the contributions of several disciplines, including economics, biology, sociology, medicine, statistics, epidemiology and social policy. And second, that many of the proposed solutions create in turn a new set of dilemmas.

The book concentrates on one particular country, the UK, and on one health care system, the NHS. Despite the fact that the NHS is in several respects an atypical system of care, many of the dilemmas it faces are common to all health care systems in industrialised countries. We assume that you may not be familiar with the way in which the NHS is organised, so in Chapter 1 we describe the basic organisational arrangements, and how they have changed since 1948. These aspects are considered in more detail in Chapters 2 and 3, which discuss the NHS, first from a national perspective and then at a local level. This involves considering the political, economic and managerial aspects of how the health service operates. In Chapter 4 we take a closer look, by examining the service that individuals receive, in particular the way staff talk, or don't talk, to us.

The NHS is only one, albeit important, part of health care in the UK. Most caring is still provided by lay people. In Chapter 5 the current policy of shifting the boundary between formal and lay care is considered. This also serves to introduce the second half of the book in which current strategies for resolving dilemmas are discussed: Chapter 6 examines the contribution of innovations; Chapter 7 discusses the various methods both for evaluating and monitoring the effectiveness, efficiency, equality and humanity of the NHS; Chapter 8 considers the contribution that screening for early signs of disease can make; and Chapter 9 assesses the opportunities for and obstacles to preventing disease and promoting health.

Up to Chapter 10, the book is largely concerned with the contribution that health care can make to improving our health. But as you have seen in other books in this course, the main determinants of health and disease lie far beyond the reach of health services — poor housing, poverty, unemployment and other social and economic factors. In Chapter 10 we consider how, in the words of the nineteenth-century health reformer Sir John Simon, it may be possible 'to make the poor less poor' through changes in far-ranging aspects of public policy.

In Chapter 11, an attempt is made to pull together the various subjects of Chapters 6–10 around a single topic — coronary heart disease. What emerges is that while each solution has a useful and significant contribution to make, it is important to avoid exaggerating the prospects of success and to retain a cautious realism. Finally, the book ends at Chapter 12 with a glance at the future, and some of the prospects that may lie ahead.

The time allowed for studying Book VIII is four weeks or 40 hours. The following table gives you a more detailed breakdown — to help you to pace your study. You need not follow it slavishly but do not allow yourself to fall behind. If you find a section of the work difficult, do what you can at this stage, and then rework the material at the end of your study of this book.

Study time for Book VIII (total 40 hours)

Chapter	Time/ hours	Course Reader	Time/ hours	TV and audiocassettes	Time/ hours
1	1¼				
2	4	Enthoven (1984)	¾	Audio sequence: Band 3, AC807	¾
3	3	Paterson (1981)	¾	TV programme 10: 'The Primary Health Care Team' Audio sequence: Band 4, AC808	1½
4	3	Jeffery (1979)	¾		
5	1¾				
6	3				
7	3¼	Cochrane (1971) Piauchaud and Weddell (1972) 'Ethical dilemmas' (1980/2)	¾ ¾ ¼		
8	1½				
9	3¼	GMBATU (1984) Hart (1981)	¾ ¾	TV programme 11: 'Asian Rickets: the English Disease' Audio sequence: Band 5, AC808	1
10	3				
11	2				
12	1½	West (1984)	¾		

Assessment There is no TMA (tutor-marked assignment) associated with this book.

Contents

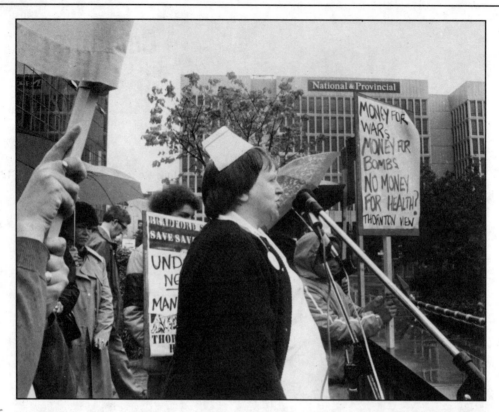

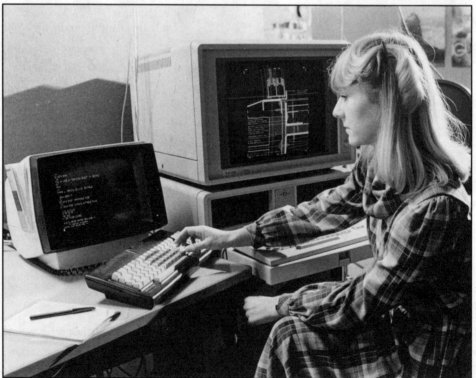

1

Introduction

This chapter takes up where chapter 10 in Book VII, *Caring for Health: History and Diversity* left off. It considers the development of the organisational structure of the NHS, building on the discussion of its creation in Chapter 5 of Book VII.

During this chapter you will be referred to the Course Reader for the article 'The structure of the National Health Service' by Gwyn Bevan (Part 4, Section 4.2). You may wish to read it at the end of the chapter, or use it to refer to during your reading of the rest of the book.

At midnight on July 5, 1948, Jean Murray was the first baby to be born into the care of the National Health Service (NHS). This book is about the achievements and performance of the NHS since then, the criticisms that have been levelled at it, the dilemmas it currently faces and its prospects for the future. While the NHS is our main concern, it is important to remember that caring for health involves not only the care provided by nurses and doctors, hospitals and health centres, but also that provided by friends and relatives, social services and charities, and, increasingly, by private facilities. We must therefore consider the NHS within this context. In addition, as our concern is not only the treatment and care of the sick, infirm and disabled but also the prevention of disease and production of health, we must also discuss the opportunities that exist to modify the social conditions and structures that influence people's health. We must, therefore, consider wider aspects of social policy, beyond that of health care.

Open any newspaper and the dilemmas facing the NHS are all too apparent:

> ### 'Millions wasted' on tonsil operations
> Huge savings could be made in the NHS if doctors spent more time assessing the real benefits of the treatment they give against the cost ... At present millions are still spent on operations to remove tonsils and adenoids from which few children really benefited, Dr Malcolm Forsythe, regional medical officer to the South East Thames Regional Health Authority said.
> (Nicholas Timmins, *The Times*, April 6, 1981)

Hospital 'danger' unit row

Health chiefs have come under fire from worried parents over the handling of plans to site a 'Broadmoor-style' secure unit in a mental hospital on their doorstep. Families living in the area claim officials have made up their minds about the unit without giving them a chance to voice a full protest.

(Danny McGrory, *Daily Express*, October 6, 1980)

Health care becomes a lottery

Mrs Jean Tremarco was at her Liverpool home yesterday hoping that she might have better luck next week if a consultant gynaecologist has another lottery to decide which patients can have an operation.

(Malcolm Stuart, *The Guardian*, October 16, 1980)

Rebel health chiefs defiant after losing case on cuts

The rebel Brent Health Authority ... moved closer to being sacked by Mr Fowler, Social Services Secretary, when it voted ... to reject the cuts.

(David Fletcher, *Daily Telegraph*, October 18, 1983)

Lack of cash 'killing' transplant patients

The confidential report on the future of heart transplants, shortly to be sent to the Social Services Secretary ... shows that sixty-eight patients have died waiting for the operation.

(Andrew Veitch, *The Guardian*, January 28, 1985)

Woman, 69, wins ban on fluoride

A grandmother from Glasgow, who has no teeth of her own, won a three-year court battle yesterday to stop Strathclyde Regional Council adding fluoride to its water supply ... in an attempt to combat what was then the worst tooth decay record in Britain.

(*The Times*, June 30, 1983)

Demand for inquiry over patients who are 'left to die'

There were calls yesterday for a Government inquiry into the treatment of kidney patients as the case of a former mental patient from Oxford who was refused further dialysis treatment focused attention on life or death decisions being made by doctors in NHS renal units.

(Charles Laurence, *Daily Telegraph*, January 9, 1985)

☐ What are the principal dilemmas for the NHS that these reports illustrate?

■ 1 The question of the *effectiveness* of health care (tonsil operations).

2 *Cost*, and the lack of sufficient resources to meet the need for care (gynaecology operations, renal dialysis and heart transplants).

3 Who *controls* and *makes decisions* about the services provided: experts or lay people (siting of a secure unit), central government or health authorities ('rebel health chiefs'); and *how* such decisions are made (gynaecology lottery).

4 Limitations of *personal rights and liberty*: the liberty of doctors to exercise their clinical freedom (tonsil operations), the liberty of individuals to challenge the introduction of public health measures (fluoridation of water), the right of individuals to receive necessary care (renal dialysis case).

5 *Inequality in access* to care (renal dialysis case).

6 *Technical and scientific developments* which cannot be afforded (heart transplant, renal dialysis).

Providing health care is beset with difficulties. Although these newspaper reports all refer to the NHS in the 1980s, they illustrate the principal dilemmas that all health care systems have to contend with. Despite both international and historical diversity in the way health care has been provided, the same problems recur.* However, the way such problems are manifested depends on the particular way in which services are organised. For example, all systems have to ration health care. Whether care is rationed on the basis of ability to pay (as occurs in a private, free-market system) or on the basis of a person's need (as, in theory at least, occurs in the NHS) depends on the type of system.

One of the great difficulties in discussing a system as massive and as complex as the NHS is deciding where to begin. Another is that no single perspective can encompass all aspects of a system. For example, if we wish to explore the problem of inequality in the availability of health care, it is necessary to consider not only the way the government allocates resources to different parts of the country, but also the way such factors as the gender, social class and ethnicity of people may affect how health staff treat them. In other words, to gain a complete view of health care we need to adopt several different perspectives, for each can reveal some key aspects that are essential to understanding the whole system.

The NHS is unique in many ways, but particularly there is one aspect that marks it out from almost all other systems of health care: its attempt to provide a national, comprehensive service. We therefore start our exploration of the NHS in Chapter 2 by considering the dilemmas that this key feature gives rise to. Given that the need for health care is potentially unlimited, but resources are always limited, how can health services be planned that are equally available to all and that attempt to meet all serious need? Not only that, but how can such a service be planned on a national basis so that it achieves a high degree of effectiveness, efficiency and humanity?

In Chapter 3, the focus shifts away from the national level and examines the dilemmas that confront those responsible for managing services locally, in the health districts. This raises such questions as who should decide how resources are spent — lay people or experts — and to what extent can services actually be planned rationally? However, even these issues are far removed from the sorts of dilemmas that the public are most aware of — those that they experience when they use the health service. Some of

these are the subject of Chapter 4, where we consider the difficulties that can arise when patients meet health service staff. What kind of service do people actually get? To what extent are they involved in decision making?

The relationship between lay people and the NHS is not confined to the public's *use* of the service. The laity and the NHS are also partners in *providing* care. Lay care is, as it always has been, the major source of care for people when they are sick or disabled. The dilemmas that arise when an attempt is made to shift the boundary between lay and formal care are considered in Chapter 5, in a discussion of the policy of 'Care in the Community'. Not only does this illustrate one of the key dilemmas facing the NHS, but it is also an example of one of the solutions that are being pursued to resolve the problems of inadequate resources. In this way, Chapter 5 both concludes the first section of the book on current dilemmas, and introduces the second, on prospects.

In Chapters 6 to 10 we consider those solutions that are currently being pursued, the contribution they might make in the future, and the dilemmas that they in turn give rise to: the development both of new treatments and new ways of organising health services (Chapter 6); the evaluation and monitoring of existing services to improve their effectiveness, efficiency, equality and humanity (Chapter 7); attempts to detect diseases earlier by screening people so that treatment may be both more effective and efficient (Chapter 8); and the wide range of strategies being pursued to prevent the onset of disease and to promote health (Chapter 9).

While all of these strategies may have a contribution to make to improving people's health, none of them explicitly addresses one of the major problems: the inequalities in health that exist between different social groups. What, if anything, can be done to reduce inequalities between males and females, higher and lower social classes, black people and white people? Chapter 10 discusses the different strategies that have been proposed and the obstacles that stand in their way.

Having, in Chapters 6 to 10, considered each of these approaches separately, Chapter 11 attempts to draw them together around a single subject — coronary heart disease — and to assess the relative prospects each approach offers. Finally, in Chapter 12, a speculative glance into the future offers some suggestions as to what the longer term prospects *might* be.

Such a wide-ranging brief requires contributions from several distinct disciplines: economics, sociology, social policy, epidemiology, political science, medicine and biology. In this respect the account of dilemmas and prospects in this book is unusual — individual disciplines usually work in isolation from one another. Unusual, but not unique. The need for a multidisciplinary approach that

*International and historical diversity in health care is discussed in The Open University (1985) *Caring for Health: History and Diversity*, The Open University Press. (U205 *Health and Disease*, Book VII.)

takes the theories, methods and findings of several disciplines into account is also the approach of *community medicine*. Since its creation in the ealy 1970s community medicine has widened its base from epidemiology, statistics and public health, to include the social sciences as well. This book is both a product of that development and, we believe, a contribution to it.

Introducing the NHS

Much of the material in this book, and especially in Chapters 2 and 3, assumes that the reader has some broad understanding of the way the NHS is organised. Even if you know nothing about its organisation, you will probably be aware that the structure of the NHS is not only complex, but also has a habit of changing. Neither fact is surprising, given the size, variety and constantly developing nature of formal health care. Traditionally, descriptions of the organisation of the NHS have dwelt in detail on the names and interrelationships of the committees and authorities, boards and councils. That degree of detail is not necessary for the subjects discussed in this book. However, without a firm grasp and understanding of the *main* features, it is impossible to enter and to take part in some of the key debates about the health service. In other words, it is necessary to understand *in broad terms* why the NHS is currently organised in the way it is. We will therefore start our account in 1948 and describe how the health service has evolved since then. There is no need to try to memorise the details, just aim to grasp the key features. One consequence of keeping the account as brief as possible is that many of the debates surrounding some of the issues are ignored. These, however, will be considered in subsequent chapters.

Although a similar pattern of services was established in Wales, Northern Ireland, Scotland and England, the detailed structure has varied. Rather than describe the development of all four structures, we shall confine our discussion to the NHS in England. A brief account of the major differences in Scotland, Wales and Northern Ireland appears at the end of the chapter.

The principal objectives in the creation of the NHS were to provide an equitable, rational and efficient system.* These were restated by the Royal Commission on the NHS in 1979 (Table 1.1). The objectives were to be achieved partly by *integrating* the management of the various existing elements: the public hospitals, which had been run by the local authorities since 1929, and included about 80 per cent of all hospital beds; the voluntary hospitals which were facing increasing financial problems; the various *community services*, such as health visiting and family planning which were provided by local authorities, under

*The creation of the NHS is discussed in greater detail in *Caring for Health: History and Diversity*, Chapter 5, *ibid*.

Table 1.1 The objectives of the NHS

To encourage and assist individuals to remain healthy
To provide equality of entitlement to health services
To provide a broad range of services of a high standard
To provide equality of access to these services
To provide a service free at the time of use
To satisfy the reasonable expectations of its users
To remain a national service responsive to local needs

(Source: Royal Commission on the NHS, 1979, p. 9)

the Medical Officers of Health; and finally, general practice, which was provided both privately and, for lower-paid workers, under the National Insurance Act of 1911 — though many were still excluded. There had been pressure for an integrated health care system for some time. In practice, the NHS that started life on the Appointed Day (July 5, 1948) was only partially integrated — this was only the start of integration, not its completion. In fact, since 1948 the NHS has been undergoing a series of reorganisations, in particular in 1974 and the early 1980s.

☐ In 1948, health care was restructured into three main parts (Figure 1.1). What were they?
■ 1 The hospitals (both voluntary and public) were nationalised under regional hospital boards, with the exception of the teaching hospitals which maintained their own boards.
2 General practice, along with dental and ophthalmic services, was organised under *executive councils*.
3 Community services and public health remained under the control of the Medical Officers of Health in the local authorities (such as city councils).

For all the significant achievements which resulted from the 1948 reorganisation, the failure to achieve a more integrated structure was to prove — so it was soon felt — to be one of the weaknesses of the system. The so-called *tripartite* (three-part) *structure* made the coordination and planning of new services difficult. Although the new structure allowed for a greater degree of coordination of formal health care, some large gaps remained: the Ministry of Health remained essentially advisory; General Practitioners (GPs) remained as *independent contractors*, that is, they were not salaried employees of the NHS but were simply contracted to work for the service as independent staff (they were and still are paid largely on the basis of the number of patients that are registered with them); and the teaching hospitals retained their freedom to select their patients for teaching purposes.

However, it would be wrong to attribute all the problems of the newly-created NHS to the tripartite

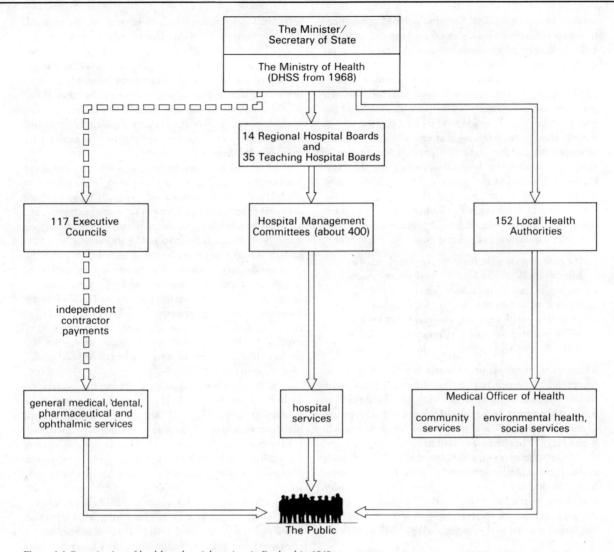

Figure 1.1 Organisation of health and social services in England in 1948.

structure. Even a fully-integrated service would have inherited all the old, long-standing problems of inadequate and inequitably distributed health services. Many of the existing hospitals had been built in the nineteenth century and were unsuited to the technical changes that had subsequently taken place in health care. Moreover, until the 1960s there was very strict financial control — virtually no new hospitals were built at all. So the new NHS had to function with old, out-dated facilities. In addition, the needs of the population were changing as many acute, infectious diseases came under control, while the population of elderly people with chronic conditions increased.

By the 1960s, after a decade of consolidation the structure of the NHS was coming under increasing

scrutiny. Widespread concern was reflected in a series of reports each of which led to changes in different parts of the service. First, the 1962 *Hospital Plan* established the model of each locality having its own *district general hospital* (DGH) which would provide all the basic acute services such as medicine, surgery, obstetrics and psychiatry. Second, during the 1960s under governmental auspices, the main health professions — doctors, nurses, social workers — reviewed both their internal and external working relationships. This led to important changes in the way these professions were regulated and structured. Third, at the start of the 1970s, Richard Crossman, the Secretary of State for Social Services (the Ministry of Health having been incorporated within the newly-established Department of Health and Social Security in 1968) commenced trying to redistribute resources away from the relatively well-off regions of the country. It was hoped that the establishment of new medical schools and teaching hospitals in areas lacking them (Nottingham, Leicester, Southampton) would contribute to this. Under the new plan, not only would each locality have its own DGH but each region of the UK would have its own medical school. Fourth, there was increasing concern about the steadily mounting demand for, and cost of, health care. During its first two decades the level of spending on the NHS increased 2.7 times in real terms and the number of staff doubled.

The final factor that gave an added urgency for reform was the decision to reorganise local government. As David Taylor, a sociologist, has pointed out:

> the time seemed right for creating complementary formats for NHS and local authority services and thus preparing the way for a better dovetailing of provisions. Some proponents of local authority control of health care may also have seen such moves as the first step towards a 'reintegration' of health with other welfare services. (Taylor, 1984, p.10)

There were, then, major pressures for the NHS to be reorganised. The debate over how to do this centred on three key topics: where should control of health services be based; what were to be the roles of experts and of lay people in control of the NHS; and what size of population should health services be organised around?

The first question — should control of health care reside at the *centre* (central government) or in the *periphery* (some form of local representative group) — had been considered in the late 1940s by the Minister of Health, Aneurin Bevan, the person most responsible for the legislation that led to the creation of the NHS in 1948.

> In framing the whole service we did deliberately come down in favour of a maximum of decentralisation to local bodies, a minimum of central approval, and the exercise of financial control through global budgets, relying for economy not so much on a tight and detailed Departmental grip, but on the education of the bodies concerned by the development of comparative costing, central supply and similar gradual methods of introducing efficiency and order among the heterogeneous mass of units we took over. (Bevan, cited in Klein, 1983, p.49)

Although the balance between the centre and the periphery has altered over the years, Bevan's view of the relationship has survived largely unscathed to the present day. It attempts to have the best of both worlds — to try to achieve equitable distribution of resources across the country while

retaining local autonomy on how those resources are used. This arrangement is a unique feature of formal health care in the UK. It represents a compromise between the two extremes, each of which is felt to have serious drawbacks: control of the NHS by central government *might* ensure a more even distribution of services across the country but would eliminate any accountability to local communities, while complete local control (such as by local government) might perpetuate significant inequalities in health care provision between different parts of the country.

The second key issue in reorganisation concerned the respective roles of experts and lay people in the control of the NHS. By the late 1960s it was generally recognised not only was there a need for greater managerial expertise, but also that health professionals, as the providers of services, must be more actively involved. However, it was also widely agreed that some degree of accountability to the local community was necessary. An attempt to resolve the competing claims of experts and lay people was the creation, in the 1974 reorganisation of the NHS, of *health authorities* made up principally of lay people (selected rather than elected) and *management teams* made up of experts (Figure 1.2). The health authorities were the decision-making bodies who were to be advised and guided by their management team.

The third issue was to decide on the size of population each health authority should cover. There were three competing claims. The 1962 *Hospital Plan* had encouraged the development of district general hospitals, each with their own catchment population. Thus one possibility was for health authorities to be based on these populations. However, the reorganisation of local authorities meant that social services and some other services relevant to health care, such as education for mentally handicapped children, were based on the new local authorities, most of which contained more than one DGH. There was therefore a strong case to make the health authorities cover the same population. Finally, there were the teaching hospitals and medical schools which had much wider catchment populations than the DGHs. Not only did they provide training facilities for staff, but they also housed the more specialised, tertiary services,* such as cardiac surgery. There was therefore a case for having a management level that corresponded to those larger catchment populations.

The strength of each claim was reflected in the 1974 reorganisation, which created what were termed 'regions', 'areas' and 'districts' (Figure 1.3). *Regional Health Authorities* (RHA) were created which covered populations of between two and six million people and

---

*Primary, secondary and tertiary services are discussed in *Caring for Health: History and Diversity, ibid.*, Chapter 9.

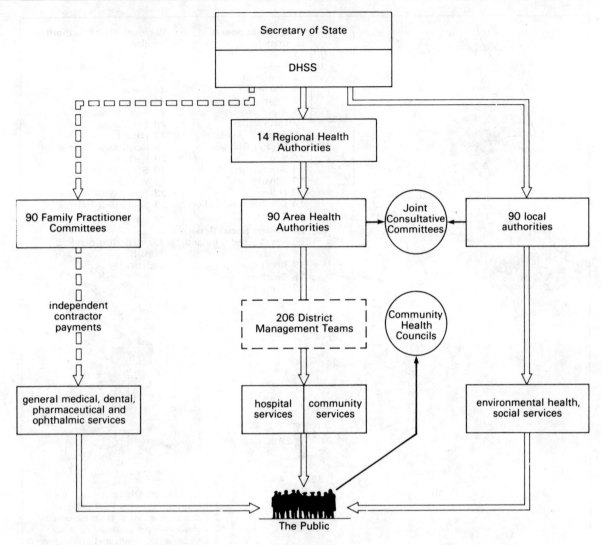

Figure 1.2 Organisation of health and social services in England in 1974.

contained at least one medical school. It was envisaged that regions would be largely self-sufficient as regards tertiary care. Below these RHAs were *Area Health Authorities* (AHA) which covered the same geographical areas as the newly-reorganised local authorities. Finally, just as regions were divided into areas, so areas were divided into *districts* based on the catchment population of each DGH. Although the districts had their own management team, unlike regions and areas, they did not have a health authority. (Some areas were not divided up into districts. In those cases the area and district functions were merged in one tier of management.) How was central government to maintain its influence over the NHS in the presence of so many health authorities? The answer lay in making use of

the *tiered system* of management: region, area and district. Each tier was made *accountable* to the tier above it and in return had *responsibility* delegated down to it. For example, AHAs delegated some responsibilities to their constituent districts which were in turn accountable to the AHA for their actions.

The executive councils (administrative bodies responsible for such tasks as the payment of GPs), which had been directly accountable to the Ministry of Health since 1948, were preserved as *Family Practitioner Committees* (FPC) with their catchment populations approximately the same as the AHAs, through whom they now received their funding. However, none of these alterations led to any significant improvement in integration between general

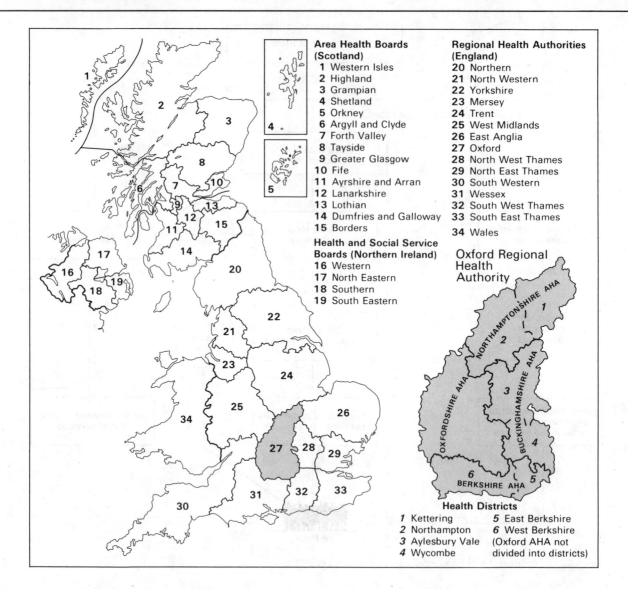

Area Health Boards (Scotland)
1 Western Isles
2 Highland
3 Grampian
4 Shetland
5 Orkney
6 Argyll and Clyde
7 Forth Valley
8 Tayside
9 Greater Glasgow
10 Fife
11 Ayrshire and Arran
12 Lanarkshire
13 Lothian
14 Dumfries and Galloway
15 Borders

Health and Social Service Boards (Northern Ireland)
16 Western
17 North Eastern
18 Southern
19 South Eastern

Regional Health Authorities (England)
20 Northern
21 North Western
22 Yorkshire
23 Mersey
24 Trent
25 West Midlands
26 East Anglia
27 Oxford
28 North West Thames
29 North East Thames
30 South Western
31 Wessex
32 South West Thames
33 South East Thames

34 Wales

Oxford Regional Health Authority

Health Districts
1 Kettering
2 Northampton
3 Aylesbury Vale
4 Wycombe
5 East Berkshire
6 West Berkshire
(Oxford AHA not divided into districts)

Figure 1.3 Geographical divisions of the NHS in 1974. The main divisions are shown (numbered 1–34). In England the Regional Health Authorities were divided into Area Health Authorities which in turn were usually subdivided into health districts (the sub-divisions of Oxford RHA are shown).

practice and hospital care. The only other aspect of personal care which was not integrated was that of occupational health care, which remained, as it always had been, the responsibility of employers.

There was one further change in 1974, which reflected the growth of consumer interest in health care. A *Community Health Council* (CHC), made up of lay people, was established in each district, to represent consumer interests.

On 1 April 1974 the reorganised NHS came into existence. Not surprisingly there was considerable con-

fusion and uncertainty about the new arrangements, but this was mixed with some optimism that it would now be possible to produce a comprehensive, integrated system of health care.

However, even as the new health authority members and management teams were being appointed, global and national economic changes were taking place which were going to undermine the potential of the new NHS to achieve its goals. Moreover, the new system proved extraordinarily complex to operate. As a result, no sooner had this fundamental change taken place than there was

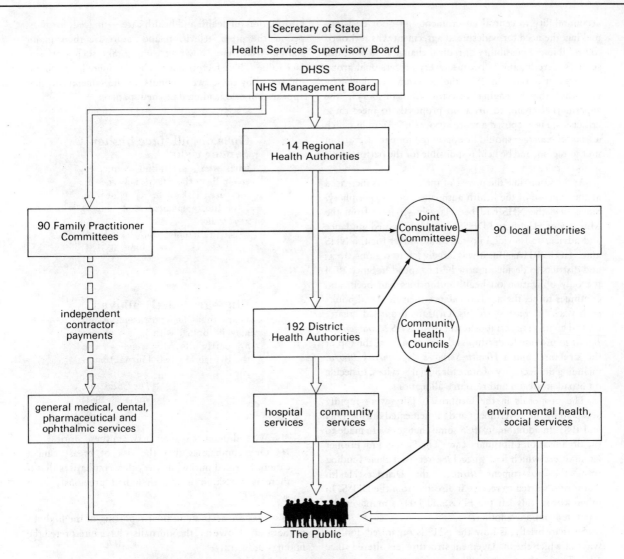

Figure 1.4 Organisation of health and social services in England in 1985.

talk of further reorganisation. During the following years the management structure of 1974 was increasingly held up as being to blame for the lack of development of services. In addition, it was felt that the NHS was not sufficiently accountable to central government. There was, however, less agreement on what changes should be made. In the event the government decided in 1982 to scrap the Area Health Authorities and replace them with health authorities at district level (DHAs) (Figure 1.4).

At the same time, the way in which services were run within districts was changed. Since 1974 many NHS staff had felt that control over their work and resources had become too distant. Previously, hospitals had had their own management committees. After 1974 many day-to-day

decisions had passed to higher levels of management, where it was felt the problems that staff had to face were not understood. In addition, it sometimes seemed as though it took several committees to decide on 'changing a light bulb'. It was with these criticisms in mind that districts were subdivided into management *units*. How services were divided up between units was left to the districts to decide; they were mostly based either on a hospital (or group of hospitals), or on a particular service, such as that for the mentally handicapped.

While these changes — scrapping AHAs, pruning formal advisory bodies, and establishing units — met some of the criticisms of the 1974 structure, they did not tackle what were seen as the key problems of a lack of accountability to central government and poor decision-making: the need for widespread agreement was reckoned to prohibit any possibility of radical change in how health services were organised because every professional group could exert a veto. In 1983 the government asked Roy Griffiths, the managing director of Sainsburys, the supermarket chain, to draw up proposals to meet these criticisms. He proposed a more autocratic system in which a *general manager* should be appointed for each tier, from unit to region, and be held responsible for the performance of the service.

At the same time the power of the centre was increased at the expense of the health authorities on the periphery. Since 1948 the NHS had been largely separate from the Ministry of Health and DHSS. The latter issued guidance and advice, and divided up the total budget for the NHS amongst the RHAs. But it was largely left to regions, areas and districts to decide on how best to spend it. Since 1974 the only obligation on health authorities had been, and continues to be, the need to balance their financial books each year. In contrast to this, Griffiths proposed greater central control: the establishment of an *NHS Management Board* to provide leadership and direction from the top of the structure, and a *Health Services Supervisory Board*, including the Secretary of State for Social Services, to decide on broad strategies and resource allocations.

The proposals in the Griffiths Inquiry were rapidly accepted by the government and implemented during 1984 and 1985. In addition, in 1985 some changes were made to the organisation of primary care. The Family Practitioner Committees which had since 1982 received their funding from the government *through* the District Health Authority, started to receive it directly from the DHSS. In other words, this left the FPCs and DHAs managerially separate from one another.

So that, briefly, is how the NHS is organised and the ways in which the management structure has altered since 1948. The key features are: the tiers of management — unit, district, region; attempts at integration and coordination of services and tensions between the centre and periphery. These issues also form the basis of an article in the Course Reader by Gwyn Bevan, 'The structure of the NHS' (Part 4, Section 4.2) in which he describes the management arrangements and other aspects of the NHS in greater detail than we have done here. You may wish to read Bevan's article now, or alternatively use it as a reference as you work your way through the rest of the book, in particular, in conjunction with Chapter 3 in which many of the dilemmas of management are discussed in greater detail.

This chapter started with a series of stories from national daily newspapers and, as you will see, many others appear throughout the book. The reason for their inclusion is that such stories are one of the major sources of information on health and health care — indeed, for most people the press, television and radio are their major source. We cannot, however, simply take such stories at face value. Three factors have to be considered. The first is illustrated by these two accounts, of the same event, that appeared in two leading daily newspapers:

Girls on pill 'face higher cancer risks'

Girls who start taking contraceptive pills in their teens may face an increased risk of breast cancer in later life, a medical study report says today.

(David Fletcher, *Daily Telegraph*, June 26, 1981)

Pill fears 'partly allayed'

Fears that the contraceptive pill may be linked with breast cancer are partly allayed by reports ... in the British Medical Journal tomorrow.

(*The Guardian*, June 26, 1981)

☐ What difference is their between these stories?

■ One emphasises that the risk of breast cancer cannot be ruled out, while the other emphasises that if there is a risk, it is less than had previously been suggested.

Both stories are accurate in their reporting of the findings of the study. However, the journalists have interpreted the findings differently.

A second factor you need to be aware of is that many news stories are actually manufactured by people other than journalists. The media are constantly fed stories by pressure groups, already written up in an appropriate form. Political parties, health authorities, government ministers, manufacturers, professions, patients' groups and trade unions all supply the media with a constant stream of press conferences and press releases. In addition, all such groups are prone to *shroud-waving* — to making unsubstantiated claims about the alarming consequences that will follow if their views are not listened to and acted upon. From a journalist's point of view, shroud-waving provides an excellent news story, and therefore tends to get greater attention than stories about the day-to-day work of the NHS.

Thirdly, it's important to remember that not everything

gets into newsprint. Just as individuals and organisations are deliberately feeding some information to the press, equally they are retaining everything else and ensuring it does not reach the press. As a result, the view that newspaper readers get is often incomplete.

Appendix on the NHS in Scotland, Wales and Northern Ireland

When the NHS was reorganised in the early 1970s, Scotland, Wales and Northern Ireland set up structures with one administrative tier less than in England. In Scotland (population 5.2 million) ultimate authority lies with the Secretary of State for Scotland, who is advised by the Scottish Health Service Planning Council. In addition, a body known as the Common Services Agency has similar responsibilities to those of the RHAs in England. The 1974 changes involved the creation of fifteen Area Health Boards immediately below the Scottish Home and Health Department (the equivalent of the DHSS in England). Below the areas, the Health Boards were free to determine how many, if any, districts they wished to establish. The areas retained more authority over the districts than occurred in England. Thus the Greater Glasgow Health Board (servicing 1.1 million people) set up five districts, while much smaller authorities like that of the Borders or the Dumfries and Galloway Boards did not establish any. Local Health Councils representing consumer interests serve the same role as the English CHCs, although the territories they serve do not usually correspond to those of entire areas or districts. Family practitioner administration is more integrated than in England, being a committee of the Area Board, rather than a separate body.

In Northern Ireland (population 1.5 million) NHS reorganisation took place in October 1973. Unlike the rest of the UK, the NHS and social services are *fully integrated* under four Health and Social Service Boards which in turn come under the Ministry of Health and Social Services. There is an advisory Central Council, and the Central Services Agency like the Common Services Agency in Scotland, fulfilling a similar role to that of RHAs in England. Each of the four boards is divided into districts with their own District Executive Teams. District Committees correspond to the English CHCs. As in Scotland, the Northern Irish family practitioners' contracts are administered by committees of the boards.

In Wales (population 2.5 million) the 1974 reorganisation followed the English pattern more closely. Eight AHAs were created, together with a Welsh Technical Services Organisation similar to the Scottish Common Services Agency. The Secretary of State at the Welsh Office has ultimate authority in the Welsh NHS.

In all three the reorganised system appeared to function relatively well during the latter half of the 1970s. One important factor in this was that the pressure on their resources has been rather less than in England (as you will see in Chapter 2). Nevertheless, all three followed England in moving to restructure their health care system at the start of the 1980s. In Wales the original districts were abolished and the AHAs converted into DHAs, except in the case of Dyfed which was split in two. Similarly, below the district level, units of management have been established.

In Northern Ireland the government decided to retain the four Health Boards but to eliminate the districts and to delegate more powers to the unit management level. Similar changes have occurred in Scotland with the elimination of the districts and the introduction of unit management.

Objectives for Chapter 1

When you have read this chapter you should be able to:

1.1 Describe the way the NHS is organised: the tiers of management (unit, district, region); the involvement of local lay people as members of regional and of district health authorities; and the change from management teams to individual managers in the mid 1980s.

Questions for Chapter 1

1 (*Objective 1.1*) What is meant by the term 'tripartite structure' as applied to the NHS before 1974? To what extent did this change with the reorganisation in 1974?

2 (*Objective 1.1*) 'All major organisations face problems in developing and pursuing integrated global policies whilst also permitting sufficient local freedom for their efficient implementation' (Taylor, 1984, p. 24). What mechanisms has the NHS used since 1974 to deal with these problems?

3 (*Objective 1.1*) During the early 1980s the form of management in the NHS was altered in an attempt to simplify and speed up decision making. What were the key changes that were made?

2
Providing a national health service

This chapter considers the NHS from a national perspective, and in particular with respect to the role of central government. A considerable amount of quantitative data on the NHS has been included, partly as a source of reference as you study the rest of the book. You are not expected to memorise the details, but rather to concentrate on the main developments of the NHS. During this chapter you will be asked to read an article in the Course Reader, 'Reforming US health care, the consumer choice health plan', by Alain Enthoven (Part 7, Section 7.5). There is an audiotape sequence in which members of several different categories of hospital staff describe their work. Details of this can be found in the Broadcast and Audiocassette Notes.

Speaking on the eve of the Appointed Day to some of the future staff of the National Health Service, Aneurin Bevan stated frankly his view of the future and in so doing revealed one of the basic dilemmas the NHS faces:

> We never will have all we need. Expectation will always exceed capacity ... This service must always be changing, growing and improving, it must always appear inadequate. (Cited in Foot, 1975, pp. 209 and 210)

Assessments of the NHS had begun within days of its creation, and have continued ever since. It has been hailed as the envy of the world, and dismissed as a tragic mistake. It has been accused of spending too much, and of spending too little. While some have argued that the only way forward lies in greatly expanded *private* health care, others have argued that the continued existence of any private health care undermines the very foundations of the NHS.

In this chapter we provide our own assessment of the changes, growth, and improvements that have occurred in the NHS since it was established, and examine some of its inadequacies and problems. We will be navigating in troubled waters, for many of the disagreements over the NHS stem from deeply-held political and ethical beliefs. These cannot be put to one side in any assessment, although they can be recognised as such and explicitly stated. But differences in beliefs are not the only source of disagreement — people also disagree about *how* the NHS should be assessed. Some argue that the appropriate method is to draw comparisons between the practical workings of the NHS and the idealised workings of some hypothetical health care system organised on entirely different principles; others claim that some ideal model of the way the NHS ought to work should be compared with an account of the way some other system works in practice. Here, we can at least make our task a bit easier by clarifying at the outset the method on which this chapter is based.

Our main concern will be to assess the NHS in the light of three of the fundamental *objectives* which you saw outlined in Chapter 1. Every Minister or Secretary of State responsible for the NHS since 1948 has had the broad duty of providing a health service that offers a *comprehensive* range of services meeting all reasonable requirements, that promotes *equality* by removing financial, geographical or other barriers to its services, and that is *planned* in such a way that it is effective and efficient.

We therefore begin by looking at the NHS as an organisation which on the one hand is meant to provide *comprehensive* health services, on the other has limited resources at its disposal, and in consequence has to *ration* in some way the services it provides. We examine what these limits are and how they are arrived at. We then compare rationing in the NHS with rationing in the USA, where the volume of resources going into health care is far greater, and consider what conclusions can be drawn from the comparison. The second part of the chapter is about *planning*. In it, we look in more detail at the way in which the NHS's resources are actually used, and at the attempts that have been made to try to plan the use of resources in order to meet the main objectives of the service. And the third part considers the extent to which the NHS has succeeded in achieving its objective of equality of health care provision.

Providing a comprehensive service

Looking back from the 1980s with the benefit of hindsight, the notion that the NHS could provide a comprehensive service, meeting everybody's needs at all times seems extraordinary, and somewhat naïve. Like any health care system, the NHS has to perform a continual balancing act: it has to balance in some way the *demands* placed upon it for health care, against the resources at its disposal to *supply* services.

> Some of us, when visiting hospitals, have discovered that by putting on a white coat and talking rudely to nurses it is easy to pass as a physician. To be mistaken for an economist is often even simpler. All one need do is nod gravely and say 'demand and supply'. (Fuchs, 1972, p.39)

The relationship between these two quantities lies at the heart of providing a national health service.

Needs and demands

'Demand' is a word with many meanings. In economics it is conventionally linked to price. Thus, if health care was bought and sold like tomatoes in a market-place, then the demand for health care would normally be defined as the amount of health care that people purchase at any particular price. In the NHS, however, with the exception of charges for particular items such as prescriptions or spectacles, people do not pay at the time they use it (it is

zero-priced). Indeed, removing financial barriers to access and providing a service free at the time of use was one of the founding objectives of the NHS. Health care, it was felt, should not be distributed according to financial means. But if the amount of health care provided by the NHS was not going to be rationed by having price barriers, just how much demand would there be for its services? How much formal health care would people want, if they no longer had to pay for it?

In 1946, nobody was entirely clear about this. One view, which can be traced to the Beveridge Report of 1942, and that laid the basis for the post-war welfare state, was that there was an untreated 'pool of sickness' in society. Financial barriers, it argued, had deterred many people from obtaining medical treatment. By offering a free and comprehensive range of treatments, the NHS would initially have to deal with a backlog of demands, but once that had been accomplished, the report expressed the hope that the NHS would be catering for a healthier population and that the cases it had to treat would fall in number eventually to reach a fixed level. Consequently, overall expenditure was projected to remain broadly constant for at least twenty years into the future.

☐ What two basic assumptions are embedded in this view?

■ The first is that the demand for the health service is *finite*; the second is that the health service will cure people and reduce illness, and therefore expenditure will be self-limiting.

In one or two areas of the service there was indeed some evidence of a backlog of demand. For example, under the old National Health Insurance scheme, only 25 per cent of the population were eligible for help to defray the cost of spectacles. Under the NHS they were supplied free, and in the three years up to 1951 the average number supplied was almost 7 million per annum. In the three years after 1951, however, this fell to around 3.5 million per annum. One explanation for this was that patient charges were introduced in 1951 to cut the cost of the ophthalmic services, but there seems little doubt that there had been a backlog of demand caused by an inability to afford glasses in the past, and that this backlog was being cleared in the first few years of the service. The same pattern occurred with dentures, and again the argument that there was a backlog seems much more plausible than the lurid tales in popular newspapers at the time that people were frantically amassing dozens of free dentures in their cupboards.

These limited exceptions apart, however, the assumptions of the Beveridge Report were rapidly exposed by events as mistaken; far from reaching any finite limit and then declining, the number of people turning up at out-patient departments, accident and emergency departments,

Table 2.1 Selected NHS activity data 1949–1983 (England)

Activity	Number ('000) in selected years					percentage increase 1949 to 1983
	1949	1959	1969	1979	1983	
In-patient cases	2 788	3 783	4 968	5 400	6 019	116
Out-patient attendances	25 080	27 768	31 801	34 100	36 500	45
Accident and emergency attendances	9 863	11 582	13 535	13 219	13 600	38
Day-case attendances	0	0	0	592	813	—
Prescriptions	188 543	199 463	245 539	304 556	315 000	67

(Source: derived from the DHSS, Health and Personal Social Service Statistics 1982 (HMSO) and DHSS, Annual Report, 1984 (HMSO))

and at dentists' or doctors' surgeries, steadily increased from year to year. So too did the numbers of people being admitted as in-patients, or being given prescriptions. In fact, using almost any measure of how much services are being used (referred to as *activity* or *process data*) the demands on the NHS have increased fairly constantly throughout its existence. Table 2.1 shows some aspects of this for the service in England.

There are a number of explanations for this turn of events. First, and most important, the demand for services from the NHS has not turned out to be self-limiting because the *need* for health care is not absolute but relative. At the heart of Beveridge's predictions, and embedded in many other discussions about the objectives of the NHS, is the notion that if somebody is ill and potentially something can be done to improve her or his condition or prevent it from becoming worse, then she or he is 'in need'. Thus one reason for removing the price barrier to health care derived from the idea that people had needs for health care which were not being met because they didn't have the money to express their needs as demands. This was not entirely wrong-headed: as you have seen, it is probable that many people needed spectacles but hadn't been able to express that need as a demand backed by money. What was wrong was the idea that the need was absolute or *fixed*: wrong, first, because the range of things that medical care can do is not fixed, and thus any innovation or development creates a new set of needs; and wrong, second, because the decision as to whether an individual has a need for health care — and if so, how much of what sort of care — is often made not by that individual alone (referred to as a person's *felt need*) but with the involvement of health professionals. Indeed the concept of the '*clinical iceberg*', that is, the notion that the population contains a submerged mass of treatable but untreated conditions, takes us even further away from the idea that need is absolute, for in this case need can be detected not by individuals themselves, but only by clinical examination. The conclusion to be drawn

from some estimates of the 'clinical iceberg' — that almost the entire population is in need of medical care, and those who appear not to be have simply been insufficiently examined — demonstrates forcibly just how relative the concept of need can be — it is, at least in part, in the eye of the beholder.*

This involvement of others — experts, administrators, researchers, or 'society' as a whole — in judgements about the need for health care is crucial to understanding how demands on the NHS are generated. By and large, patients initiate contact with the NHS themselves, for example, by calling or visiting a general practitioner. But having done so, they are largely in the hands of the doctor, and it is therefore the doctor who makes decisions about what forms of treatment they need and what further demands are placed on the resources of the NHS. It is the GP who decides whether to refer someone to a consultant, the consultant who decides whether hospital in-patient care is required, what pathology tests to order, what drugs to use, and how long to keep the patient in hospital. The doctor, whose role is to *supply* care, is also cast in the role of *demanding* care on the patient's behalf. Supply can therefore create its own demand (hence the expression '*supplier-induced demand*') and the demand for health care is constantly pressed against the limits of what is supplied.†

There are other factors influencing the demand for health care in the UK, which are to some extent independent of changing definitions of need or the existence of supplier-induced demand. Trends in tobacco and alcohol consumption, in factory and road safety, may all result in a change in the demand for health care, as may

*The 'clinical iceberg' is discussed in more detail in *Caring for Health: History and Diversity*, Chapter 6, *ibid*.

†Supplier-induced demand is discussed in more detail in *Caring for Health: History and Diversity*, Chapter 8, *ibid*.

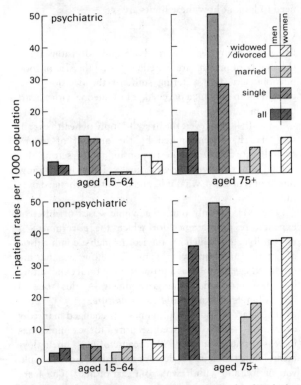

Figure 2.1 Rates of admission to hospital in England and Wales by age, sex and marital status, 1971. Based on data from OPCS. (Source: *Public Money*, 1984, p.61)

long-term changes in overall patterns of disease. And changes in the *demographic structure* of the population have also had an effect.

  □ Why might this be the case?
  ■ The demand for health care is not spread evenly throughout the population, and therefore if the proportion of the population in high-demand groups increases, the overall level of demand will rise.

Figure 2.1 shows variations in *in-patient rates* (the number of patients in hospital per 1 000 population) by age, sex and marital state, for England and Wales on the census night in 1971.

  □ What does Figure 2.1 reveal about, for example, the non-psychiatric* in-patient rate for married men compared with widowed or divorced men aged 75 or over?

*Routine data on the NHS usually distinguish between *psychiatric* hospitals for the care of the mentally ill and mentally handicapped from *non-psychiatric* which includes all general, maternity and specialised hospitals.

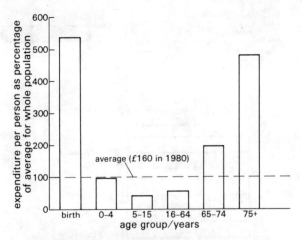

Figure 2.2 Cost of providing hospital and community health care to different age groups in England, 1980. (Source: DHSS, 1983a, p.11)

  ■ The in-patient rate among widowed or divorced men is around three times that of married men.
  □ So if the proportion of widowed or divorced men aged 75 or over rose, and that of married men fell, what would be the likely consequence for non-psychiatric hospital demand, all else remaining constant?
  ■ It would rise.

In fact, the most important aspect of demographic change for the health service in recent years has been change in the *age-structure* of the population. As Figure 2.2 shows, the use made of the NHS by different age-groups varies enormously. In England in 1980 the NHS spent an average of £160 on each person. However, whereas it spent around half the average to provide care for people aged between 5 and 64 years, it spent twice the average on people aged 65–74 and five times the average on those aged 75 years and above. A similar pattern exists in the use of primary care. As a result, as the proportion of the population who are old or very old rises, so too do the demands placed on the NHS.

We will return to the effects of these demographic pressures in a moment, but first we need to consider an important point that relates to the earlier discussion of the shifting definition of need. Figure 2.3 shows the *percentage change* between 1965 and 1979 in the average length of time spent in hospital by people in Scotland. As you will see, this is measured in *bed-days*. Around midnight every day all NHS hospitals conduct a *bed-count*. The count records the number of beds *available* for the reception of patients (this may vary because of staff shortages or ward maintenance) and the number of available beds that are *occupied* by patients. In a year, each bed can therefore in theory provide 365 bed-days.

  □ Looking at Figure 2.3, what change took place

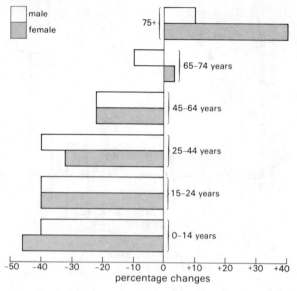

Figure 2.3 Changes in the use of hospital beds by different age–sex groups in Scotland, 1965–1979; expressed as percentage changes in average number of bed–days per person per year in non-psychiatric, non-maternity hospitals.
(Source: Registrar-General for Scotland, and Scottish Hospital In-Patient Statistics)

between 1965 and 1979 in the use of hospital beds?

■ It shows that the average lengths of time spent in hospital changed markedly, falling by 40 per cent or more among the young and rising by up to 40 per cent among the old.

In other words, the demand for hospital services by the elderly has increased not only because the age-structure has altered, but also because the average demands made by elderly people have increased. The latter has arisen as a result of such technological changes as the availability of new anaesthetics which make it safe to operate on old people. *New needs* have gradually been created, increasing the level of demand placed on the NHS by the elderly.

These new demands have been much more significant than alterations in the demographic structure *per se*, and return us to an earlier question: if demands for health care are constantly increasing, and if many of those demands are being induced by doctors, then what is to stop the entire economy from gradually becoming an extraordinarily elaborate health care system? The answer, of course, is that the government, the health departments and the health authorities and boards are also involved in making decisions about just how many demands are to be met: they have to decide what level of resources to *supply* to the health service. Before looking at the way in which doctors come to terms with having to work within these limits we

need to look at how these limits are set.

Supply

Every day, many people in the NHS make decisions about the supply of health care, whether this be the size of food portions served by catering staff, or the decision by a consultant to implant a pacemaker in someone with a heart condition.

Since 1948, however, the overall supply of health care in the NHS has been limited by the amount of money available in any year. The responsibility for setting this annual limit rests with the government. Let us look at how this limit is decided, what it is, and how it has changed over time.

The NHS is only one of a whole series of different expenditure programmes for which the government is responsible, and which are funded through a combination of taxation and borrowing. Figure 2.4 shows expenditure on the NHS since 1950 as a proportion of total expenditure by UK central and local government — this total is normally referred to as *public expenditure*.

The share of some programmes has changed markedly over time — that of social security, for example, has increased sharply in the 1980s because of mass unemployment, while the share for defence has halved since the cold war period and withdrawal from east of Suez. The share

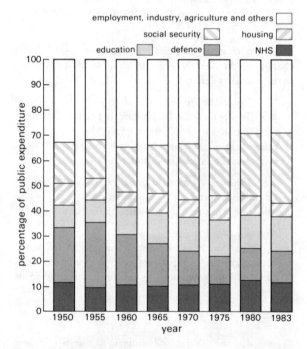

Figure 2.4 Shares of UK public expenditure by different programmes, 1950–1983.
(Source: CSO, *National Income and Expenditure*, various years)

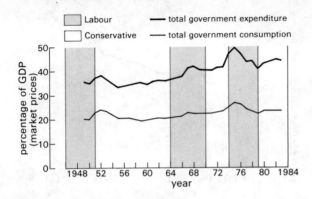

Figure 2.5 Changing level of UK government expenditure and consumption as a percentage of GDP (market prices), 1949–1983. (Source: as Figure 2.4)

taken by the NHS, however, has been fairly constant at 9.5 to 12.5 per cent of the total since 1950.

Before focusing on NHS expenditure, we must mention another aspect of public expenditure — its size in relation to the economy as a whole. Two ways of looking at this are shown in Figure 2.5.

The top line shows total public expenditure since 1949 as a proportion of the UK's *Gross Domestic Product* (GDP), which strives to measure the value of all the goods and services produced by UK residents each year. The public expenditure proportion has fluctuated but generally rose from about 35 per cent of GDP in the 1950s to around 45 per cent by the 1980s. All governments have some general policy towards what total expenditure should be quite apart from the policies towards programmes within the total, and have sought either to increase or reduce it for various reasons. From 1941 to the 1970s, for example, successive governments manipulated the total level of public expenditure in an attempt to regulate the economy as a whole. In consequence, individual programmes were affected by wider national economic policies and events. In 1976, for example, an economic crisis resulted in the International Monetary Fund requiring the government to reduce spending across the board; the NHS, like other programmes, experienced a squeeze.

But a large part of total public expenditure is not actually spent by government on goods and services, such as on frigates or nurses; rather, it simply involves transferring money through the taxation system from one person to another *without any goods or services being exchanged*, as part of policies aimed at redistribution. Expenditures of this sort are known as *transfer payments*, and because they don't involve any additional claims on the nation's resources, but rather a redistribution of different people's ability to make claims on resources (a pensioner rather than a professor, for instance) they are normally

excluded from assessments of *cost*. The bottom line of Figure 2.5 shows public expenditure excluding all transfer payments: known as *consumption*.

□ How has consumption changed over time?
■ This figure has represented a fairly constant 20–25 per cent of the country's GDP since the war.

In general terms, therefore, the decision about how much money is made available to the NHS is part of the government's wider economic policies and its attitude towards what the level of *total* public expenditure should be. Within this context, how are NHS expenditures determined?

In 1948, just as there was doubt about how many demands would be placed on the NHS, so there was no definite view as to how much it would cost to run. For some services, for example, the family practitioner services, it was decided that no definite figure could be set in advance; expenditure would simply have to be *demand-led*, and the bill picked up afterwards. But for the bulk of services, the only way to proceed, argued Bevan, was in the first place to provide enough money to maintain the existing services, that is, to continue to run the buildings and pay the staff that the NHS had inherited. The best way to view the whole matter, he suggested in a letter to *The Times* in November 1949, was as 'a gigantic *transfer* of expense from the private pocket to the public purse'. The level of expenditure would be determined largely by what that level had been in the past.

In the first few years of the NHS, there was a great deal of confusion over precisely how much the NHS was costing and whether the amount was changing.

□ What reason can you think of that might make it difficult to compare the cost of running the NHS over different years?
■ The main difficulty is *inflation* — a sustained rise in the general level of prices — which makes it necessary to distinguish expenditure in current money prices from expenditure adjusted to take account of changing money prices: usually known as expenditure in *constant prices* or *real expenditure*.

This confusion over the NHS's expenditure had begun within months of the Appointed Day, and by February 1949 the leader of the opposition, Winston Churchill, was accusing the government of 'the most wild miscalculations ... an enormous addition to the burdens of the nation ... the grossest carelessness' (cited in G. Bevan, *et al*, 1980, p.17). In 1953 it was found necessary to appoint a Cambridge economist, Claude Guillebaud, to lead a full investigation into the whole matter.

In fact, the Guillebaud Report, published in 1956, found that expenditure had increased very much less than

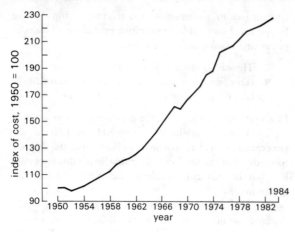

Figure 2.6 Change in the cost of the NHS in terms of volume, 1950–1983.
(Source: Royal Commission on the NHS, 1979, Table E7, p.432)

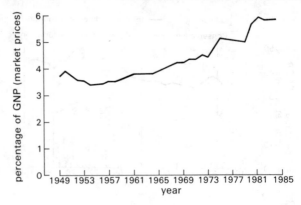

Figure 2.7 Expenditure on the NHS as a percentage of GNP, 1951–1984.
(Source: Office of Health Economics, 1985a. Note: the OHE is not a government agency, but an organisation sponsored by the Association of the British Pharmaceutical Industry)

generally thought, and that a basic reason for this was not just that general inflation had been ignored but that the rate of inflation experienced by the NHS was higher than the general rate. This still causes a great deal of confusion, but is basically quite simple to explain and important to understand. The general rate of inflation is normally measured by the *Retail Price Index* (RPI), which measures the changes in price from year to year of a 'basket' of goods and services — food, drink, tobacco, clothes, energy, transport, housing — bought by an average consumer. But some items change in price more rapidly than others, for example, energy prices in the 1970s, and so anybody buying a 'basket' of goods and services that isn't average may experience a higher or lower rate of inflation than that measured by the RPI. The 'basket' bought by old-age pensioners has tended to have a higher than average rate of inflation, as has the 'basket' bought by the NHS. So to measure the change in expenditure on the NHS in such a way as to exclude price changes and record only changes in the *volume* of goods and services it uses, the RPI is no use; what is required is a special price index for the NHS.

Figure 2.6 shows expenditure on the NHS as an index starting at 100 in 1950 that has been calculated to show changes in the volume but not the cost of goods and services. After the first few years, as the post-war austerity period gave way to a long period of fairly continuous economic growth in the UK and the world economies, real expenditure on the NHS began to rise. So too did the share of the UK's *Gross National Product** devoted to it (Figure 2.7).

Throughout the 1960s and early 1970s the whole

business of deciding what to allocate to the NHS was fairly relaxed: government ministers gathered in the views of regional hospital boards about requirements and future developments, and then discussed with the Cabinet and the Treasury the amount of money likely to be available, all within a tacit understanding that the economy was growing and some real increase in NHS funding would be forthcoming. Because there was growth in the economic system as a whole, there was no necessity to make painful decisions about the relative priority of one area of government expenditure compared to another; and within the NHS, there was little inducement to think about the relative priorities of different parts of the service.

In the 1970s, however, the growth of the economy slowed down; government control over its expenditure programmes began to tighten, and the whole relationship between central government and the NHS began to change. This has continued into the 1980s. What have been the changes, and what have been the consequences? Since the 1960s the government's financial system has operated on the basis of five-year plans. These are 'rolled forward' each year, so the plan always stretches five years into the future. The whole process of arriving at a spending plan starts with the Treasury, with Cabinet approval, issuing to each government department detailed instructions on the overall limits within which departmental spending plans must be submitted. Each departmental submission must cover the following five years. The health department's plans are then collated alongside all other departments' plans by the *Public Expenditure Survey Committee* (PESC), and its report is discussed and amended by the Cabinet before being published in the autumn or winter each year as the Public Expenditure White Paper. The *Main Estimates* of expenditure presented in the White Paper are voted through

*GNP is the same as GDP except that it includes income from abroad and excludes income moved abroad.

Parliament in the spring, and are thereafter referred to, in the case of the health service, as the *NHS Votes*.

Until 1974–75, these Votes included allowances for the predicted level of inflation, but if wages subsequently rose by more than predicted, extra money was voted through Parliament as *Supplementary Estimates* to cover the increases. This is a process known as *volume planning*, because it allows the volume or quantity of services to be maintained despite any changes in prices. But in the mid-1970s, as the rate of inflation increased and became more unpredictable, this procedure changed, and in 1976–77 a fully-fledged system of *cash limits* was introduced. This consists in fixing a limit on the Supplementary Estimates so that unpredicted inflation is not automatically compensated, the result being that if inflation turns out to be higher than allowed for, the volume of services has to be reduced. By 1985, cash limits were being applied to all NHS spending except for the family practitioner services, which remained 'demand-led'.

What effect have cash limits had on the NHS? By far the largest single item of expenditure in the NHS is the salaries and wages of staff in the hospital and community services, accounting for two-thirds of all health authority expenditure. It is precisely this item that has created the most controversy in relation to cash limits.

> ## Patients will suffer 'if pay norm is broken'
>
> Health authorities which fear industrial action by unions determined to break through the Government's 4 per cent ceiling in the current pay round warned yesterday that a higher level of settlement would almost certainly lead to cuts in services to patients.
>
> (John Ardill, *The Guardian*, January 8, 1982)

In effect the ability of people working in the NHS to bargain over wages has increasingly been pre-empted by guidelines laid down in the cash limits by the Treasury or the Cabinet. For example, if it is laid down in advance that 4 per cent has been allowed in the cash limits for price changes, but inflation turns out to be 6 per cent, then the NHS as an employer cannot agree to settle with any NHS occupational group for a pay rise of more than 4 per cent unless it takes the money away from another group, cuts back on services, or tries to squeeze more out of its resources by improving efficiency.

The control which the Government holds over the purse-strings of the NHS is the main way in which it sets

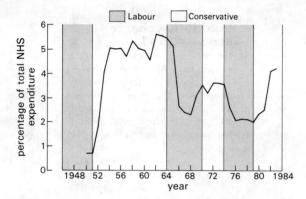

Figure 2.8 Proportion of total cost of the NHS raised by patient charges, 1950–1983.
(Source: CSO National Income and Expenditure and Annual Abstracts of Statistics, various years)

limits on the demand for health care. But the Government also has at its disposal a more direct control over the level of demand for the NHS — by setting *charges* for services. The Government raises the money to fund the NHS from three main sources. The great bulk is drawn from general funds raised through taxation, duties, excises and so on (known as the Consolidated Fund). Eighty-four per cent of NHS funds came from this source in 1983. Another source is the National Insurance contributions deducted from wages and salaries, a portion of which is set aside for the NHS, largely as a hangover from the days of the National Health Insurance Scheme which ran from 1911 to 1948. Twelve per cent of NHS funds came from this source in 1983. The third source is from charges to patients for services. These have always been a source of controversy, and their introduction in 1950–1951 led both Aneurin Bevan and Harold Wilson to resign in protest from government posts.

The attitude of different political parties to health service charges has varied, as Figure 2.8 shows. Although these charges have never raised more than 6 per cent of the total cost of the NHS, they are not evenly spread across its services; the dental service (excluding hospital dentistry), for example, raises around 25 per cent of its costs through charges. The main argument for charges is that they may reduce the 'trivial' use of services. The main argument levelled against charges is that they reintroduce financial barriers which may discourage people from seeking health care, and although research on their disincentive effects on patients has not produced unanimous findings, and although many patients are in principle exempt, the arguments against them were felt by the Royal Commission on the NHS to be sufficiently strong to recommend their abolition. In practice, they have increased sharply since the Royal Commission reported in 1979.

Consequences

You have now seen that on the one hand, the overall amount of health care supplied through the NHS is limited, in the last resort, by central government, and on the other hand how there appears to be no limit to the potential demands for NHS services. *Rationing* is the inevitable result. How in practice does this occur?

Let us turn first to a study entitled *The Painful Prescription: Rationing Hospital Care*, in which two Americans, Henry Aaron, an economist, and William Schwarz, a physician, examined the differences in the provision of a range of services between the NHS and American health care. Their starting-point was the observation that the per capita expenditure on hospital patient care in Britain was barely a half (53 per cent) of that in the USA. Their objective was to explore the way in which rationing occurred in these circumstances, by selecting ten different forms of hospital treatment and comparing the rates of use in the two countries.

In three of their ten case-studies — treatment of haemophilia (failure of the blood to clot), megavoltage radiotherapy for cancer patients, and bone-marrow transplants — approximately the same level of treatment was provided in Britain as in the USA. In another instance — chemotherapy for cancer patients — there was no clear pattern. But in the remaining six examples they studied, the levels of provision in Britain were markedly lower than in the USA. These included X-ray examinations, carried out half as often in Britain; the treatment of chronic renal (kidney) failure, where the dialysis rate was one-third that in the USA, but the transplantation rate was similar; and coronary artery surgery, * performed in Britain at one-tenth the rate of that in the USA. Similarly, the CT scanning† capability of Britain was found to be one-sixth that of the

*Coronary artery surgery is discussed in Chapter 11.

†CT scanning is discussed at more length in Chapter 6.

USA, and the number of intensive-care beds relative to population in Britain was only 10 to 20 per cent of the number in the USA.

Putting this another way, to increase the provision of just these ten forms of treatment in Britain to the same rate as in the USA would involve increasing the total hospital budget of the NHS by 18 per cent. Moreover, in the instances where rationing in the NHS seems most clearly marked, as in dialysis treatment for kidney failure, resource limits are not necessarily mentioned by GPs or others when explaining their rationing decisions to a patient (or to her or his family):

> I would say that mother's or aunt's kidneys have failed or are failing and there is very little that anybody can do about it because of her age and general physical state, and that it would be my suggestion or my advice that we spare her any further investigation, any further painful procedure and we would just make her as comfortable as we can for what remains of her life. (Cited in Aaron and Schwarz, 1984, p.37)

Age, diabetes, physical disability, mental illness, hepatitis and lack of facilities for home dialysis are all incorporated to some degree into the decision whether or not to provide treatment. Moreover, GPs become attuned to the likelihood of patients being accepted or rejected if they are referred to a renal specialist, and therefore adjust their referral patterns accordingly. Rationing thus becomes part of accepted standards of clinical practice.

The second point to note is that the difference between the NHS and the USA is not uniform: some treatments are provided at very much lower rates, others at almost comparable rates. Aaron and Schwarz deduced from these observed variations a set of seven factors that appeared to result in less rationing:

1 Age: for children than adults (particularly the elderly).

2 'Dread' disease: for diseases inspiring fear.

3 Visibility of illness: if suffering is severe and obvious.

4 Advocacy: if organised pressure groups exist.

5 Aggregate cost: if the total cost of a programme seems negligible.

6 Need for capital funds: if capital outlays are fairly low.

7 Cost of alternatives: if the costs of not treating exceed the costs of active intervention (for example, providing hip replacements may be much cheaper than caring for people with osteoarthrosis of the joint).

But there is a third point which can be drawn from this study's method of comparing one set of resource constraints with another: the systematically higher levels of provision in the USA make it tempting to conclude that, there, health care is not rationed. However, if the NHS was compared to health care services in, say, Bangladesh, then the temptation would be to see the NHS, not as a heavily rationed system, but as a model of the *absence* of rationing, and to draw a range of conclusions about the way accepted standards of clinical practice in Bangladesh have been altered to accommodate the lack of resources. The whole point is that rationing is only useful as a concept which summarises a *relationship* between supply and demand. The existence of a higher level of supply of health care in the USA must therefore be placed in the context of the level of demand in the USA. When this is done, two facts emerge.

First, there has been a long-standing concern in the USA that some treatments are *over-supplied* relative to their demonstrated effectiveness, or to the level of need for them;* this is partly because the economic structure of American health care provides powerful incentives for supplier-induced demands — many doctors' incomes increase the more operations they perform or the more drugs they prescribe. Second, in some respects the American health care system also rations, but in different ways from the UK. In particular, the absence of universal health insurance in the USA results in rationing of health care by means of *price barriers*, and, in practice, around 18 million people, or 8.6 per cent of the population, are permanently uninsured, and a further 16 million people, or 7.5 per cent of the population, are temporarily uninsured for part of any year.

We will return to the second point in a moment, but first let us look in more detail at the problem of *over-supply* in the USA. An analysis of this problem, and a suggested way of dealing with it by the organisational reform of American health care on the principles of *Health Maintenance Organisations* (HMOs), is contained in an article in the Course Reader by Alain Enthoven, an American health economist, 'Reforming US Health Care: the Consumer Choice Health Plan' (Part 7, Section 7.5). You should read this article now.

☐ How would you summarise Enthoven's diagnosis of the problems of American health care?

■ The system insulates almost all concerned from the cost implications of their actions, providing few incentives to economise and many incentives to increase demand. The result has been a very rapid growth in spending.

☐ What does Enthoven claim to be the key advantage of HMOs?

■ They have certain built-in incentives for economy, and are claimed to maintain quality of care while reducing costs by roughly 25 per cent.

☐ What is the essential principle that Enthoven claims would provide these incentives for economy?

■ The proposed system would be based on the principle of fair *economic competition* between provider organisations, with consumers exercising choice between them.

The principle of fair economic competition has proved extraordinarily difficult to enforce in many other industries. Also, while universal membership of HMOs would provide health care for everyone, they would *not be* the same as a system such as the NHS, in which central government has the power to plan services on a national, integrated basis. It would therefore have difficulty in overcoming the wide regional inequalities and duplication of services that are a feature of American health care. Nevertheless, as Enthoven remarks towards the end of the article, the proposal must be judged realistically against alternatives in the USA.

While the pros and cons of HMOs are debated, some 16 per cent of the US population continue to have inadequate insurance coverage. Some effects of this on the use of health services in the USA are shown in Table 2.2. In general, as the two American economists who collated these statistics observed,

> those fortunate enough to be employed by large, unionized, manufacturing firms are also likely to be fortunate enough to have good health insurance coverage. Those who are poor, those who live in the South or in rural areas, and those who are black or minority group members are more likely to bear the personal and economic effects of lack of insurance and the consequent financial barriers to health care. (Davis and Rowland, 1983, pp.158–9)

The point is not, therefore, that health care in the USA is unrationed, but that rationing takes a different form from that in the NHS: financial means is an important criterion of access to health care. This is also incorporated into accepted standards of clinical practice, as the following two cases reported in *The Lancet* in 1984 demonstrate:

> A 36-year-old Cuban refugee was taken to a private hospital emergency room in California after being beaten. He lapsed into a coma as two neurosurgeons refused to respond to the emergency physician's calls for assistance because the patient lacked health insurance. After transfer to a public hospital, a skull fracture and irreversible brain damage due to intracerebral bleeding was discovered.

*The example of hysterectomy is discussed in The Open University (1985) *Medical Knowledge: Doubt and Certainty*, Chapter 7, The Open University Press (U205 *Health and Disease*, Book II).

Table 2.2 Rationing health care: USA (1977)

Physician visits per person under 65 years of age, per year		(i) Uninsured	(ii) Insured	Ratio of (ii) to (i)
Total		2.4	3.7	1.5
South	white	2.3	3.7	1.61
	black/other	1.5	2.8	1.87
Non-south	white	2.7	3.8	1.41
	black/other	1.9	3.5	1.84
Hospital patient days per 100 persons aged under 65, per year				
Total		47	90	1.91
South	white	33	100	3.03
	black/other	40	119	2.98
Non-south	white	51	81	1.59
	black/other	89	119	1.28

(Source: Davis and Rowland, 1983, Table 6, p. 163)

A woman of 21 was hit by a truck and taken to the nearest (private) emergency facility. Despite multiple leg, ankle, pelvic, and rib fractures, and a rapidly falling haematocrit [evidence of severe bleeding], she was transferred 30 miles to a public hospital because she was uninsured. A ruptured aorta was diagnosed, and she was transferred to another private hospital for surgical repair because the thoracic surgery programme at the public hospital had been closed several years earlier. (Himmelstein and Woolhandler, 1984, p.392)

Thus, whatever the level of overall resources, and whatever the system of health care, the services provided inevitably finish up being rationed, but in very different ways and according to widely differing criteria.

Let us therefore return to the NHS and explore further aspects of the way it rations health care. One of these is the existence of queues or waiting lists for treatments.

8 yr wait for some in hospital queue of 600,000

More than 600,000 patients are on hospital waiting lists for operations and some have had to wait for as long as eight years the Department of Health said yesterday.

A report into waiting lists for orthopaedic surgery — 131,000 are awaiting operations — said that better management of resources could reduce waiting lists substantially.

But the report admitted that the shortage of nurses, caused by the 2½-hour cut in their working week and the ten bank holidays they enjoy each year, was a major problem.
(David Fletcher, *Daily Telegraph*, March 18, 1981)

What is a *waiting-list*? Before admitting non-emergency cases to hospital, the NHS operates a system of placing people on a list from which people waiting are drawn. One reason for this is to try to ensure that people have some advance notice of admission, another is to obtain a mix of patients that is relatively even; for example, to avoid having a large number of minor operations one day and complicated operations the next. The length of waiting lists can, however, be manipulated by consultants or departments trying to obtain extra money from their health authority, by increasing the rate at which out-patients are seen so that the rate of additions to the waiting-list exceeds the rate at which people are admitted for treatment.

A survey of in-patients conducted for the Royal Commission on the NHS found that 20 per cent of in-patients were caused some inconvenience or distress by waiting for admission, and among those waiting for out-patient appointments almost half of the 17 per cent who had had to wait six weeks or more were in consequence 'distressed, in physical pain or discomfort, or anxious'.

Waiting problems are greatest for non-emergency in-patient surgery, and it is in this area that the *private sector* has experienced the biggest growth. Figure 2.9 shows the

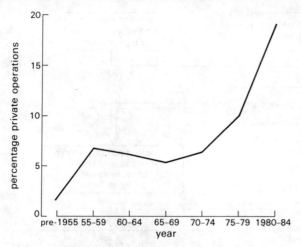

Figure 2.9 Percentage of eight common surgical operations performed privately, 1955–1984. Based on a study of 6 000 adults living in Oxfordshire in 1984; operations included hernia repair, hysterectomy, D & C, appendicectomy, breast operations, varicose veins, cholecystectomy, oophorectomy, thyroidectomy and prostatectomy.
(Source: McPherson, Coulter and Stratton, 1985, Table 1, p. 798)

trend over time in the proportion of all operations for people living in Oxfordshire performed by the private sector.

Nationally, the activities of the private sector are very unevenly spread. The Royal Commission noted:

> ... considerable geographical variation in the proportion of women obtaining an abortion in the NHS, ranging from nearly 90 per cent in the Northern Region to about 22 per cent in the West Midlands Region ... this suggests that lack of availability of NHS facilities, rather than real desire for private treatment, is the major factor in most cases where the full cost of treatment has to be met by the patient. (Royal Commission on the NHS, 1978, p.286)

In the late 1970s the private sector expanded rapidly, and the number of people covered by the three main insurance companies (British United Provident Association (BUPA), Private Patients Plan (PPP) and Western Provident Association (WPA)) rose from 2.2 million in 1977 to 4.1 million in 1981. Less than 9 per cent of the increased number of subscribers enrolled as individuals, the vast majority being in company or employee schemes. Most of the increase cannot be attributed directly to a rapid increase in problems of availability in the NHS, but rather to a shift in government policy: tax changes made it cheaper for companies to offer private health insurance as a fringe benefit.

As an essentially profit-making activity, the private sector can only offer a limited range of services to a limited range of people. It concentrates primarily on providing non-emergency surgery to low-risk people who are basically fit and healthy and will not therefore need prolonged after-care. However, the rapid expansion noted above drew a larger proportion of higher-risk patients into private schemes, upsetting the calculated margins of profitability: in 1977 the benefits paid out by insurers were only 71 per cent of subscription income, but by 1981 this had risen to 96 per cent. Consequently, rates of growth in this part of the private sector were not sustained.

The private sector, therefore, is partly a guide to areas of severe rationing in the NHS, and partly also a reflection of government policy on the NHS. In both respects, it raises the issue of how the NHS actually goes about planning and providing comprehensive health care.

Planning from the centre

Even if it will never be possible to provide a comprehensive *amount* of health care to meet all needs, it may be possible to plan a comprehensive *range* that reflects the full spectrum of need. But what is meant by *planning*? In the words of Harry Eckstein, an American political scientist:

> the purpose of planning, in a word, is to 'rationalise' the activities on which planning is imposed: to make subject to calculation what was previously left to chance, to organize what was previously unorganized, to replace spontaneous adjustment with deliberate control. (Eckstein, 1958, p.262)

In his study of the NHS, Eckstein noted that those responsible for planning faced three main difficulties. First, he observed that the objectives of the NHS are to a degree *mutually inconsistent* (for example, providing fully-comprehensive care without restriction *and* operating within fixed budgets) and thereby ambiguities and inconsistencies are likely to enter into planning decisions. Second, he drew attention to the *psychological burden* carried by planners, in that having assumed control they are inevitably held responsible for almost every conceivable aspect of the NHS's activities:

> to decide between the relative weight of an improvement of the mental health *versus* the tuberculosis services or between the demands of the Newcastle *versus* the Manchester region, and to be aware of the human issues involved, may try emotional stability as much as the calculating intelligence. (Eckstein, 1958, p.272)

Or, as Bevan once commented, comparing his position to that of St Sebastian pierced by a thousand arrows, 'for every mistake you make I shall have to bleed'. Third, Eckstein emphasised the *lack of control* exercised by

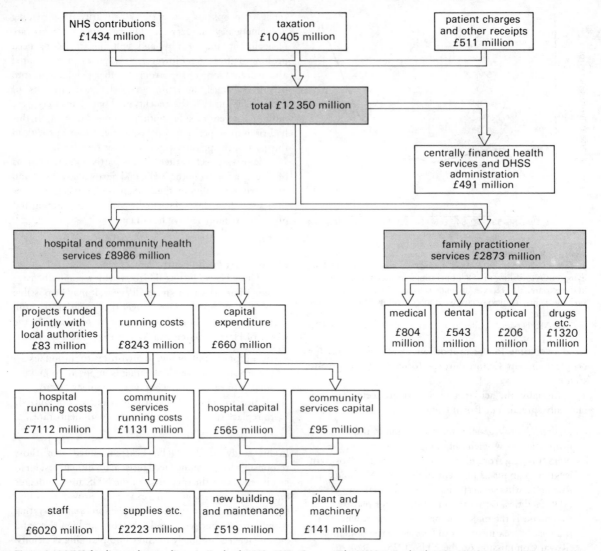

Figure 2.10 NHS funding and expenditure in England, 1982–1983. (Source: *The NHS in England*, 1984, HMSO, Annex B)

planners over factors bearing upon their decisions, and in particular the fact that the level of funding and annual changes in that level, are outside their control, making long-range planning extremely difficult. As you will see in Chapter 3, most NHS planning takes place in the districts and regions. However, there is, in addition, a role for central or national planning; inevitably this tends to concentrate on long-term issues, an example of which we will consider in a moment — that of the 1962 Hospital Plan. First, we need to consider what the ingredients of a health service are.

The production of formal health care requires labour, an assortment of non-labour items ranging from bandages and electricity to buildings and land (about 50 000 acres are

occupied by the NHS). Figure 2.10 gives a rough idea of the relative importance of different items in terms of expenditure.

The first item under the total — centrally financed services and DHSS administration — covers such services as the heart transplant programme, the research and production of vaccines, the special hospitals such as Rampton and Broadmoor, and the Health Education Council. Only 0.5 per cent of the total budget is spent on central administration. This remarkably low figure gives an indication of the extent to which the detailed planning of the NHS is delegated to the lower tiers of the organisation — the regions and districts.

The family practitioner services account for less than 25

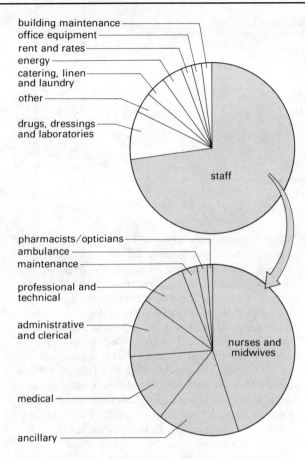

building maintenance
office equipment
rent and rates
energy
catering, linen
and laundry
other

drugs, dressings
and laboratories

staff

pharmacists/opticians
ambulance
maintenance

professional and
technical

administrative
and clerical

nurses and
midwives

medical

ancillary

Figure 2.11 NHS expenditure by Regional Health Authorities in England, 1982–1983.
(Source: DHSS Annual Report, 1984, p.79)

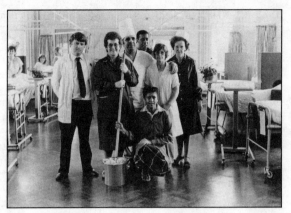

Figure 2.12 Hospital staff — porters, domestic, catering, maintenance and nursing.

☐   Figure 2.11 shows the main revenue items. How would you summarise the overall pattern?

■   The bulk of revenue (almost three-quarters) is spent on paying staff, and of that, almost half on nurses and midwives.

So, in expenditure terms, the NHS is not only a largely hospital-based service, but one which devotes most of its money to the staff it employs (Figure 2.12). Who are these staff, and what do they do?

The first distinction to make is between whole-time and part-time workers. In 1982, 74 per cent of the NHS's employees worked whole time, 26 per cent part time. Rather than simply adding them together, official statistics frequently measure part-time workers in terms of *whole-time equivalents*; that is, if two part-time nurses each work half the weekly hours of a whole-time nurse, then they are counted as one whole-time equivalent (WTE). Table 2.3 shows some broad aspects of NHS employment over the ten years up to 1982.

☐   What are the two largest occupational groups?

■   Nurses and midwives, accounting for almost a half of all employees, and ancillary staff (porters, domestics, laundry, catering) accounting for around a quarter.

The table also shows that the numbers in different occupational groups increased at different rates. Professional and technical staff (including physiotherapists, radiographers and laboratory workers) and administrative and clerical staff increased by over 40 per cent, while ancillary staff hardly increased at all. But measured in whole-time equivalents the numbers are a bit misleading: over time, in the NHS as elsewhere, the average hours worked per week has been falling while holidays have been increasing. But hospitals are a twenty-four hours a day, seven days a week, business; they cannot be closed

per cent of the NHS's total cost, and the bulk of this is attributable to the general practitioners' pay and the pharmaceuticals they prescribe. That leaves the bulk of NHS expenditure being used by the hospital and community services,* a dominance that has steadily increased since 1948. The NHS is, above all, a national *hospital* service.

As Figure 2.10 shows, expenditure on the hospital and community services can be split into three broad items: (a) running costs (or revenue), (b) capital expenditure, and (c) a small amount for the joint funding of projects with local authorities (discussed in more detail in Chapters 3 and 5). It can be seen that revenue expenditure is the main item: in 1982–1983 it was about twelve times greater than capital expenditure.

*Routine statistics amalgamate hospital with community services. The latter is a small proportion of the combined total.

Table 2.3 NHS staff, 1973 and 1982 (whole-time equivalents), Great Britain*

	1973 Number (%)	1982 Number (%)	Percentage growth, 1973–1982
Medical and dental	35 864(4)	46 406(5)	29
Nursing and midwifery	370 595(47)	481 873(48)	30
Professional and technical	80 208(10)	113 270(11)	41
Administrative and clerical	87 406(11)	124 863(13)	43
Ancillary, ambulance and others	219 955(28)	231 221(23)	5
Total	794 028(100)	997 633(100)	26

*Excluding Family Practitioner Committtee staff.

(Source: derived from HMSO, Annual Abstract of Statistics, 1984, Table 3.32, p. 66)

down for weekends, bank holidays or at night, unlike banks, shops or factories. So the NHS has had to employ more people just to compensate for falling hours of work, and this has accounted for perhaps a third of the growth shown in the table.

Until 1984, the growth in the number of people employed by NHS had been entirely in the hands of the health authorities. As long as the revenue was available, the health authorities were free to employ whom they wished (with the exception of some medical posts which were, and still are, subject to central government approval and control). This changed in 1984 when the government imposed *manpower controls** — the number of staff a health authority could employ was to be specified by the government. This represented another restriction on the freedom of health authorities to determine their own policies and a further increase in the centralisation of control of the NHS. One consequence of the imposition of manpower controls was that a health authority could find itself in the position of having funds to provide a service but not able to use those funds to employ staff to carry out the work. This led at least one district health authority to pay a private hospital to treat patients who were on an NHS waiting list. Such consequences have led some critics of government policy to suggest that manpower controls were deliberately introduced to assist the private sector of health care.

Statistics such as those in Table 2.3 are cold and stark, and within them are concealed many variations and complexities. For example, the NHS contains a very large number of women workers — 75 per cent in 1982. But they are not spread evenly across all occupational groups — 91 per cent of nurses are women and 67 per cent of ancillary staff. In contrast, only 24 per cent of medical and dental staff are women. And *within* occupational groups there are

*Government and NHS publications use the term 'manpower' despite the majority of NHS staff being women.

also differences: at the bottom of the medical hierarchy, for example, 36 per cent of house officers are women; in the middle of the hierarchy, 20 per cent of registrars are women; but at the top, the proportion of women consultants is only 11 per cent. Similarly the 9 per cent of nurses who are men tend to be concentrated in the top jobs. There are also large variations in pay and conditions: for instance, a consultant at the top of the profession can earn more in a month than a laundry worker in a year.

What is it like to work for the NHS? To answer this, a group of hospital staff were interviewed in 1985, and their views, opinions and attitudes are contained in an audiotape sequence (Band 3, Audiocassette AC807). You should now listen to this sequence, having first read the accompanying audiocassette notes.

Having sketched the components of the NHS we can now consider the extent to which the objective of a nationally planned system can be, and has been, achieved. To do this we will look in more detail at capital expenditure. Figure 2.10 includes some indications of what is included under capital expenditure.

☐ Comparing the definitions with the items of revenue expenditure shown in Figure 2.11, what problems of definition can you detect?

■ Maintenance is included under both headings, and office equipment could be difficult to distinguish from plant and machinery.

There are great difficulties, therefore, in defining precisely what is meant by '*capital*': one health service treasurer giving evidence to the Royal Commission on the NHS defined it simply as 'anything you can see from the road', and in practice his comment actually gets quite close to what we will be referring to here — the buildings and fabric of the NHS. It is in this area that we can observe the longest-running attempts by the NHS to plan services, which is one reason for taking it as our example. It is also important for another reason: although revenue expenditure is very much larger, the way it is spent depends to a large extent on previous capital spending. For example, building a new operating theatre may cost £500 000, but once it is built it has to be staffed, cleaned, heated, lighted, and generally run from revenue expenditure. In the same way, the existing pattern of revenue expenditure in the NHS is influenced strongly by capital expenditure in the past, sometimes from as long ago as the eighteenth or nineteenth century.

Capital expenditure is necessary for two main reasons: one is that the existing capital stock is always depreciating because of wear and tear — a hospital like any other building will not last indefinitely; and second, new methods of medical care may be impossible to introduce unless new buildings are provided. For example, old hospitals tend to be built with open *'Nightingale' wards* that have a long row of beds down each side, whereas current styles of care and attitudes to privacy encourage a series of small rooms containing four or fewer beds.

In the first few years of the NHS, capital expenditure was extremely low — in fact, well below its replacement level. As Figure 2.13 shows, it rose quite sharply in the 1960s, and the reason for this was the *Hospital Plan* of 1962 (actually separate plans were published for England and Wales and for Scotland).

The plan proposed a 10-year programme of hospital building and, as you have seen in Chapter 1, the creation of a new institution as the basis of hospital services: the District General Hospital (DGH). In England and Wales, the plan envisaged 90 new DGHs being built, a further 360 existing hospitals being extended to become DGHs and 1 250 of the existing 2 750 hospitals being closed down. As the Plan noted:

In recent years there has been a trend towards greater interdependence of the various branches of medicine and also an increasing realisation of the need to bring together a wide range of facilities required for diagnosis and treatment. Hence the concept of the district general hospital ... which provides treatment and diagnostic facilities both for in-patients and out-patients and includes a maternity unit, a short-stay psychiatric unit, a geriatric unit and facilities for the isolation of infectious diseases ... The size of the hospital this concept implies would normally be of 600–800 beds serving a population of 100 000–150 000. (Ministry of Health, 1962, para.20)

It was reckoned that the whole scheme would cost around £500 million over ten years, doubling previous levels of capital spending. These new DGHs were considerably larger than the average-sized hospital of the time, and the Plan expressed the hope that bigger hospitals would be more efficient that the smaller hospitals they would replace because of *economies of scale*. Economies of scale are said to exist when the average cost of producing a unit of output — for example, a car in a car factory — is reduced by an expansion in the level of total output; if, for example, a car factory producing 100 000 cars a year can do so at a unit cost of £4 000 per car, whereas another factory producing 20 000·cars a year can't get its unit costs below £6 000 per car, then the former factory is experiencing economies of scale.

Economies of scale are known to be widespread in many manufacturing and commercial activities, and are one reason why the world is increasingly dominated by very large companies. But do they exist in hospitals? The answer to the question is crucial, because the NHS is hospital-based; if they do, then a more efficient health service could be created by gradually building hospitals big enough to take advantage of economies of scale; if they don't, then the reasons for having big hospitals are weakened, as indeed are the reasons for perpetuating such a strongly hospital-based health service. Figure 2.14 shows the results of one

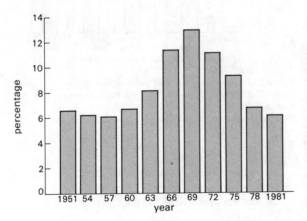

Figure 2.13 Capital expenditure on hospitals as a proportion of total hospital expenditure in Scotland, 1951–1981.
(Source: Summarised accounts, NHS (Scotland), various years)

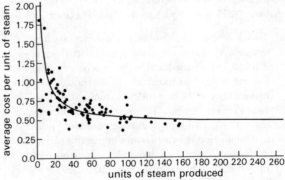

Figure 2.14 Variation in the cost of steam production in hospital boiler houses by size of boiler house, 1971–1972.
(Source: Hurst, 1979, Figure 3.7, p.88)

study, which examined one aspect of hospitals, that of boiler-houses.

☐ Do economies of scale exist with boiler-houses?

■ It shows clearly that hospital boiler-houses running at high levels of output had lower average unit costs than those running at lower levels of output — economies of scale exist.

☐ But now look back at Figure 2.11. What proportion of hospital running costs is devoted to energy, which includes boiler-houses?

■ Only 4 per cent.

A great deal of research has been done to try to find out whether economies of scale exist in hospitals, taking into account all their costs and not just a small part of them. The results have been inconsistent, with some research suggesting the costs are lowest in hospitals with 25 beds, others that the best size is 880 beds, and most finding no conclusive evidence one way or the other.

The fact that economies of scale have not been proven conclusively in hospitals can be interpreted in different ways. Perhaps the most important point to note is that it is extraordinarily difficult to isolate and measure something that represents the hospital's *output*. Ideally, this would be a measure of the improvement in health of the patients — a notoriously difficult task which is discussed further in Chapter 7. Instead, hospitals' performance tends to be judged on process or activity data such as the number of patients treated, irrespective of the outcome of their treatment.

Although the confidence of the 1962 *Hospital Plan* in economies of scale turned out to be misplaced, it need not be concluded that the planning process which resulted in the decision to go ahead with it was therefore shown to be deeply flawed. In a case-study of the events surrounding the acceptance of the Plan, David Allen has argued that planning decisions must always be dependent on the political circumstances pertaining when they are taken, and that the DGH was 'an idea whose time had come'.

To ask why hospital building rather than another alternative was chosen as the appropriate thing to do, is to ask the wrong question. It conceives the decision-making process far too abstractly, as though decision-makers choose the best solution from a selection. Policy makers are busy people, they are confronted by many things to do, by conflicting pressures for action and conflicting information about the alternatives available to them. Hospital building presented an opportunity to be grasped, it was acceptable to the NHS employees, to the medical profession, to the Ministry of Health, it was an improvement over the current circumstances and above all the Treasury was

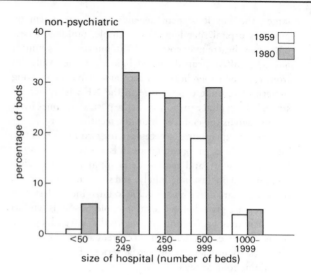

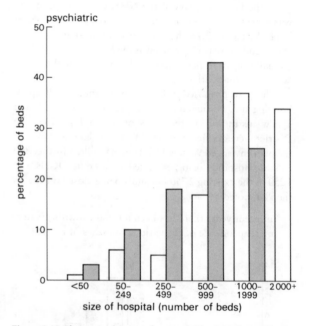

Figure 2.15 Change in the size of non-psychiatric and psychiatric hospitals in England between 1959 and 1980 as measured by the number of beds.
(Source: *Health and Personal Social Service Statistics*, 1982, Table 4.2)

not against it; it was financially feasible. There was consensus about the initiative with no evidence of any conflict. An opportunity too good to miss. (Allen, 1981, p.15)

As a result, as Figure 2.15 shows, the distribution of beds by hospital size changed markedly between 1959 and 1980:

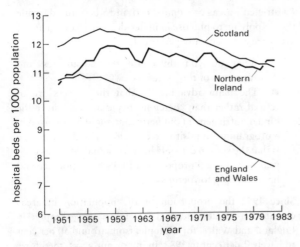

Figure 2.16 Change in the number of available beds (psychiatric and non-psychiatric) per 1 000 resident population in Scotland, Northern Ireland, and England and Wales, 1951–1982. (Source: Annual Abstract of Statistics)

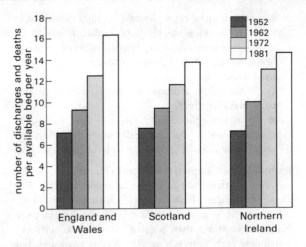

Figure 2.17 Discharges/deaths per available bed per year in Scotland, Northern Ireland, and England and Wales, 1952–1981. The number of episodes of in-patient care are measured by counting patients when they leave rather than when they are admitted to hospitals — hence, the use of beds is measured in discharges and deaths, and not in terms of admissions. (Source: as Figure 2.16)

the very large psychiatric hospitals of over 2 000 beds (which housed one-third of all psychiatric beds in 1959) had vanished by 1980, while in non-psychiatric hospitals the 500–1 000-bed hospitals that became standard after 1962 increased their share of beds markedly.

Thus the capital decisions of the past exert their influence on the present, for although the notion behind the *Hospital Plan* of more large, single-site, multi-speciality, custom-built hospitals has now been abandoned, and although the levels of capital spending in the 1980s are again low, the pattern of hospital services, and thus of a large part of the NHS, is set for the present and foreseeable future around DGHs. As regards the question of whether or not it is possible to *influence* the NHS from the centre through national planning strategies, the example of the 1962 *Hospital Plan* clearly demonstrates that such an approach is possible — at least in the field of capital planning.

However, before leaving capital planning it is important to realise that many of the developments in the *use* of the capital stock have not been planned in any systematic way. This can be seen in Figures 2.16 and 2.17 which show that while the number of hospital beds has fallen in relation to the population, particularly in England and Wales, the number of cases passing through each bed has approximately doubled, because the average length of time that patients spend in hospital has gradually fallen. The alteration in lengths of stay was not planned or even predicted, but has resulted largely from changes in what is regarded as acceptable clinical practice by doctors.

As you will see in Chapter 3, the issues involved in revenue planning, which take place locally in health

districts, present a rather different range of problems from those of capital planning, and illustrate another set of dilemmas. Meanwhile, let us consider a third objective of the NHS — the pursuit of equality. This also serves as another example of the power and scope of national planning.

The pursuit of equality

The 1944 White Paper on the NHS stated that one objective of the NHS would be to ensure that everyone 'shall have equal opportunity to benefit from the best and most up-to-date medical and allied services available'. To what extent has 'equal opportunity to benefit' been achieved in the NHS? Let us start by noting some different interpretations of the phrase. *'Equality'* might refer to some comparison between individuals, or between different social groups: social classes, sexes, age groups, disease groups, or groups in different regions of the country. Opportunity to benefit might mean having *access* to health services, making *use* of health services, or trying to get everyone onto the same *level of health*.

☐ Suppose this objective of the NHS was interpreted as equality of levels of health between different social classes. How would this fit in with other interpretations of 'equality', or 'opportunity to benefit'?

■ First, it would implicitly exclude inequalities that exist in addition to those of social class: a good example would be the gender inequalities in health that exist within each social class.* Second, it might mean that in trying to attain equal levels of health, it would be necessary to create deliberately *unequal* access or use of health services, so that those in poorest health received most health care.

□ What other assumptions are contained in this particular objective?

■ It assumes that health care can have significant effects on health, and that health inequalities between social classes can be tackled through the health service.

Each different interpretation of this objective of equality contains a different set of implications for the NHS. For example, if equality of *use* of services is sought, should the NHS actively seek out people who might benefit from health care, rather than waiting for them to turn up? Expanding such 'outreach' services has its advocates, but how far should it go before it becomes an authoritarian intrusion rather than a service?

Perhaps because there are so many difficulties associated with different ways of defining 'equality', the NHS has tended to devote most attention to just one particular aspect: the availability of services in different regions of the country. To a lesser extent, it has sought to reduce differences in the standard of care offered to different patient groups. How much has it achieved?

In 1948, one of the most glaring aspects of the regional maldistribution of health services was the availability of GPs. The situation was typified by the findings of a study of GPs published in 1944:

the number of residents per GP was twice as great in Kensington as in Hampstead, thrice as great in Harrow; four times as great in Bradford, five times in Wakefield, six times in West Bromwich, and seven times in South Shields. (PEP, 1944)

The attempts that have been made to tackle this situation are of interest not least because they allow us to look at one aspect of the NHS's *central manpower machinery*: the apparatus at the disposal of health ministers to plan the deployment of medical labour in the NHS. When the NHS began, doctors were free to set up in general practice wherever they pleased, but within three years national agencies called *Medical Practices Committees* had been established. Their purpose is to classify different areas of the country as relatively over- or under-doctored, and GPs wishing to set up practice have to apply to the committees for permission. Those applying to practise in over-doctored

('restricted') areas are almost certain to be refused, while those applying to practise in under-doctored ('designated') areas are automatically permitted.

□ What do you think are the advantages and disadvantages of this system?

■ The main advantage is that the powers are of refusal rather than coercion: they don't constitute the kind of infringement of liberty that might be involved in a programme of positive redirection. The disadvantage is that the system can only have a gradual effect, as each year only a small proportion of GPs enter practice and have to apply for permission.

Since 1952 the proportion of the population in areas classified as under-doctored has fallen very sharply; in England and Wales, for example, from around 50 per cent to barely 2 per cent in 1982. In important ways, therefore, the scheme has proved successful although *within* the areas classified by the Medical Practices Committees, the distribution of GPs can still be highly uneven. In particular, access to primary care is very poor in many inner-city areas. In other words, planning has largely achieved one objective, but must now be refocused onto smaller areas.

Plans to alter the distribution of hospital services took longer to appear, and throughout the 1950s and 60s the resources distributed to different regional hospital boards (see Table 2.4), continued to reflect the historical inequalities. Regional resource allocation was largely

Table 2.4 Revenue allocation per resident for Regional Hospital Boards in England, 1960/61

RHB	£ per resident
SW Metropolitan	10.4
NE Metropolitan	9.4
SE Metropolitan	9.3
S Western	8.9
Liverpool	8.8
Wessex	8.6
NW Metropolitan	8.1
Newcastle	7.6
Manchester	7.6
Oxford	7.3
Birmingham	7.0
East Anglia	6.6
Sheffield	6.5
Leeds	6.4

(Source: 1961 Census; and Digest of Health Statistics for England and Wales, 1969, HMSO)

*This and other parameters of inequality are discussed in The Open University (1985) *The Health of Nations*, Chapter 9, The Open University Press (U205 *Health and Disease*, Book III).

Table 2.5 Regional variations in health services, 1965–1967, (England and Wales)

Measure	Situation in:		Difference (larger as percentage of smaller)
	best-off RHB	worst-off RHB	
Population per consultant	4 425	8 932	202
Available beds per 1 000 population	13.59	7.54	182
Discharges/deaths per 1 000 population	120.7	85.3	141
Persons on waiting lists per 1 000 population	8.1	14.6	180
Expenditure on psychiatric hospitals per person per year (£s)	4.7	1.7	278
Expenditure on all hospitals per person per year (£s)	10.20	7.22	141
Anaesthetists per million population	23.6	13.6	172
Gynaecologists and obstetricians per million female population	22.6	11.0	205

(Source: derived from Cooper and Cuyler; in Hauser, 1972, p. 45–7)

determined by the existing level of services. The more hospital facilities a region had, the more funding it received, and vice versa. By the late 1960s pressure was growing to do something, and in 1970 the Secretary of State for Social Services, Richard Crossman, introduced a formula aimed at ironing out the regional differences in expenditure on the hospital services (Table 2.5). The formula contained three components that were intended to assess each region's *need* for hospital services, the existing *supply* of hospital services, and the *demand* being met for hospital services.

☐ What are the *simplest* ways of measuring these three aspects of hospital services that you can think of?
■ The level of need could simply be based on the total size of the population in each region; supply by the amount of hospital services available, for example, the total number of beds in the region; and demand by the number of people using the hospital services, for example the number of hospital cases treated each year.

Although the 'Crossman formula' had some statistical refinements, the underlying method was as simple as that. Each region's resource requirements were calculated on the basis of their populations, number of beds, and caseload, and then this requirement or *target* was compared with the actual resources each region received. If they were below requirement, they would get extra resources each year until they reached the target; if they were above requirement, their allocation of resources would be held back. There would not be any actual cutback, rather some regions' allocations would grow less rapidly than others; neither was it to be too sudden, instead the adjustments were to take place over a ten-year period.

In his diaries, Crossman recorded that the chairmen of the Regional Hospital Boards were initially extremely hostile to the idea, but the formula did begin seriously to alter the status quo for the first time since the NHS had begun. Between the mid-1960s and the mid-1970s hospital expenditure per person in each region moved significantly closer to the national average.

The Crossman formula was replaced in 1976 with another formula based on the research of the *Resource Allocation Working Party* (*RAWP*). The RAWP formula, like its predecessor, only covered the regions of England, not the UK as a whole. Among the many details of the RAWP formula — a topic of almost endless debate — a key innovation was that each region's need for hospital services would partly be assessed by calculating its standardised mortality ratio (SMR).*

Figure 2.18 illustrates the progress of the fourteen English RHAs towards the RAWP target between 1977 and 1983.

☐ How would you describe the pattern in Figure 2.18?
■ Generally, the distance from the target allocations have been reduced, but only Mersey and Oxford regions are approximately on target. Progress towards equalisation seems to have slowed since the 1970s.

The RAWP procedure raises many complex issues: it is only altering the funds given to regions, not the services

*SMRs are discussed in The Open University (1985) *Studying Health and Disease*, Chapter 5, The Open University Press (U205 *Health and Disease*, Book I).

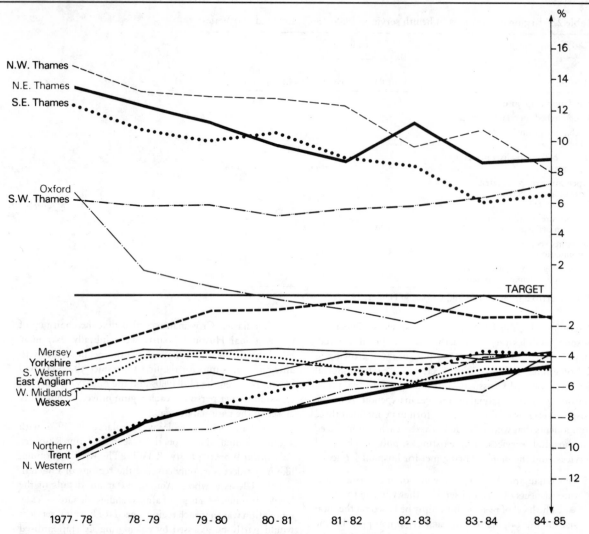

Figure 2.18 Resource allocation to the English Regional Health Authorities, 1977/8 to 1984/5, in terms of the region's distance from its target allocation. The distance is expressed as a percentage of the region's total allocation, e.g. in 1984/5 North West Thames received 8 per cent more than its target allocation.
(Source: *The NHS in England*, 1984, HMSO, Figure 2)

themselves; some regions may be more efficient than others in the way they use their resources; and many important inequalities in provision lie *within* regions. It has also been suggested that the private sector should be taken into account in RAWP calculations, a move that would result in services for the 92 per cent of the population not participating in the private sector being determined in part by the existence of services only available to the 8 per cent who are privately insured.

The procedure has raised two other issues, one recent and one ancient. The RAWP formula, like the Crossman formula, was devised on the assumption that no region would actually *lose* anything: the idea was that continued

growth in the total NHS budget would make redistribution painless, through a gradual levelling *up* of resources. During the 1980s, however, this assumption has been severely strained by tight restrictions on total NHS spending. Increasingly, it has seemed that regional inequalities can only be reduced if some regions, for example, Oxford and the four Thames regions, have resources taken away to be given to others. Levelling *down* is a very much more painful exercise than being held constant.

The dilemma it poses is whether having an explicit formula gives a spurious air of objectivity to resource allocation decisions and disguises an inevitably political element in such decisions, or whether an explicit and consistently applied formula is at least an improvement on implicit and almost certainly inconsistent yardsticks buried deep in the decision-making process.

The RAWP procedure has also exposed a much older issue.

☐ Think of the geographical area covered by RAWP. What does it exclude?

■ The RAWP procedure only covers resource allocations between regions *within* England. It does not deal with the differences between England and other parts of the UK.

Scotland, Wales and Northern Ireland have all busily produced their own formulae for distributing resources between their own Areas, and have even come up with more resonant acronyms for their formulae than 'RAWP' — the Scots have 'SHARE', the Northern Irish 'PARR', the Welsh, alas, could only come up with 'SCRAW'. But there is no explicit formula for deciding how much the Scots should get compared to the English, or the Welsh compared to the Northern Irish. In fact, the way different parts of the UK are treated remains a deep mystery, lurking in the shadowy recesses of the public expenditure process. It has been suggested that in 1891(!) the Census showed that Scotland accounted for eleven-eightieths of the UK's population, and that this figure became frozen into a Treasury rule-of-thumb for dispensing public spending until the 1970s, long after Scotland's population share had fallen (to around seven-eightieths by 1981). This rule-of-thumb even has its own name — the 'Goschen formula', after George Goschen, a Chancellor of the Exchequer who also happened to be the last President of the Poor Law Board. Whatever the reason, it was evident by the 1970s that wide disparities existed in the level of health funding between the four parts of the UK. In an attempt to pin down these differences more exactly, two economists, Alan Maynard and Anne Ludbrook, calculated how much the Scottish, Welsh and Northern Irish health services would receive if they were 'RAWPed', that is, if the RAWP formula was applied to them as if they too were regions of England. The results are shown in Table 2.6.

Here, certainly, the political element in resource allocation decisions is on display, for some Scots and Northern Irish would regard such differences as compensation payments for political union. The Welsh, however, appear to be compensating the English.

So much for service provision between different parts of the UK and between English regions. What about between patient or disease groups?

Table 2.6 Effects of applying the RAWP formula to UK health care budget, 1977–1978

Country	NHS allocation in 1977/8 (£ million)		Indicated change to reach target (%)
	Actual	RAWP target	
England	3 430.1	3 499.4	+ 2.0
Scotland	485.2	418.4	− 13.8
N. Ireland	144.1	126.4	− 12.3
Wales	210.3	225.4	+ 7.2

(Source: Maynard and Ludbrook, 1980, p.86)

Brave little Hollie dies after 18 days

Tiny Hollie Roffey, the world's youngest heart transplant patient, left a legacy of hope when her brief life flickered out yesterday. The millions who prayed for her survival now mourn her.

(Robert McGowan and Clare Dover, *Daily Express*, August 18, 1984)

In the late summer of 1984, newspapers were carrying reports on two stories involving the NHS, one in which one person died, the other in which twenty-seven people died. One story was about a baby called Hollie Roffey, who received a heart transplant in the London National Heart Hospital at the age of ten days, and died eighteen days later. The other was about an outbreak of food poisoning in the Stanley Royd Hospital in Wakefield, West Yorkshire, a psychiatric hospital occupied largely by elderly women. The stories received very different amounts of coverage.

In many ways the media treatment of these two stories reflects the fact that not every patient in the NHS receives equal *priority* in treatment or attention, and perhaps also that the public is more interested in some types of patient and illness than others. Once again this raises the issue of the NHS's objective of 'equal opportunity to benefit': how can this be ensured for different kinds of patient, and what has been achieved so far?

Many of the hospitals the NHS inherited in 1948 had been built in the nineteenth century. This was true of almost two-thirds of psychiatric hospitals, including the Stanley Royd Hospital. In 1954, when Parliament debated the subject of mental health for the first time in twenty-four years, much of the debate consisted of a catalogue of deficiencies: there were shortages of beds, suitable buildings, staff and money. 'There was serious overcrowding in many mental hospitals. Sometimes beds were placed in the corridors, or crammed up in the wards no more than nine inches apart...' (Jones, 1972, p. 290). Kenneth Robinson MP pointed out that although mentally ill and mentally handicapped patients occupied 42 per cent of the NHS's beds, they had attracted only 16 per cent of all NHS capital investment, and a miserly 1 per cent of the £80 million the Medical Research Council had spent on research over the previous eight years. Despite this there was little immediate response: £1 million extra was set aside for the following year (1955), a sum that came to be referred to as the 'mental million'.

In 1962 the Hospital Plan made a declaration of intent to halve, in fifteen years, the number of hospital places for mental illness, and in their place provide some beds attached to DGHs and an expanded system of community care. But three weeks later a Ministry of Health circular to the Regional Hospital Boards spelling out the policy implications provides a good illustration of long-term strategic planning creating a short-term expedient response:

> ensure that no more money than is necessary is spent on the upgrading or reconditioning of mental hospitals which in ten to fifteen years are not going to be required. (Cited in Jones, 1972, p.322)

During the late 1960s, a fresh wave of criticism of the low priority being given to patients in psychiatric, geriatric and psychogeriatric hospitals was set in motion by the publication of a book entitled *Sans Everything — a Case to Answer* (Robb, 1967). Seven separate inquiries into hospital conditions were launched as a result of allegations and testimonies contained in the book. When the results of an enquiry into conditions at the Ely Hospital in Cardiff for geriatric patients was published in 1969, Richard Crossman, who was the responsible Secretary of State, made the following entry in his diary:

> Wednesday March 12, 1969
> At 12.30 this afternoon we had the critical meeting on Ely in my room at Alexander Fleming House with about twelve people round the table, Bea Serota [a government whip in the House of Lords] came ...'
> One of the most dramatic moments of this meeting was when I referred to our not knowing anything about it and Bea said, 'Didn't we? You ask the Chief Nurse what she knows about it'. Dame Kathleen said, 'Oh yes. We used to have people going down there, regularly visiting'. I said, 'Did they report?' 'Yes'. 'When was the last report?' 'Three or four years ago'. 'Have you got it?' Bea had arranged to have it and she threw it across the table at me. It was a deplorable report, admitting scandalous conditions, bad nursing, the basis of all the *News of the World* revelations that Geoffrey Howe had confirmed. I asked what had happened to this when it came in and the answer was that it had gone on file. (Crossman, 1979, pp.592–3)

The Ely Hospital inquiry, and others at the time, did not fix the blame solely on lack of money. Local hospital problems were also cited, as were management difficulties arising from the tripartite division of the NHS. However, it was clear that the problems could not be solved without additional money. At this point, Crossman collided with another information problem: the accounting system of the NHS was entirely geared up to keeping track of items being purchased, but could reveal almost nothing about the

Table 2.7 Hospital and community current expenditure on priority and non-priority services in England, 1975/6 and 1981/2

Priority services	Expenditure (£million) in 1981/2 prices, in 1975–1976	1981–1982	Percentage change 1975–1976 to 1981–1982
Mental handicap in-patient	365.7	388.6	+ 6
Mental handicap out-patient	0.3	0.5	+ 67
Mental illness in-patient	733.3	764.7	+ 4
Mental illness out-patient	35.0	46.7	+ 33
Geriatric in-patient	580.7	663.2	+ 14
Geriatric out-patien.	3.4	5.1	+ 50
Other	543.1	678.1	+ 24
Total	2 261.5	2 546.9	+ 12.6
Non-priority services			
Acute in-patient	2 586.5	2 713.3	+ 5
Acute out-patient	704.7	790.9	+ 12
Obstetric in-patient	334.5	342.5	+ 2
Obstetric out-patient	42.7	49.7	+ 16
Other	1 035.2	1 139.0	+ 10
Total	4 703.6	5 035.4	+ 7.1

(Source: Green *et al.*, 1984)

different purposes to which these items were being put. Thus, it was quite possible to obtain accurate figures on total NHS purchases of split peas or safety-pins, but impossible to state how much in total was being devoted to the mentally ill, the mentally handicapped or any other group of patients. This deficiency led to a gradual reorganisation of the way in which financial information in the NHS was collected and presented. The concept of the *programme budget* was introduced, in which the activities of the NHS were grouped under different programmes of care related to patient groups.

In 1976, the DHSS published its first *priorities document* — a general review of existing patterns of expenditure on different patient groups, and how it wished to see these patterns of expenditure alter in the future. In particular, it identified a list of priority groups which became known as the '*Cinderella services*' because of their traditional low level of funding:

the central proposal in this document is that much of the available 'growth money' should be concentrated on services used mainly by the elderly and the physically handicapped, the mentally ill and handicapped, and children. (DHSS, 1976a, p.27)

A series of further documents was issued in 1979 and 1981, and also by the health services in Wales, Northern Ireland and Scotland. In these documents, although there have been some important changes of emphasis over the years, there

has been one consistent underlying theme: a general agreement that the 'Cinderella services' require priority. To what extent have these intentions been put into practice since the mid-1970s? Table 2.7 shows the priority ('Cinderella') and non-priority services in the NHS, and the change in expenditure on them between 1976 and 1981.

☐ In Table 2.7, looking first of all at the *size* of the budgets of the different services, which part of the service dominates the overall expenditure?

■ Acute in-patient care which consumes over a third of the total expenditure on hospital and community services.

☐ How much evidence does the table give for a shift towards priority services?

■ Between 1975/6 and 1981/2 the priority services as a whole grew more rapidly, but the growth of money was fairly evenly split between priority and non-priority services — around £300 million in each case.

The generally slow progress towards changing priorities in the NHS has raised a number of questions. In the first place, the priorities documents have only been advisory, and there has until recently been no mechanism for forcing regional or district health authorities to follow them. Some health authorities have made more progress than others, but it is not clear that any sanctions can be imposed on those that are not following the advice.

There are other problems. Altering priorities is an

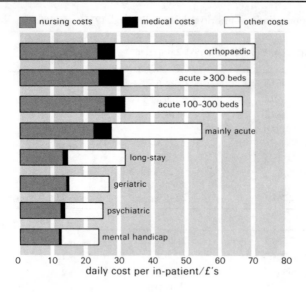

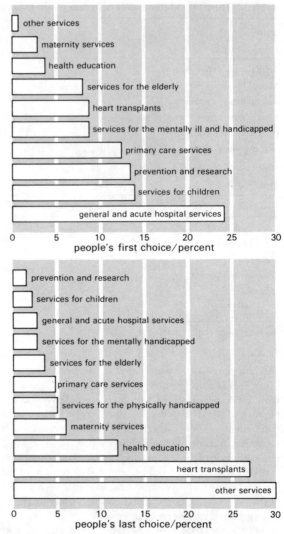

Figure 2.19 Daily costs for in-patient care in different types of hospital in Wales, 1980–1981.
(Source: DHSS Hospital Costing Returns, 1981)

exercise affecting many groups of health service staff, whose own priorities seem in some instances to be contrary to the government's departments. For example, there exist long-standing difficulties in getting nursing staff to work in 'Cinderella services', and this, coupled with a lack of resources, is reflected in the low nurse-staffing levels in such hospitals. Figure 2.19 shows the cost of a hospital in-patient day in different types of hospital in Wales in 1980–1981. Between two and three times as much is spent per in-patient day in the hospitals providing non-priority services as in the hospitals providing priority services, and this order of difference is reflected in the amounts spent on nursing care. It is also reflected in many other aspects of hospital care: for example, in long-stay hospitals standards of catering generally remained lower than in short-stay hospitals.

Figure 2.19 also shows that the amount spent on medical care is very much lower in hospitals providing priority services. This partly reflects the fact that doctors can make little in the way of an effective contribution to the care of such patients compared with nurses and other therapists (e.g. occupational therapists, physiotherapists and psychologists). The lack of a medical role is reflected in the career preferences and choices of medical students who tend to attach low status to working with such patients. This in turn is reflected in the distribution of *distinction awards* for consultants — salary increments awarded for 'meritorious' service. Whereas the percentage of consultants with awards in 1980 was 63 per cent in cardiothoracic surgery, 61 per cent in neurosurgery, and 53 per cent in neurology, only 28 per cent of consultants in psychiatry

Figure 2.20 Public choices of priorities for health services: (a) services given highest priority, and (b) services given lowest priority.
(Source: Trent, 1981, Figures 2 and 3, p.667)

held an award, 24 per cent in geriatrics, and 21 per cent in mental handicap. So the officially-designated priority areas in the health service are not by and large the priority areas for some occupations.

A further problem is that the policy guidelines contained in the priorities documents do not only affect the NHS. In particular, the emphasis on increasing care to dependent groups 'in the community', rather than in hospital or other residential accommodation, requires the close participation both of local authorities and lay carers. We will examine this in more detail in Chapter 5.

In examining the attempts that have been made by the NHS to alter priorities, we have focused on the problems arising from occupational attitudes, funding arrangements, organisational obstacles and the inherited fabric of health services. But to what extent is it possible for the NHS to set priorities independently of the attitudes of people outside the health service? What is the public's opinion on the subject? There been few studies conducted, but one by Sheffield Community Health Council asked people to state which care groups 'should have first call upon extra funds that become available over the next few years'. Figure 2.20 shows the percentage of first choice and last choice indicated by the respondents.

☐ How do these responses compare with the official priority statements of governments and the NHS?

■ Highest priority seemed to be given to the official low-priority acute hospital services, while officially high-priority services were well down the list.

It might of course be that most people are generally unaware of the prevailing standards of care for different patient groups, and would modify these priorities if they had more information.

☐ But think back to the question posed in this Sheffield survey. Why might it be seen as posing a 'soft option?'

■ The question was not about taking money away from some groups to give to others, but rather about what to do with *extra* resources.

If the question of choice between groups had been presented more explicitly, the priority rankings expressed in the survey might have become not less but more pronounced.

Priorities, regional resource allocations, plans, financial and manpower controls and other aspects of NHS planning raise many issues for management in the NHS. Planning may be a co-operative activity, but it can also create conflicts of interest and opinion. Plans may involve closing local hospitals, opening health centres, providing more care for some groups of patients and less care for others. Plans may affect people's lives in many different ways, and consequently the exercise of planning in a health service paid by and run for the population as a whole is very much more than a technical issue. The responsibility for planning services within broader national plans and taking such difficult decisions as shifting resources from one group of services to another, rests in the main with the district health authorities in England and Wales, and the health boards in Scotland and Northern Ireland. It is to them that we must turn our attention if we wish to understand how those decisions are taken.

Objectives of Chapter 2

When you have read this chapter, you should be able to:

2.1 Explain what is meant by need, demand and supply, and the relationship between them.

2.2 Outline the main aspects of the financial development of the NHS, its main sources of funding, and its broad pattern of expenditure.

2.3 Contrast the main consequences for the availability of health care between three different systems of funding — the NHS, fee-for-service private care, and health maintenance organisations.

2.4 Discuss some of the problems in defining the 'equality' objective of the NHS, and describe the policy steps that have been taken to improve geographical equality.

2.5 Discuss the existence of varying standards of care for different patient groups and the difficulties of creating a new set of priorities.

Questions for Chapter 2

1 (*Objective 2.1*) One of the newspaper stories at the beginning of Chapter 1 reported the deaths of sixty-eight patients who were awaiting a heart transplant, an operation that has only been available in the UK during the 1980s. Describe this story in terms of need, demand and supply.

2 (*Objective 2.2*) What effect has the change from volume planning to cash limits had on the provision of hospital services? Has the introduction of cash limits affected the provision of general practitioner services?

3 (*Objective 2.3*) Why is rationing inevitable in any system of health care? In what way is health care rationed in (a) the NHS, (b) fee-for-service private care, and (c) HMOs?

4 (*Objective 2.4*) How did significant geographical differences in NHS funding arise (a) within England, and (b) between England and Scotland? Why has it proved so difficult to reduce the differences between English regions?

5 (*Objective 2.5*) Despite a commitment by central government to give priority to 'Cinderella' services, such as those for the mentally handicapped, only slow progress was made during the late 1970s. Why has this been so?

3

Democracy, politics and management

Every organisation needs some kind of decision-making body to plan and to guide its actions; it needs, in other words, a *management* — and alongside this it also needs an *administration* to implement the management's decisions. The NHS is no exception; indeed, because the service is so large it has several tiers of management ranging from the Secretary of State through Regions and Districts, all the way down to Units. It is the Districts which (in England at least) actually shape the day-to-day activity of the health service — they run the hospitals, organise the health visitors and provide family planning clinics. It is for this reason that the Districts are the principal focus of this chapter.

Management is often looked upon unfavorably in the health service. Its practitioners are dismissed as bureaucrats obsessed with red tape and remote from the reality of actually providing health care. To some people the very word 'management' conveys an aura of the business world which they find wholly inappropriate to the task of providing health care. And despite the management costs of the NHS consuming a smaller proportion of its total resources than any other health care system in an industrialised country, its management is commonly portrayed as extravagant and wasteful. Not only that, but many hold that its constitution is far from democratic.

In this chapter we shall therefore attempt to answer two broad sets of questions: first, how far is the management of the NHS inefficient or weak or bureaucratic; and second, how far are its problems a consequence of the unparalleled complexity of the service it provides? No other organisation or industry serves so many different people, each with their own needs and views, and no other organisation employs so many types of staff, each of which holds a valuable, but different perspective on the provision of health care.

The District Health Authority

We shall begin with one person's perspective — that of David Steel, a lecturer in politics, who also served as a member of a District Health Authority (DHA) in the early

During this chapter you will be asked to read an article contained in the Course Reader entitled 'Food-work: maids in a hospital kitchen' by Liz Paterson (Part 5, Section 5.2). There is a television programme on primary health care associated with this chapter (TV10 'The Primary Health Care Team') with an accompanying audiotape sequence (Band 3, Audiocassette AC808).

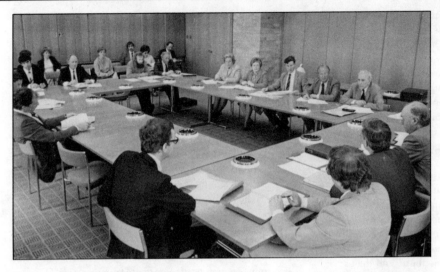

Figure 3.1 Milton Keynes District Health Authority meeting. DHAs usually hold meetings about once a month. The meetings are open to the public and press who can be seen at the far end of the room.

1980s. As you have seen, there are 192 DHAs in England. Their membership is largely composed of lay people, and it is they who are responsible to the government for the way the NHS is managed locally (Figure 3.1). The DHA has a team of *executive officers* (usually including a medical officer, nursing officer, treasurer and administrator), who are the full-time, professional managers.

Despite the fact that there are over 1 600 DHA members in England, the account that follows of one member's experience accords with the views of many others. He begins his account with the official description of the powers and responsibilities of DHA members.

> Department of Health and Social Security circulars state that each authority is responsible for 'the planning, development and management of health services in its district within national and regional strategic guidelines.' Members are enjoined to:
> Determine policies and priorities for their district within national and regional guidelines and on the advice of their officers;
> Review and, where necessary, challenge proposals by the district management team and to make effective arrangements for the implementation of the authority's decisions;
> Appoint and monitor the performance of their officers ... As the direct employer of a large number of staff, concern themselves with their working conditions, general interests and welfare (but not pay and conditions of service, which are determined nationally). (Steel, 1984, p.37)

So these are the formal duties of DHAs as laid down in the early 1980s by the Secretary of State. It is here that local power in the health service mostly resides. But we still need to know several more things. Just who are the members and how do they conduct their business? Who do they represent — the Secretary of State, the local population, local business, the professions? How are they chosen? What are their real as opposed to their nominal powers — just how do members really direct the NHS? Do they actually pay much attention to central government guidelines, or do they go their own way, or are they perhaps in the grip of the very people whom they are formally meant to be controlling?

Let us start by considering the membership and routine work of one particular DHA in the early 1980s:

> Exeter Health Authority has a chairman, and 17 other members. In common with all such authorities, these can be divided into three groups: the 'professionals' (three doctors and one health visitor); the local authority appointees (two county councillors and three district councillors); and the eight generalists, who are expected to provide a balance of age, sex, geography, and — where appropriate — race, but one of whom must be a nominee of the trade union movement.
> The authority meets formally once a month. At the outset, members decided that these meetings should be devoted primarily to a discussion of policy, and that its agendas should be drawn up with this in mind. During the first year, we considered papers by

the officers setting out existing policy for each of the major services: mental illness, mental handicap, community, district general hospital, health education, and so on. Major new developments and reports on progress continue to form the main items on our agendas. Two meetings are devoted to examination of the operational plan (now called the annual programme); in the first we examine a draft document paragraph by paragraph, in the second the comments received during the consultation process. In addition, we receive monthly reports from the treasurer on the financial position, quarterly reports on complaints and the action taken to deal with them, and more recently upon manpower; we also deal with various issues that may be referred to us by the chairman, or by officers, or occasionally raised by members themselves (for example, the question of whether to 'buy British', drug abuse, and the use of management consultants). Generally, however, agendas have been kept short and meetings rarely last more than two hours.

Health authorities are statutorily required to meet in public but can resolve to exclude the public for certain items. In Exeter, only limited use has been made of this provision, and the closed part of meetings is normally confined to the ratification of the decisions of appeals panels (all of which relate to individual cases) and to the registration of nursing homes. In practice, the local press is always represented, but very few members of the public take advantage of the opportunity to attend.

In order to be able to contribute to the authority's work, members need to be well-informed both about national and regional policies and about local services. With no secretariat or back-up staff to help them (at least in Exeter), they have to do that for themselves. Visiting hospitals and other NHS institutions is also extremely important, since it familiarises members with the services being provided; it enables them to meet staff and to discuss problems informally; and, as far as long-stay hospitals are concerned, it is an important safeguard that standards of care are being maintained. In addition to attending meetings and making visits, members are involved in appointing senior staff (usually chairing the selection committee), in hearing disciplinary and grievance appeals, and in sitting on mental health review panels in relation to compulsory detention orders. There is no question, therefore, that a member who is willing and able to do so can spend much more than the two to four days a month on authority business which is mentioned at the time of appointment. In practice, their interest and commitment vary, with some

spending about a day a week but others significantly less. (Steel, 1984, p.38)

The members of a health authority, who are all unpaid (with the exception of the chairperson), therefore have a major set of responsibilities. How are they chosen? The key point is that unlike their nineteenth-century predecessors, the Guardians of the Poor Law,* members are *selected* from among, rather than *elected* by, the local community. Selection is conducted, directly or indirectly, by two distinct bodies. On the one hand, there are *local authorities* (both county and district councils) who choose representatives from among their councillors. On the other hand, there is the involvement of the Secretary of State. She or he appoints those who chair the DHAs, while all the other members, apart from those selected by the local authorities, are vetted by the Regional Health Authority members, who are in turn vetted by the Secretary of State. But what determines *which particular people* are selected? This was Steel's experience.

In 1979 I was nominated for appointment by a university colleague who was a member of the South West regional health authority and who knew of my interests in public administration and in the NHS. For my own part, all that was required was the completion of a short form concerning my personal background, education, employment and experience of public and voluntary service. Some months later, I received a formal letter of appointment from the regional authority. The process of selection at that time was entirely closed. The only clues that I have been able to elicit as to the reasons for my appointment are, first, my experience as a teacher and researcher in public administration and second, my relative youth (I was then 31). Health authority members are unpaid and do not receive attendance allowances, and so it is always difficult to find young people who are able to devote time to this sort of work during working hours.

On appointment in 1979, I received from the regional authority three (DHSS) circulars — on the structure of the NHS, on the system of appointments to health authorities, and on their functions. They were followed by copies of the authority's standing orders and of various current papers, including the three-year operational plan, and the NHS Handbook, produced by the National Association of Health Authorities. As far as training was concerned, a one-day seminar was organised by the authority's officers

---

*The Poor Laws are discussed in *Caring for Health: History and Diversity*, Chapter 4, *ibid*.

with some external input for those new members who wished to attend. Otherwise, I was expected to learn on the job. (Steel, 1984, p.37)

☐ Is the method of appointing members a democratic or an undemocratic system?

■ 'Democracy' is a word with several meanings (we shall explore some of these later). In one sense, the method is undemocratic — the local community does not elect the authority members. But they can vote for local councillors, some of whom are on the health authority, and they can also vote in parliamentary elections and influence from which political party the Secretary of State is drawn — and he or she in turn influences the selection of members of the health authorities. So there is a measure of local democratic control, though it is *extremely* indirect.

Apart from the local councillors a variety of *interest groups* are represented. Some of these have considerably more representation than others: doctors do particularly well, comprising about one quarter of all the members — a fact which goes against the strong recommendations of a 1950 government report. The Jones Report on financial management in the NHS forcefully argued that the entire membership of the hospital boards and management committees that existed at the time should be drawn from the laity:

In any democratic organization it is axiomatic that, whilst due attention must be paid to the advice of technical experts, if there is the slightest suspicion that such experts have a pecuniary or other self-interest in any matters they should not be a party to the making of decisions thereof. (Cited in Klein, 1983, p.49)

☐ Why do you think that doctors and nurses have, nevertheless, been included within the membership of health authorities?

■ A basic political principle on which the NHS is run would seem to be that of *incorporation*. Although the government tries to retain ultimate control of the NHS, any local interest group, such as doctors or trade unionists, which might want a say or might cause trouble, is officially incorporated within the organisation.

Let us turn now from the composition of health authorities to look at their functions and performance, and to consider the extent to which members live up to the responsibilities expected of them in government circulars. A '*circular*' is the term for a letter sent to health authorities and boards by ministers and civil servants in London, Edinburgh, Cardiff and Belfast. Circulars generally contain either official advice or simply information about any changes in centrally controlled aspects such as wage levels. Occasionally, circulars may contain instructions. So, how well does Steel think that he and his colleagues fare in their attempt to manage the local service?

District authority members ... operate within parameters set by the Department and by the regional authorities, and these have tightened in recent years, but they still enjoy considerable discretion in determining the character of local services. The initiative locally lies primarily with officers and with doctors rather than with members but, working in partnership rather than in competition with the professionals, members have the opportunity to make a modest but significant contribution. The Department's job-description is reasonably accurate provided that it is not interpreted too literally. Members do contribute to the determination of policies and priorities for their district; they do review proposals emanating from management and occasionally they challenge them; they do appoint the officers and are in a position to monitor their performance; and they do become involved in matters affecting NHS staff.

Without doubt, members' impact would be greater if they were elected. This would give them much greater legitimacy to challenge the judgement of Ministers, officers and doctors. However, quite apart from the major practical problems involved in either establishing separate elected health authorities or in adding the NHS to the responsibilities of existing local authorities this option lies outside the realm of practical politics because of the deeply entrenched opposition of the medical profession.

The present system of appointed authorities seems likely, therefore, to persist, at least for the time being. It is not perfect, but it incorporates doctors and, to a lesser extent, nurses into policy-making, it provides some link with local authorities, and it brings into NHS decision-making a few members of the local community.

Moreover, despite their limitations, health authorities act as a restraint upon both centralisation and professional power. Without doubt, their effectiveness could be increased if more effort was put into recruiting members who are keen to work in this kind of environment, and into providing training and other resources to assist them in undertaking their duties. (Steel, 1984, p.40)

It seems that members are caught between three powerful forces: from above — government and Regional Health

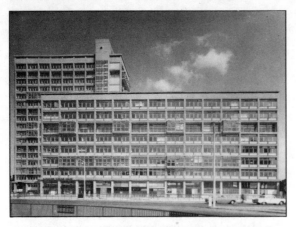

Figure 3.2 Alexander Fleming House: one of the main buildings of the Department of Health and Social Security in London.

Authorities — comes increasing pressure from their political, financial and administrative masters (Figure 3.2), while from below the members have to contend with the expertise both of the executive officers and of the medical profession. The untrained, unpaid, largely amateur members lack even their own secretariat to advise them. Despite this, there is still room for members to exert some influence:

> Neither the DHSS nor the region is equipped to run the service on its own, and lacks the information about local conditions needed to do so. Moreover, any decisions either may want to impose have to be implemented locally, through what is in effect a *highly complex political system*, comprising community health councils, local authorities, doctors and other staff groups, and local pressure groups. Implementation has perforce to be left to the discretion of individual health authorities or their managers. (Steel, 1984, p.39, our emphasis)

☐ To what extent do you think it is possible to understand how decisions are made in the NHS at district level by simply studying the formal management arrangements?

■ Steel's description suggests that such an approach would be severely limited as it would fail to consider many aspects of local politics, both within and outside the NHS.

Instead, we must go well beyond those who are formally charged with responsibility at this level and examine the links the NHS has with other services, to delve into the workings of the officers who serve the authority, to consider the clinicians and their many powers, and to inspect the entire management strategy and the nature of planning. In short, to understand what goes on, we must

follow the lead Steel has given us and explore both the *internal* and the *external environment* of management.

The internal environment contains both the members and their executive officers; the external environment is everything beyond — the government, the DHSS, the public, the NHS staff and so forth. Some idea of the complexity of the external environment is given in Figure 3.3, which sets the DHA in the context of the many outside forces which impinge upon it. As it illustrates, far from there being just one centre of power there are many, each of which exerts its influence upon the health service. This is not peculiar to health care. In the words of the political scientist A.F. Bentley, writing at the turn of the century:

> All phenomena of government are phenomena of groups pressing one another, forming one another and pushing out new groups and group representatives (the organs or agencies of government to mediate the adjustment). (Bentley, 1908; cited in Richardson and Jordan, 1979, p.3)

In fact, Figure 3.3 is really far too simple — the various groups are also connected with one another and such links come in a multitude of both formal and informal ties: friendships, enmities, old girl/boy networks, liaison committees, business lunches, and so on.

Let us now explore the three main elements of this complex external environment: formal health and welfare services not managed by the DHA; the local community; and occupational associations in health care. (The fourth main element, that of the role of central government, has already been discussed in Chapter 2.) When we have considered these we will return to examine further the internal environment, for only when we have understood the external reality with which it must deal, can we understand why management behaves as it does.

Formal care — divisions and links

As you have seen in Chapter 1, the management of formal services which provide health care and social welfare in England is only partly integrated. While the hospital and community health services are both organised by the DHAs, the GPs are administered by a separate body — the Family Practitioner Committee. Also each individual GP is independently contracted to work for the NHS rather than being a salaried employee of the organisation. This independence is something that most GPs value highly.

☐ Why might DHAs wish to control the activities of GPs?

■ Primarily because the GPs partly control the demand for secondary care (i.e. hospital services). In addition, if the DHA is trying to plan health services for

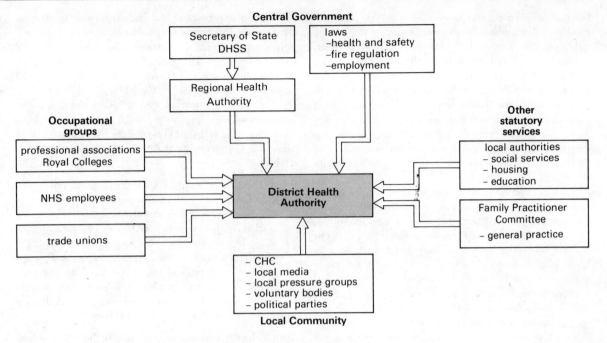

Figure 3.3 The political and organisational environment of a District Health Authority.

the local population, then it is desirable that such plans include primary (i.e. GPs) as well as secondary care.

As the DHAs do not formally control the GPs they have tried to integrate them in other ways. For example, between 1974 and 1985 GPs were included in all District Management Teams. In addition, many DHAs have provided custom-built *health centres* for GPs, in which DHA-employed staff, such as health visitors, district nurses and therapists, could work alongside the doctors. So while the GPs are independent and nominally self-employed, they have increasingly been integrated into the rest of the system, becoming part of *primary health care teams* in the new health centres. This has led to a major reshaping of primary care.*

The other formal services that have a direct bearing on health, but which are also organised separately from the NHS (i.e. part of the external environment) are those run by the local authorities: in particular, social services (known as social work in Scotland), environmental health and housing.

☐ Which country in the UK differs significantly from the English arrangements as regards social services, and in what respects?

■ Northern Ireland, where the management of health and social services has been fully integrated since 1973.

Social services include the management of *residential care*, such as homes for the elderly and for the mentally handicapped; of *day care* — an institution which takes people such as the elderly, but only during the day; of all kinds of *domiciliary services*, such as home helps and meals on wheels; and finally, of the fieldwork or casework side of social work in which the social worker tries to solve a great variety of individual or family problems, such as financial, criminal and psychiatric ones.

☐ Why might DHAs be interested in these services?
■ There is clearly considerable overlap between health needs and social needs. Any shift from hospital to 'community' care — such as the long-term programme to run down the large psychiatric hospitals — is premised upon the assumption that parallel services will be developed partly by the local authorities. Likewise, any shortages in the services provided by local authorities may increase the demand for hospital care.

For example, hospital consultants commonly complain that hospital beds intended for acutely ill patients are being widely used for reasonably fit elderly patients who no longer require medical care, but are not yet fit enough to return home without domiciliary care. The lack of sufficient social services means that they have to remain in

*Primary health care teams and health centres are the subject of a television programme (TV10) and associated audiotape sequence.

hospital, a phenomenon known in the NHS as 'bed-blocking'. Any cutback, expansion or change in plans by either side can therefore have serious effects for the other; lightening the load here, dramatically increases it there. One central feature of the 1974 reorganisation was an attempt to provide greater formal coordinating mechanisms between the health and social services. *Joint Consultative Committees* were set up; special funding was allocated for joint projects; a *joint planning system* was created; local councillors were appointed as members of DHAs; and, for a few years at least, there was an attempt to make the geographical boundaries of the local authorities and the NHS the same (known as *co-terminous*), through the area tier of management.

Such attempts at liaison between the two authorities have, however, not proved very successful for a number of reasons: hospital services are delivered at district, not area level; just as hospital and GP services are separately managed in the NHS, so the services managed by local authorities (environmental health, social services, education, housing, etc.) are similarly divided; the officer and member/councillor relationship within each body is different, as are their budget cycles; and the representatives of each authority on the joint committees have different degrees of responsibility and power in their own organisation and therefore different abilities to promote change. The difficulties of liaison were further increased in 1982 with the abandonment of the area tier by the NHS. The joint planning of services has proved to be exceptionally cumbersome, with decisions often requiring the approval of both authorities separately. For example, in Torbay in Devon, eighty-four formal meetings were required between health and social services before a Community Mental Health Centre could be opened!

Perhaps even more important as regards the possibilities for liaison between the NHS and social services has been the absence of much financial inducement. All of the money made available for jointly planned services comes from the health authority, but it is only to fund a relatively brief period, such as the initial few years of a new service (although this period has gradually been extended since 1974). After the period of initial funding, the local authority is expected to subsume financial support. But at a time of increased financial uncertainty, local authorities have had difficulty in making expenditure commitments for several years hence. This has seriously impeded progress in joint planning between the two authorities; and for most services, where there was no money available at all, no one took joint planning seriously anyway. Indeed, overall, the amount of joint planning has been merely 'vestigial'.

While the organisational divisions between the DHA, the GPs and the local authorities present health service management with dilemmas in planning and organising

services, there is no clear evidence that greater integration of these services would necessarily be a solution; for if it solved some problems, it is possible that integration would give rise to others. The question of how much to integrate and how much to divide functions is one that confronts all large organisations, not just the NHS.

The divisions just discussed take place between *statutory* bodies — public agencies of the state such as local authorities and DHAs. This is not the case with several of the other key groups in the external environment of the DHA.

   □   Looking at Figure 3.3, which groups are not part of the official machinery of government?

   ■   There are two main groups to consider: those based in the *local community* including pressure groups, voluntary bodies (such as Age Concern), political parties, and the mass media; and *occupational* groups such as trade unions and professional associations. (Whether community health councils are or are not part of the official machinery of government is a delicate question to which we shall return later).

Although a diverse range of groups, all of them are involved in trying to influence decisions taken by DHAs. The elaborate organisation used by government to manage the NHS is counterposed by many other organisations, each of which is striving for some degree of influence and claiming to be acting on behalf of NHS employees and the public. It is these groups that we must now consider.

The local community

The DHA may find its actions opposed by *pressure groups*; these may focus on a particular subject — such as the National Childbirth Trust's interest in maternity care — or they may be concerned about a particular locality, or, as is often the case, a group may represent both sorts of interest.

Hospital 'danger' unit row

Health chiefs have come under fire from worried parents over the handling of plans to site a 'Broadmoor-style' secure unit in a mental hospital on their doorstep.

Mr Ken Dennis, chairman of the Thorpe Residents Action Committee, said: 'There are 10,000 people living alongside that area and many parents are worried for their children's safety'.

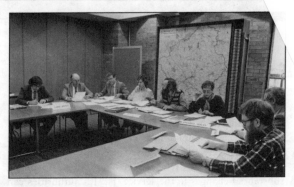

Figure 3.4 Milton Keynes Community Health Council meeting.

With an emphasis, during the 1980s, on shifting care from large institutions into the community, this sort of public response may play a significant part in limiting the options available to health authorities.

Another example of the way in which public action can modify DHA plans is the raising of large sums of money by public appeal to purchase expensive items of high technology equipment. During the early 1980s these appeals have mostly been for highly sophisticated CT scanners (the development of which is discussed in Chapter 6). In several instances, health authorities have found themselves in the ironic position of trying to reject an offer of help from the community it is serving. This arises for two reasons. First, the health authority my have made a positive decision not to buy the piece of equipment on the grounds that it was seen as a lower priority than other developments. Second, many of the public appeals only raise money for the capital cost of the equipment and not the revenue for its consequent maintenance and use. Even when the authority has accepted the gift of equipment, there may be difficulties between the appeal organisers and NHS managers.

equipment they have purchased. In contrast, the health authority consider it their role to determine how the health service is organised and managed as they are responsible for allocating resources and ensuring that overspending does not occur.

Faced with so much external pressure from organised public groups how do health authorities react? Just as official links have been formed between health authorities, GPs and local authorities, so the NHS has tried to create official links with those who try to pressurise it. The best example of this is the Community Health Councils (CHCs) that provide a formal channel of communication between the public and the DHA (Figure 3.4). Half the CHC membership are local councillors, while most of the remainder come from local voluntary bodies and pressure groups such as MIND and Age Concern. The character and activities of CHCs are as varied as their members. Some CHCs maintain a low profile, confining themselves to assisting and advising individuals who have complaints about the NHS while, in contrast, others mount high profile campaigns of public criticism and denunciation of their DHA.

☐ What is the basis of this conflict?
■ The organisers of the public appeal wanting to decide, or at least influence how the NHS uses the

National Childbirth Trust has already won 1,500 signatures.
(Paul Lewis, *Reading Evening Post*, October 18, 1980)

During the 1980s much of the activity of CHCs has concentrated on fighting hospital closures not only because this has been a common and recurrent decision of health authorities, but also because the only management decisions that the CHC can veto are those involving substantial changes in the service. Health authorities can ignore the opinion of the CHC on all non-substantial matters. If the CHC does object to a hospital closure, the DHA has to refer the issue to the next tier of management — the RHA — which in turn may have to seek the intervention and decision of government ministers if they cannot get the DHA and the CHC to reconcile their differences. So the CHCs are granted a little power — which encourages people to serve on them — but at the same time their members too, like the members of the DHAs, are incorporated to some extent within the system.

Occupational associations

To concentrate on pressure group campaigns ... is in a real sense to misunderstand the nature of the bulk of group influence. Pressure groups are about relationships. Campaigns are the currency of unsuccessful groups; permanent relationships are the mode of the successful. (Richardson and Jordan, 1979, p.123)

The relationship between authorities and clinicians is not mentioned by the Department in its circulars but of course it lies right at the heart of the health service. (Steel, 1984, p.38).

So far we have considered groups and organisations that lie someway beyond the health authority's remit — social services, general practitioners, pressure groups of various kinds. We now turn to the staff who make up the service which it is the authority's duty to manage. As you have seen in Chapter 2, every authority employs a bewildering variety of staff. Even in 1948, there were no less than fifty-five separate trade and professional associations with members in the NHS. There are doctors in endless variety, nurses of many kinds, laboratory technicians, cleaners, porters, drivers, and so on. Health care is *people-work* (i.e. work with people, as is social work, for example) and people-work is labour intensive. Over 70 per cent of expenditure is on wages and every health authority is a major employer — the average sized DHA has around 6 000 staff. Thus the primary task of NHS management is the management of people.

Managing people presents two main kinds of problem. First, there is the official task of management, which is to make decisions: to decide what jobs need doing, to arrange them so that they fit together, to choose the right people to do the right job, to motivate them to work, to find ways of measuring their performance, and to check that the job has been done. All these are difficult tasks in themselves. But they are made far more difficult by a second problem — there is an inherent conflict between management's desire to control the work that is done and an equally strong desire by the workforce to control the work they do. This latter desire potentially gives rise to yet another form of democracy. Just as there is the democracy by election and democracy by pressure groups, so there is the democracy of workers' control.

☐ On the basis of Steel's account of Exeter DHA is the health service an example of workers' control?
■ No. Although doctors do have some autonomy they too are subject to a fair degree of control by management. Other groups of workers have little or no control.

The Department's circulars don't mention medical power, for they operate within the world of *formal* management structures — like the formal charts of NHS organisation in Chapter 1; but this is not, however, a sign of doctors' weakness. Medical power is mostly part of the *informal* side of the organisation. This makes it no less formidable. Doctors still control the NHS at most of the key points of delivery, and are consulted at every twist and turn of policy-making and implementation. Indeed, their power to influence extends way beyond the narrow confines of the health authority, affecting the public in ways that then further constrain the actions of their managers:

Not merely do the practitioners, by virtue of gaining admission to the charmed circle of colleagues, individually exercise the license to do things that others do not, but collectively they presume to tell society what is good and right for the individual and society at large. Indeed, they set the very terms in which people may think about this aspect of life. (Hughes, 1971, p.288)

Doctors' power has very striking effects as regards the management of the service. For example, the Royal College of Obstetricians and Gynaecologists normally insist on a minimum of twenty-five beds if an obstetric unit is to qualify as suitable for doctors training in the speciality. Other Royal Colleges (Figure 3.5) set similar kinds of standard and since every district general hospital relies heavily on student nurses and on junior doctors who are training to be consultants, health authorities are forced to comply — even where they feel there is little justification in

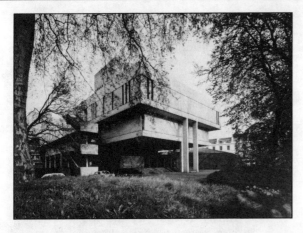

Figure 3.5 The Royal College of Physicians in Regent's Park, London. The building was designed by award-winning architect, Denis Lansden, and, like other Royal Colleges, houses lecture and seminar rooms, an extensive library, dining facilities, administrative offices, a wine cellar and a collection of paintings.

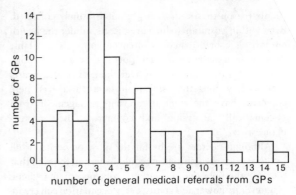

Figure 3.6 Variation in the number of referrals to general medical outpatient clinics made by GPs. Based on 65 GPs in full-time practice, over a 13 week period in 1977. (Source: Dowie, 1980, p.8)

Table 3.1 Variations in consultants' operation rates for tonsils and adenoids on children under 15 years within one Scottish health region (1970)

	Number of cases referred from GPs for possible operation	Percentage actually operated upon
Surgeon 1	374	54.0
Surgeon 2	372	60.8
Surgeon 3	83	45.8
Surgeon 4	128	81.2
Surgeon 5	555	84.5
Surgeon 6	77	57.1

(Source: derived from Bloor, Venters and Samphier, 1978, Table V, p.796)

terms of patient need. Moreover, doctors not only shape the size and general staffing levels of the service — for every extra bed also requires extra nurses, cleaners and so forth — but they also enjoy huge individual liberty to conduct their own work as they see fit: they enjoy the *clinical freedom* to exercise their *clinical judgement*. Health authorities do not tell doctors how to treat their patients. The result is an extraordinary variation in the way which doctors actually carry out their work as Figure 3.6 and Table 3.1 demonstrate. NHS doctors may have to work within the overall constraints of a limited budget but within that they have complete clinical freedom to treat patients in whatever way they may choose. By contrast, in a fee-for-service system such as in the USA, doctors have no total budget to constrain them, but their clinical freedom is severely limited. The way they treat patients, the length of time they keep patients in hospital and other aspects of clinical care are carefully monitored and regulated. As one American observer has concluded:

> The English doctor who is not in a training grade is in many ways more independent than his American counterpart. The consultant receives, in effect, a lifetime appointment and cannot be disciplined or removed except for major transgressions. The GP has independent contractor status, but unlike most contractors his performance is not reviewed periodically. (Fox, 1978, p.10)

Thus, for example, GPs who prescribe more than 75 per cent above the regional average are contacted by DHSS officials. (In the late 1970s, this affected 6 to 7 per cent of GPs each year.) The officials, however, are powerless to do any more than pass on the information to the GP — it is left to the doctor to decide what to do. However, in 1985 the first compulsory restriction on the prescribing habits of GPs was introduced by central government.

A wide variety of commonly used medicines, such as laxatives and cough medicines, are available for doctors to prescribe. There is considerable variation in the price of the different preparations. In an attempt to reduce the NHS drugs bill the government introduced a '*limited list*' which restricted the varieties of drugs that doctors could prescribe to the cheaper ones. This action, which curbed the clinical freedom of doctors in the NHS, was met with a howl of outrage from the medical profession and the pharmaceutical companies. It represented a radical new move by central government to control the activity of doctors, and in particular GPs.

As regards other matters, such as GPs' rate of referral of patients for specialist opinions, their hours of availability or their use of laboratory tests, no action is taken for the simple reason that such data are not routinely collected. Even within hospitals (which are directly under the health authority's control) there is often no routinely available data on such activities as each doctor's use of pathology tests and X-rays. Data are only available on in-patient care, such as how long they stay in hospital, and even here clinicians have the right to prevent management from systematically analysing and comparing their performances.

Although doctors are by far the most powerful of all health service occupations, it would be wrong to think that they are the only one to present problems for managers. Whatever its power and status, every occupation can create difficulties, kitchen-maids as much as doctors. To consider this further, you should now read the article in the Course Reader by Elizabeth Paterson, a sociologist. Like David Steel's article this one is based on personal experience — the author worked in a hospital kitchen for several months.

☐ What are the 'good organisational reasons' for kitchen work being badly organised?

■ One obvious point is that kitchen-maids are badly paid — but this can't be the only reason; if it were, doctors would always perform splendidly. There are other important factors besides: the work is poorly supervised and most kitchen practices are invisible to others. It is also poorly scheduled — it just is not possible to fit in special dietary requirements. In addition, the work itself is demeaning, hard, repetitive, sometimes dangerous and, above all, personally unrewarding. The maids get little pleasure out of preparing food in bulk and little if any possibility of thanks from those who consume the product of their labours.

☐ In what ways do the maids try to control their work?

■ They work hardest on the tasks that are most visible to outsiders (such as washing lettuce); they take illegal breaks; they sometimes act sullenly and answer back; but, above all, since their power is so limited, they try to distance themselves from their work — to imply that this is not the real them, merely something that they are paid to do.

Managers are therefore faced with a huge variety of occupations each of which require synchronising and monitoring, and each of which is also trying to control its own labour as best it can. And, for all their differences, all these trades use the same basic set of weapons in their struggle. Each tries to band together in trade associations to negotiate with their employers and each engages in *restrictive practices*. Just as in some hospitals no one is allowed to change a plug except a qualified electrician —

thus preserving jobs — so the GPs and the consultants have carved up the medical trade between them and jointly agreed to prevent patients seeing a consultant unless they have first seen a GP — another *demarcation agreement* that preserves jobs.

Such agreements are, however, rarely reached easily; indeed, just as management has to struggle with each occupation, so it must also contend with the disputes that break out between different occupations as each tries to better its conditions.

Doctors prescribe too many drugs, say nurses

Family doctors in Northamptonshire have come under fire for prescribing tranquillizers as a 'cure for everything'. The attack comes from top nurses in the county who were shocked to hear that the annual National Health bill for drugs has almost reached a staggering £800 million. They say that in many instances GPs are guilty of prescribing too many drugs at a time. And sometimes they prescribe when patients really need someone to talk to.

(*Northampton Chronicle and Echo*, September 29, 1981)

So great is the power of doctors, that a key part of the struggle between health service trades is, in reality, a struggle by other trades against the doctors. These groups are, however, far from united in their attempts to win more power. Some of them have tried to follow the doctors' route by seeking the status of a licensed *profession* with its own standards of training and examination, and a register of all those who are properly qualified. Indeed, so many health occupations have tried this, both in Britain and elsewhere, that in America in the early 1970s the federal authorities placed a ban on the creation of new health professions (by that time there were well over a hundred).

The other occupations have a long way to go to catch up with doctors: the scientific basis of medical training has been developed over several hundred years and is developing more rapidly than ever. British doctors (or some of them) have enjoyed a legal monopoly since the sixteenth century; even the more modern form of the profession dates from as far back as 1858, and finally, unlike some other trades, such as nursing, doctors enjoy the advantage of being relatively few in number.

Nurses press for exclusive treatment over pay

The Royal College of Nursing conference gave unanimous and emotional support yesterday to demands that the nurses and mid-wives pay review body, promised as part of last year's pay settlement for all nursing staff, should cover only qualified nurses and students.

It backed the demand already pressed by the college's leaders to the Government with a plea that the country's 120,000 unqualified auxiliary nurses should have their pay negotiated alongside cleaners and porters in the ancillary staff's Whitley Council.

(John Ardill, *The Guardian*, April 14, 1983)

□ What advantages might there be for nurses if they negotiate their pay separately from the nurse auxiliaries?
■ They are more likely to gain larger pay awards as a smaller number of staff will be involved in any settlement.

Given the many difficulties involved in professionalisation, health service occupations have banded together in the alternative form of occupational association — the trade union (though it is important to note that the professions, such as medicine, have also formed trade unions, with great

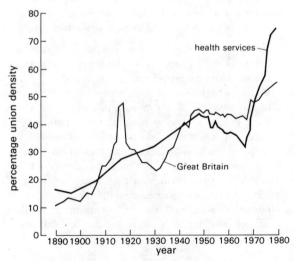

Figure 3.7 The changing extent of unionisation in the health service and in the entire British labour force.
(Source: based on data from Bain and Price, 1980)

effect). Kitchen-maids might strive for professional status by recasting themselves as trainee chefs, but simply joining a trade union is easier. During the lifetime of the NHS, increasing numbers have followed that route. Between 1968 and 1979 the proportion of health service employees in a union increased from 33 to 70 per cent (Figure 3.7), resulting, after a long period of industrial peace, in a wave of industrial disputes. During the 1970s virtually every group of NHS employees took industrial action — one of the first groups being the doctors. Such action has continued into the 1980s.

Health union calls strikes

More than 250,000 health service workers were asked by their union yesterday to ban non-emergency admissions, hold a series of two-hour strikes, and stop servicing private patients. The measures in protest at the Government's insistence on limiting pay rises were drawn up yesterday by the action committee of the Confederation of Health Service Employees.

(Donald Macintyre, *The Times*, April 14, 1982)

□ With a system of cash limits, what would be the potential effect on an authority's services to patients of (1) a pay award which satisfied the employees, and (2) a pay award within the Government's (then) 4 per cent ceiling?
■ (1) A reduction in services because the health authority would have to find the extra money for meeting the award by cutting services. (2) A reduction in services as a result of industrial action taken by employees.

Increasing unionisation has posed yet further problems for health service managers. How have they coped? Having explored much of the health authority's external environment, it is time to delve within and explore the inner processes of management.

Internal environment

For all the dilemmas that the external environment poses for management, might it be that the more serious problems are those to do with the internal environment — the way management is structured, the methods of coordination between staff groups, the quality and ability of the managers, and the way decisions are made? Broadly speaking, management can either adopt a *cooperative* approach in which managers attempt to gain agreement for any decision, or a *conflict* approach in which managers are autocratic, that is they take decisions without necessarily seeking the agreement of those people who will be affected. In practice, few organisations make *exclusive* use of either. Cooperation and conflict can be thought of as the extremes of a spectrum with most organisations at some point in between. So where do health authorities lie on this spectrum? Until 1980 the dominant theme was cooperation. However, during the 1980s the management arrangements have altered, as already described in Chapter 1, to a more conflict oriented model. To what extent does each approach create or resolve some of the dilemmas facing management? Let us start by considering the case for a cooperative approach.

This was the approach embodied in a government document published in 1972 entitled *Managerial Arrangements for the Reorganized Health Service* — more snappily known, after the colour of its cover, as 'the Grey Book'. This formed the basis of the management arrangements for the reorganised NHS after 1974. Throughout the service, the keyword was *teamwork*. Once everyone was more involved in the overall problems of the service then, so it was hoped, there would be a chance to steer it in a more promising direction. To this end, the NHS was filled with *professional advisory committees* (groups of doctors or nurses with a special interest in one part of the service), while at the very core of the new health authorities a new type of body was created to advise the members — the *district management team* (DMT). That team involved not only the newly created executive officers (administrator, treasurer, nursing officer and medical officer) but also a representative of the hospital consultants and of the GPs.

Like the security council at the United Nations it was explicitly based on the *consensus* model of decision making, in which everyone had to agree, or failing that, no one disagreed so strongly as to veto the decision. By gathering several different occupations together, and by providing everyone with a veto, the hope was that a new and much more binding form of consensus would emerge.

The new multidisciplinary management teams included a new actor — the *community physician*. It was felt that an integrated service required a manager who would be able to assess the needs of the whole community and the priorities for service development. To achieve this a new body of doctors was required with a much broader training than any doctors had previously received: one that integrated (hopefully) epidemiology, management and social sciences with their established knowledge of clinical medicine.

There were, however, problems for the new discipline. They might be doctors — and thus within the medical pecking order — but they occupied a lowly position,

somewhere near psychiatry, geriatrics and general practice. And what was the NHS to do while waiting for several hundred such doctors to be trained? In practice, hundreds of community physicians metamorphosed overnight from Regional Hospital Board medical administrators and local authority Medical Officers of Health.

One further ingredient of the cooperative approach was a new emphasis on *rational planning*, to replace the 'muddling through' or '*crisis management*' of the pre-1974 NHS in which managers simply dealt with whatever was at the top of the pile or was most pressing; there had been little attempt to take the long-term view into account, to plan for the future, to think systematically about the main directions the service should move in and try to shift resources in those directions. As a result, policy making had consisted of what has been termed *incrementalism*. There was no real policy, instead the service just responded to whatever pressures or opportunities arose on a wholly piecemeal basis — adding little bits or 'increments' as it went along. All this was to change, or so the '*paternalistic rationalisers*' (as Rudolf Klein, the political scientist, has dubbed them) hoped.

> The politics of administering the status quo gave way to the politics of technocratic change. At long last the paternalistic rationalisers — those who in the years before 1946 had seen the creation of a national health service as an opportunity to apply expert knowledge to dealing with need in a planned and systematic way — came into their own. (Klein, 1983, p.62)

The government and DHSS were to set the basic guidelines for the direction the service should move in (after consulting with the service), and then the health authorities would prepare more detailed *strategic* (long-term) *plans*, outlining the stages by which change would take place.

> ☐   What difficulties can you see with the managerial doctrines of cooperation, teamwork, consensus decisions and integrated strategic planning?
> ■   If the health service is rife with conflict, then is any of this possible? Will teamwork prove possible where some groups are vastly more powerful than others? How long will it take to reach agreement and will the sorts of decisions made simply reflect the lowest common denominators? Is it feasible to expect so many people scattered throughout such a vast organisation actually to be able to agree? And if professionals hold a power of veto, will the key question of medical effectiveness ever be raised, or will this be dismissed as necessarily a matter of individual professional judgement?

In short, the philosophy of communication and cooperation pays relatively little attention to the equally

The Calf Path
(edited version)
Sam Walter Foss (1895)

One day, through the primeval wood,
A calf walked home, as good calves should,
But made a trail all bent askew,
A crooked trail as all calves do.

The trail was taken up next day,
By a lone dog that passed that way;
And then a wise bell-wether sheep,
Pursued the trail o'er vale and steep,
And drew the flock behind him, too,
As good bell-wethers always do.

And from that day, o'er hill and glade,
Through those old woods a path was made;
And many men wound in and out,
And dodged and turned and bent about,
And uttered words of righteous wrath
Because 'twas such a crooked path.

This forest path became a lane,
That bent and turned, and turned again;
This crooked lane became a road,
Where many a poor horse with his load
Toiled on beneath the burning sun,
And travelled some three miles in one.

The years passed on in swiftness fleet,
The road became a village street;
And this, before men were aware,
A city's crowded thoroughfare.

Each day a hundred thousand rout
Followed this zig-zag calf about;
And o'er crooked journey went
The traffic of a continent.
A hundred thousand men were led
By one calf near three centuries dead.

A moral lesson this might teach,
Were I ordained and called to preach;
For men are prone to go it blind
Along the calf-paths of the mind,
And work away from sun to sun
To do what other men have done.

But how the wise old wood-gods laugh,
Who saw the first primeval calf!
Ah! Many things this tale might teach —
But I am not ordained to preach.

important facts of power, size, time and conflict. As such, the new managerial approach ran into problems almost as soon as it was implemented: there was conflict between areas and districts as to their respective roles; the professional advisory structure proved unwieldy; health authorities continued to ignore a high proportion of what became a tidal wave of ministry circulars; there was relatively little evidence of a shift towards many of the new priority areas; and the new planning system ran into immediate problems. Many managers found they spent all their time preparing the next plan and had too little time implementing the existing one. There were also complaints that the quality of the planning staff was poor. Neither of these problems were surprising given the lack of staff preparation for the task. Above all, perhaps, the new approach was based on the 1960s assumption of steady economic growth, an assumption that no longer held true by the 1970s. As you have seen in Chapter 2, major changes in direction are much easier to achieve if they can be produced largely by extra money. For example, instead of cutting other services to make more money available for geriatrics, one keeps other things as they are and just gives more to geriatrics.

In consequence, rational planning largely failed; crisis management continued as before with the most powerful clinicians continuing to dominate incremental decision making. Indeed, since the NHS was undergoing a dramatic alteration in industrial relations, crisis management was, if anything, on the increase. A study of planning both in health and in local authorities, both of which had experienced the attempt to introduce rational planning, found little sign amongst the staff of belief in its utility, nor indeed of teamwork and cooperation.

Officials and professionals expressed goals in terms of departmental expansion. They viewed individuals as engaged, like themselves, in an extended game whose prize was more resources. Planning was seen as a strategy for convincing fund holders of your department's need for more money. (Glennerster, Korman and Marslen-Wilson, 1983, p.263)

So what of the alternative approach based on conflict management introduced in the mid 1980s? In place of multidisciplinary teamwork, the DHAs have a single *general manager* with personal responsibility to the health authority. In addition, as you have seen in Chapter 1, the general manager is appointed by and accountable to his or her health authority, the chairperson of which is appointed by the Secretary of State. In addition, government ministers have taken an active role themselves in the appointment of general managers both at regional and district level. In other words, a management structure exists that allows government ministers to exert much more influence and control on the NHS than has previously been so.

Whitehall to vet shortlists for 200 NHS posts

Health authorities have been ordered to keep secret from their own members and officials short-lists of candidates for over 200 general manager posts until they have been personally approved by Mr Norman Fowler, the Social Services Secretary. At West Lambeth health authority, a job was offered to an applicant who was subsequently vetoed by ministers.

(David Hencke, *The Guardian*, January 18, 1985)

Once in post, the general managers are free to create a management structure to their own liking. Thus, instead of formally recognised positions and roles in a standard structure, general managers are free to create informal groups of people, including the executive officers, to advise and help him or her — people whose views can also just as easily be ignored if the manager so wishes. Unlike a team approach no members of these informal groups possess a veto; power lies almost entirely with the general manager who in turn is on a short-term contract to the health authority. Finally, just as a single manager now rules the officers so there is some evidence that the power of the chairperson of the DHA is also increasing. Consensus as a means of coordination has been replaced by control.

What effect will this have on the management of the NHS? The American historian George Rosen, writing of related but slightly earlier manifestations of the same process in American medicine commented as follows:

One may say that the Industrial Revolution has finally caught up with medicine and that the medical practitioner is being brought into the 'factory' (the hospital and the whole bureaucratic complexity for the provision of medical care) where he is being subjected to the necessary 'labour disciplines'. (Rosen, cited in Guest, 1972, p.289)

In this context the following contemporary news story makes interesting reading:

NHS team set for purge on doctors' perks

The heart unit at Guy's Hospital which grabbed the headlines recently after over-spending its budget is a particular point of contention. 'If they [the surgeons] use public uproar as an alternative to co-operating with the management, we will have to get them to realize that they will get nowhere', Clarke [the Minister of Health] said. 'In the last resort the place will shut ... At the end of the day, it comes down to resource allocation', said Paige [the general manager of the NHS in England and ex-chairman of the National Freight Corporation]. 'That is the ultimate discipline over doctors as it is over everyone else'.

(Brian Deer and Tim Rayment, *Sunday Times*, March 17, 1985)

☐ In what way might difficulties arise for conflict management?

■ Just as to run an organisation on the assumption of consensus is to ignore the very real conflicts that often occur, so conflict management in its turn may ignore the cooperation without which management is also impossible.

One particular source of future trouble may lie in the effect conflict management has on local control. Although the NHS is nationally organised, it has preserved at least some measure of local influence. The members of health authorities may not be elected or representative of the local community — white, middle-class, middle-aged to elderly males are the norm — but they still have important ties to the neighbourhood, and there is still a good deal of local variation in the health service. If, however, power is now being removed from most members and officers — and even, to some extent, from the clinicians — and if, instead a far greater *central* control is exerted, how will localities react (Figure 3.8)? Of course, centralisation of power and control is not just a phenomenon of the 1980s, it has been going on since 1948.

☐ What elements in this centralising programme have been mentioned so far in this book?

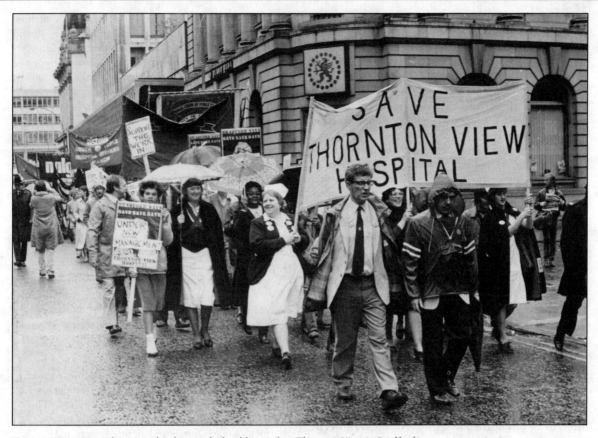

Figure 3.8 Protest march against the closure of a local hospital — Thornton View in Bradford.

■ The imposition of a ceiling on total NHS expenditure; the *Hospital Plan* (for the DGH); the creation of health authorities; the development of national priorities; attempts to achieve geographical equality of provision; attempts to devise a standard planning system; the recent marked increase in the powers of the chairperson and her or his accountability to the Secretary of State; the introduction of general managers at regional, district and unit levels; the creation of an NHS Management Board in England (and similar bodies in the rest of the UK) under the control of a general manager.

The methods by which centralisation has been pursued have varied over the years: there have been several major tactical changes, but the broad strategy has remained unchanged despite occasional shifts in governmental rhetoric. Indeed, in the testimony of Enoch Powell, the minister who introduced the *Hospital Plan*, central planning is implicit in the very concept of a national health service. On his account, whatever the feelings of the particular government of the day, the NHS imposes its own centralising logic:

> To have been obliged, in order to plan the development of the hospitals, to settle upon a standard pattern for the provision of hospital services was bad enough. I would have hated to produce a standard pattern for community care. Yet that is the responsibility which presiding over a fully monolithic NHS entails upon the Secretary of State for Health and Social Services. (Powell, 1976, p.78)

While centralisation may, as Powell has suggested, be an inevitable consequence of having a *national* health service, the extent of that central control is largely determined by the government. The 1980s have witnessed an increasing degree of central interference in local decision making, both through direct and indirect means. The direct approach has focused on the establishment of *accountability reviews*: annual meetings in which each tier of management has to account for the performance of the services it is responsible for, to the tier above it. Thus, the units are reviewed by the district, the districts by the region, and the regions by the ministers. Any changes in health services that the ministers wish to see implemented can therefore be conveyed to districts and units through this process. In subsequent years the ministers can check on what progress has been made to meet their wishes. To assist the reviews, the government requires all districts to collect similar information about the performance of its services — another example of the increasing central control on local services.

So much for direct measures by government. Of equal importance are the indirect measures, two examples of which illustrate the power of central government. The first is that of manpower controls which as you saw in Chapter 2 were introduced into the NHS in 1984. Control on the number of staff a DHA can employ has led to the situation in some districts of funds being available to provide services but the authority not being able to spend them on employing staff.

The second example also concerns finance: that of the *privatisation* of NHS services such as laundry and catering. In response to complaints of a lack of finance by DHAs, the government has decreed that the authorities should make savings by contracting out some services to private companies. The main reason why the latter can be cheaper than the in-house NHS staff is that many private contractors use fewer staff, do not provide holiday or sick pay, do not perform such a thorough job and pay lower wages to their non-union labour. While many DHAs are happy to use private contractors, others are not. However, the latter are faced with an impossible choice: if they defy the government and continue to employ their own staff, they end up having to reduce the clinical services they provide to patients. Faced with such consequences, many DHAs have reluctantly accepted privatisation as the lesser of two evils. Both this and the preceding example illustrate how effectively central government can exert control on DHAs simply by issuing a circular.

But just how far can central government extend its control? Health services are important to people and they have grown used to regarding them as theirs. Clinicians might just, unite with patients in the defence of their local service. There might even be strong demands to return health services to local authority control (as components were before 1948) or to a directly elected health authority. Such a shift might also preserve the power of health professionals which is under increasing threat. But, at the time of writing, this is both speculative and sketchy, for the shift from cooperation to conflict management is still in its infancy.

The art of the possible

Throughout this chapter we have avoided addressing directly the key issue in management: what is its *role*? Why

have managers? Hidden beneath all the issues of how management should be structured and how it should function lies the question as to what management is for. There are two distinct views: one that management's role is to *support* the activity of all the clinical staff, and the other that its role is to *control* their activity.

In most sectors of the economy, managers are at the top of the organisational hierarchy, *controlling* those who carry out the main work — whether it be car-workers or social workers. The workers are down at the bottom, with less power, less prestige, and less pay (Figure 3.9a). Those who progress up the hierarchy have progressively more of these things but less and less contact with conditions on the ground. In medicine, however, the reverse is true: senior clinicians, however powerful, still engage in regular patient care. For most doctors, it is only the front-line work which has the real prestige. Managers, on this account, are mere *support* staff who simply facilitate the work of the doctors, making sure that patients, potions and ancillary workers are in the right place at the right time for the doctors' convenience. In short, as Figure 3.9b illustrates, the organisational pyramid is turned upside down. To quote further from the newspaper story cited earlier:

'The concept of the NHS was to provide an administrative system within which doctors treated patients in the light of their professional judgement', said Paddy Ross, the consultants' spokesman. 'The NHS is just the system that pays the bills and provides the hospitals and all that.' (Deer and Rayment, *ibid*.)

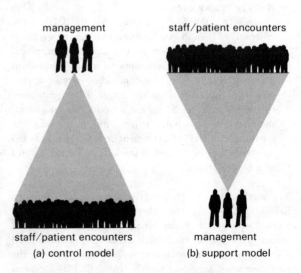

Figure 3.9 Two views of the function of management: control or support?

This view is in direct contradiction to the view of government in the 1980s which wishes to turn the pyramid back, and to treat the NHS like other commercial organisations. How and to what extent this will actually be carried out is, at the time of writing, unclear. So too is the manner in which both doctors and the public may respond. What is certain, however, is that the present struggle to stand the health care pyramid on its base will prove difficult.

Finally, we end this discussion of the dilemmas of management on a cautionary note. Rosemary Stewart, who has made extensive studies both of management in general and NHS management in particular, has made the following observation:

> There is rarely a solution to an organizational problem that does not create fresh difficulties. Usually it is a question of finding the best balance between the advantages and disadvantages of different forms of organization. (Stewart, 1970, p.ix)

Just as this proved true of consensus management in the 1960s and 70s, so too it may do so for 80s conflict management. Whichever way up the pyramid ends, one thing is clear: the key element in health care will remain the front-line workers along the base. Regardless of whether the management structure is supporting or controlling them, the delivery of clinical care will remain of central importance. It is to the front line that we must now turn our attention.

Objectives of Chapter 3

When you have read this chapter, you should be able to:

3.1 Discuss several key aspects about control of the NHS: the extent to which there is local democratic control; the relative contributions of experts and lay people; and the balance of power between central government and local DHAs.

3.2 Describe the different management approaches (crisis intervention and rational planning); the different relationships that can exist between managers and the managed (support and control); and the different forms of decision making (conflict and consensus).

3.3 Describe some of the many external groups whose views a DHA has to take into account when managing the health service.

3.4 Describe the similarities in the way each health occupation tries to control its work and the problems this presents for managers; the differences between professions and trade unions; the extent to which, and some of the reasons why, doctors have had far more success than other health occupations in controlling their work.

Questions for Chapter 3

1 (*Objective 3.1*) To what extent is there local democratic control of health services? You should consider the composition of DHAs and the extent to which DHAs are free of central government control in making decisions.

2 (*Objective 3.2*) The following extract is taken from a definition of the manager's role by a leading American management writer, Peter Drucker:

> There are five basic operations in the work of the manager. Together they result in the integration of resources into a viable growing organism. A manager, in the first place sets objectives ... Second a manager organizes. He or she analyses the activities, decisions and relations needed. He classifies the work. He divides it into manageable activities and further divides it into manageable jobs. He groups these units and jobs into an organisation structure. He or she also selects people for the management of these units and for the job to be done. Next a manager motivates and communicates. He or she makes a team out of the people that are responsible for various jobs ... The fourth basic element in the work of the manager is measurement. The manager establishes targets and yardsticks ... He or she sees to it that each person has measurements available which are focussed on the performance of the whole organization and which, at the same time, focus on the work of the individual. The manager analyses, appraises and interprets performance ... Finally a manager develops people, including himself or herself. (Drucker, 1979, p.20)

Which of the following styles of management does Drucker's analysis fit best: (i) rational planning or crisis intervention; (ii) management as support or management as control; or (iii) management through conflict or management by consensus?

3 (*Objective 3.3*) Drucker's account assumes that the manager controls all the relevant jobs and activities. But health authorities do not employ GPs, nor do they control local authority services. Why are these services important to them?

4 (*Objective 3.4*) In what ways does the management of the NHS conform to Drucker's analysis of its five 'basic' tasks (consider each in turn)?

4

Customer service

In this chapter you will be asked to read 'Normal rubbish: deviant patients in casualty departments' by Roger Jeffery (Part 5, Section 5.3) in the Course Reader. You will find that consultations between health professionals and patients included in television programme TV 8 'Customer Service' is relevant to the subjects discussed in this chapter. You may wish to listen again to the audiotape that accompanied that programme (Band 1, Audio-cassette AC 808).

In every hospital recognized by the Medical Council as a place of instruction for medical students, the treatment of the patients is entirely subordinated to the instruction of those students ... Quite recently, I heard a railway signalman make a request. It was four o'clock and he had been waiting since twelve ... the visiting surgeon had given a long demonstration on him and was then discussing an entirely different question ... When the surgeon stopped speaking and began to draw diagrams on the board — diagrams which had nothing to do with the case in question — the man mildly and politely asked if he might go as he was wanted 'on duty'. He was instantly told to 'shut his mouth'. For forty minutes did the man wait and then the surgeon said, 'Dear me, how late it is! We must get on' and to the signalman: 'All right don't stand there, you can go' ... This is a very common occurrence. (Anon. 1905; cited in Ferris, 1967, p.200)

All trades take liberties with their customers at times. This particular description is a fairly old one, coming in fact, from a gentleman's magazine at the turn of the century. At that time, teaching hospitals offered free treatment to the poorer members of society in return for their use as 'teaching material'; a bargain which led to considerable abuse, at least according to the doctor who wrote this description. Are there any modern equivalents to this story? To what extent has the creation of the NHS done away with such problems? Are there any other perhaps more subtle forms of mistreatment which are in need of serious reform? If so, how should this be done? To try to answer these questions, this chapter considers the interaction between the health care trades and those whom they serve — the public in their capacity as patients. Such occasions — bed-baths, home visits, out-patient consultations or *encounters** between patients and staff — are often referred to as the 'coal-face' of formal health care, for it is here that the most direct and personal kinds of formal

---

*A more general discussion of encounters is contained in *Studying Health and Disease*, Chapter 7, *ibid*.

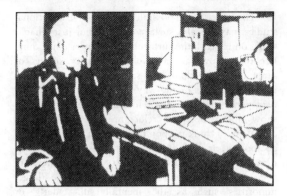

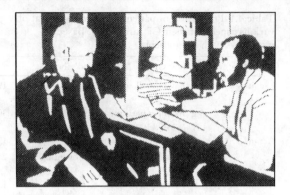

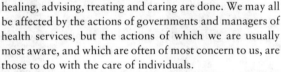

healing, advising, treating and caring are done. We may all be affected by the actions of governments and managers of health services, but the actions of which we are usually most aware, and which are often of most concern to us, are those to do with the care of individuals.

In the NHS, personal care is carried out on the most enormous scale: on average, people consult their general practitioner four times a year — making more than 200 million such consultations annually; there is a huge array of hospital out-patient consultations — 37 million in 1982; and there are over 6 million admissions to hospital every year. During their stay in hospital, patients meet many different staff — cleaners, doctors, porters, nurses and so forth — and for some patients the hospital will come to constitute almost their entire world. For example, despite the policy of community care, 40 per cent of the patients in hospitals for the mentally handicapped have been there at least twenty years. Twenty years represents a lot of interaction with medical staff. Finally, since formal health services reach out into the home, there too, a myriad of health care encounters take place: as health visitors see young mothers and their babies; as district nurses care for the elderly — 7 million people a year are seen in this way.

With so many different types of staff, patient, setting and medical condition, not to mention personality, the nature and quality of the interaction varies enormously. No generalisation about these matters will ever prove universally true. None the less, in those areas that have been explored by researchers — mostly encounters with doctors — certain regularities have emerged.

How do patients fare in the NHS? From one point of view things look quite good. There are still occasional gross scandals concerning the mentally handicapped and the elderly, just as there were a hundred years ago. But a variety of reports suggests that most other patients are satisfied with the treatment they receive. For example, research which directly observes what goes on in staff–patient encounters has shown that, with relatively few exceptions, most are calm, even-tempered affairs — at least overtly.

Perhaps, however, patients have rude things to say when out of the staff's hearing?

Hospital patients find appointment systems keep them waiting

One in three out-patients have been kept waiting in hospital, despite the appointment system, according to a Gallup Poll conducted for the *Daily Telegraph*. Hospital food keeps its reputation as the least satisfying aspect of hospital care, with only one in four completely satisfied. On the whole, the public remains appreciative of National Health Service hospitals' care, ... the overwhelming majority (93 per cent) of in-patients are generally satisfied with the way they are treated.

	medical care	nursing staff	food	hospital cleanliness
Very satisfied	64	69	25	63
Satisfied	28	24	42	30
Not very satisfied	4	5	17	3
Not at all satisfied	1	1	11	0
Don't know	2	2	5	3

(*Daily Telegraph*, October 22, 1984)

A more detailed survey of general practice by two sociologists, Ann Cartwright and Robert Anderson, suggests that there too, the patients are fairly happy. Again, around 90 per cent said they were satisfied with the general quality of the care they received. Moreover, though they did have some criticisms when asked about specific features

Table 4.1 Proportion of patients who were critical of various aspects of their GP care (1977). Based on interviews with 836 patients.

Percentage who felt their GP was 'not so good' about:

Facilities	— having well-equipped, up-to-date surgery	19
	— having a pleasant, comfortable waiting room	30
Action	— always visiting when asked	13
	— keeping people waiting in waiting room	21
Treatment	— examining people carefully and thoroughly	13
	— sending people to hospital as soon as necessary	8
	— only sending people to hospital when necessary	3
Communication	— taking time and not hurrying you	14
	— listening to what you say	7
	— explaining things to you fully	23

(Source: Cartwright and Anderson, 1981, p.7)

of that care, the impression is one of reasonable contentment (Table 4.1).

☐ What do GPs do best, and what are the worst features of their practice according to Table 4.1?

■ The really good aspects of the service according to the patient survey are that GPs only send people to hospital when necessary (only 3 per cent had complaints) and that they send them as soon as it is necessary (only 8 per cent complained). They also listen to what patients have to say (only 7 per cent felt otherwise). The worst feature, of which 30 per cent complained, was the lack of a pleasant waiting-room, while 23 per cent felt that things were not always explained fully, and 21 per cent felt they were kept waiting too long.

Some other findings seem to fit this general picture. A study carried out for the Royal Commission on the NHS in the late 1970s found that a similar proportion of people (25 per cent) were dissatisfied with the information they received about their progress as hospital outpatients (Table 4.2) as occurred in general practice (Table 4.1). And yet, although there are many millions of consultations between doctors and patients, in 1983 there were only 8 323 formal complaints laid against doctors. Encounters between staff and patients are it seems, in the main, a success. But can this story be entirely true?

☐ What doubts, if any, might you have about the argument?

■ There are several possible problems. Observational studies may reveal a surface calm — but just what is going on beneath the surface? And is *every* clinic quite like this? How far can we trust survey studies of satisfaction — perhaps high satisfaction merely reflects low expectations or the way the question was asked? And perhaps the levels of formal complaints merely show that people are reluctant or even afraid to complain, or think it's pointless, or don't know how to go about it, or don't even know it's possible? And even if many encounters are satisfactory, perhaps there are some which are not. What happens to the (large) minorities such as the mentally ill, elderly or handicapped who are normally excluded from surveys of patient satisfaction? Have we any real idea how they feel? And, what about the enormous range of criticisms that are commonly made about health services on television, radio and in newspapers?

You have already seen in Chapter 2 that many kinds of illness are never formally identified (the 'clinical iceberg'). In addition, there are fears about the impersonal nature of (total) institutions; arguments about medically-induced disease (iatrogenesis); worries about class, gender, age and ethnic stereotyping; concerns about unwarranted medicalisation, as well as claims that many treatments are ineffective.* Are these mostly without foundation? In short, although there are some reasons for thinking that almost everything in the interaction is creditable, there are equally reasons for thinking otherwise — reasons which we shall now explore.

Table 4.2 Aspects of the hospital service with which more than 10 per cent of outpatients were dissatisfied. Based on a survey of 2 267 people of all ages. Percentages exclude those giving 'no answer'.

Aspect of service	Percentage dissatisfied
Information about progress	25
Length of time spent at the hosptial	19
Adequacy of space in waiting room	18
Length of wait before seeing doctor	16
Difficulty understanding medical terminology	15
Other difficulty in understanding doctor	15
Appearance of waiting room	14
Number of seats in waiting room	11

(Source: Royal Commission on the NHS, 1978, Table 13.2)

*These topics have been touched on in The Open University (1985) *Experiencing and Explaining Disease*, Chapter 13, The Open University Press (U205 *Health and Disease*, Book VI) and *Caring for Health: History and Diversity, ibid.*, Chapter 6.

Analysing staff–patient encounters

Consider the following transcript of a consultation between a male GP and a female patient. It is taken from a study by a general practitioner, Patrick Byrne, and a psychologist, Barry Long, in which data were gathered from seventy-one GPs who, with their patients' permission, tape recorded their consultations — around 2 500 in all. This particular example is typical of a style used by many GPs.

DOCTOR   Come in, please, come in and sit down. No better?

PATIENT   I don't know what was the matter, but I've had a fortnight in bed.

DOCTOR   With what?

PATIENT   With flu.

DOCTOR   Flu?

PATIENT   I lost my balance.

DOCTOR   And how did this flu affect you?

PATIENT   I was sweating and sneezing, I couldn't stop sneezing.

DOCTOR   Any aches and pains?

PATIENT   Well, I was all aching, all over.

DOCTOR   Any cough?

PATIENT   Yes, I had a cough.

DOCTOR   Bad?

PATIENT   Well, it was really like bronchitis. I got a lot up, it was that greeny colour.

DOCTOR   No blood?

PATIENT   Oh, no.

DOCTOR   Has that cleared now? The phlegm.

PATIENT   Well, no, not quite, it's still loose on the chest.

DOCTOR   You still get it up? Still green?

PATIENT   Yes.

DOCTOR   ... [indistinct]

PATIENT   Rusty again.

DOCTOR   Are you taking those tablets I gave you?

PATIENT   Oh, yes, I'm still taking those tablets.

DOCTOR   Have you got any pain in your chest?

PATIENT   No. There's no more pain.

DOCTOR   Are you short of breath?

PATIENT   Oh, yes, I get that. You see, when I was short of breath before, I used to get the pain.

DOCTOR   Gone completely has it?

PATIENT   Yes.

DOCTOR   That's something.

PATIENT   But during the night, sometimes, I can feel it like catarrh at the back of my throat. But that looks brown.

DOCTOR   Does it wake you? Your chest.

PATIENT   Well, it's not these last few nights.

DOCTOR   These little white tablets, have you any left?

PATIENT   No ...

DOCTOR   What's your weight doing now, steady?

PATIENT   Well, as a matter of fact, doctor, we were weighing ourselves last night, my husband and I, and he said, 'What weight are you?' and I said, 'According to those I'm only eight stone', and we put it past the zero and it was only eight stone odd.

DOCTOR   ... [indistinct]

PATIENT   So I don't think ... [indistinct] the scale for a while. I think I was eight stone two when you weighed me last.

DOCTOR   You were eight stone four, you have lost a bit.

PATIENT   Yes, I have.

DOCTOR   That's reasonable, because the thyroid tablets ... I'll make a note of that. Well, keep on the white tablets, one a day. I'll give you some tablets and medicine to clear your chest, the instructions will be on the bottle.

PATIENT   ... everyone has a cold.

DOCTOR   It's a bad time of year; you take the tablets four times a day and the medicine according to the instructions, I think you'll find that will clear it. There is enough there anyway for about a week. If you are not 100 per cent certain, you must come back. But the little white tablets you must take permanently. So see how you get on and if you're not happy come back in a week.

PATIENT   I see Andrew's had a bad cold, hasn't he?

DOCTOR   Has he?

PATIENT   He's still sniffly.

DOCTOR   Well, it's the time of year for it, you can't expect ...

PATIENT   ... but I could have done with trying those flu injections ...

DOCTOR   It's too late this year now.

PATIENT   Yes, it's too late.

DOCTOR   About November.

PATIENT   I'll come in then.

DOCTOR   Well, last year was a good year for flu and this year isn't so good.

PATIENT   My throat is a bit ...

DOCTOR   When you get an infection you will always get this rustiness ...

PATIENT   I noticed that ... Dr — told me I had a relaxed throat. I had to not speak as much and stop singing so I can't get the high notes now. All my notes have gone.

DOCTOR   Bye now.

(Byrne and Long, 1976, pp.91–3)

Now consider some short extracts recorded by another researcher, this time a nurse, Jill Clark. She asked nurses (all female) on surgical wards to wear a small microphone clipped to their uniform. The extracts below illustrate what she found.

NURSE   How are you feeling this morning?
PATIENT   Hungry.
NURSE   Ah well, I'm afraid there's nothing we can do about that, just at the moment.
PATIENT   But...
NURSE   You can have any fluids you like — but just stick on the fluid diet at the moment.

NURSE   How do you feel?
PATIENT   A lot better thanks.
NURSE   Do you?
PATIENT   Yes, surprising as it was quite painful. I feel a lot better today.

NURSE   There we are dear, OK? [gives tablet]
PATIENT   Thank you. Do you know, I can't feel anything with my fingers nowadays at all.
NURSE   Can't you?
PATIENT   No, I go to pick up a knife and take my hand away and it's not there anymore.
NURSE   Oh, broke my pen! [moves away]

NURSE   Did they find you an interesting case?
PATIENT   They did, yes.
NURSE   That's nice. Can I just rub your bottom then?
PATIENT   But they um...
NURSE   One, two, three...up. Not getting sore, sitting here, are you?
PATIENT   Well I am a little bit sore.
NURSE   Are you walking around a little bit with your [colostomy] bag so you don't get too sore?
           (Clark, 1981, pp.15–16)

As these extracts may suggest, nursing interaction is typically far briefer than that with GPs, even though the normal GP consultation lasts on average only between five and six minutes. By contrast, a study of traditional types of medical practice in India by the medical geographers A. Ramesh and B. Hyma showed that the Indian average was over ten minutes and no less than 35 per cent took between twenty to forty minutes.*

☐   What else did you notice about the interaction? Can you spot any similarities between (a) the doctor and the nurses, and (b) the various patients?

*This study 'Traditional Indian medicine in practice in an Indian metropolitan city' can be found in the Course Reader (Part 4, Section 4.3).

■   (a) The doctor asks a lot of quick-fire questions, seventeen in all, which produce short, snappy answers. He moves rapidly from one topic to another as do the nurses, who also have a quick-fire style composed of questions, comments and instructions. Both the doctor and two of the nurses interrupt remarks by patients and you may also have noticed that in two of the extracts staff end the interaction while patients are still trying to talk. Indeed, neither the doctor nor the nurses respond in a particularly inviting way to patients comments and questions (except for the nurse in the second nursing extract).

(b) In contrast to the very precise manner of staff, patients have a far more conversational, even rambling style on occasions, in which some things are described in an anecdotal, story-telling fashion. For example, 'Well, as a matter of fact doctor, we were weighing ourselves last night, my husband and I, and he said...' Note also that the patient consulting the doctor does not ask nearly so many questions, nor, like the other patients, does she object when her remarks are over-ridden. Finally, you may have noticed that relatively little technical information is passed on from staff to patient.

What can be made of all this? The doctor cited above felt that his particular style was essential to proper doctoring:

The doctor's primary task is to manage his time. If he allows patients to rabbit on about their conditions then the doctor will lose control of time and will spend all his time sitting in a surgery listening to irrelevant rubbish. Effective doctoring is characterised by a 'quick, clean job'. (Byrne and Long, 1976, p.93)

Not everyone, however, may see it this way. Two sociologists, Gerry Stimson and Barbara Webb, conducted informal group interviews with women in South Wales, letting the women talk freely amongst themselves. For these women, talking with the GP could sometimes be a difficult and frustrating experience:

I very often go in and I feel sometimes I've forgotten what I was going to ask him [the doctor] in the first place — not the main problem, but if I'm going to see him about something else at the same time. I come away and think 'Oh, he's put me off again', you know. (Stimson and Webb, 1975, p.34)

Sometimes you go in there and he's so charming you know, and other times, you go in and you think 'Oh, let's get out of here quickly, because you feel a nuisance, you know'. (Ibid. p.33)

In short, some patients, can find it very difficult to express their real fears and some are easily put off. Staff have large numbers of other patients to see and lots of other things to do. They are also highly skilled in formulating problems in concise medical terms, for these are matters they deal with every day. But most patients lack practice in such matters, while to them their problems are unique, not merely one in a series of such problems to be dealt with. What to the patient is a personal problem which can prove hard to express is to the provider of health care simply a form of *work*. As such, like most work it becomes a matter of *routine*.

Workers in most occupations, whether secretaries, truck drivers, plumbers, or nurses, develop routine ways of doing their work. However, in jobs that are based on contact with people, workers face special problems. Clients are a constant challenge: they make time-consuming demands and some think — sometimes, but not always, rightly — that they know better than the experts. In such jobs, staff develop standard ways of maintaining a distance between themselves and their clients. There is thus a marked tendency for the work of all service industries to become impersonal. The routines that staff learn in order to cope are developed by repetition and enforced by habit. Moreover, staff doing similar jobs tend to develop common routines. There is, for example, the change in personal demeanour which accompanies the transformation from nursing or medical student to fully-qualified nurse or doctor. (The differences in Table 4.3 may well reflect this.)

Table 4.3 Duration of nurse–patient conversation

	Average number of minutes per 2 hours	Average length of each conversation	Median lengths
Student nurses	21.72	2.01	1.13
Trained nurses	16.24	1.43	1.05

(Source: Clark, 1981, p.14)

Byrne and Long's study of doctors found only a small range of personal styles, and Clark noted that many of the encounters between nurses and patients took a similar form.

We can look at another consequence of viewing health care as work. Health care has a highly specialised *division of labour*, which means that the work is split up and shared among a number of different occupational roles oriented to different tasks. For some patients this can result in extraordinarily fragmented care, as can be seen in Figure 4.1, which illustrates the range of agencies involved in the care of the disabled. Even within a single institution such as a hospital this has important effects. Different staff have different rights to give information to the patient about the illness. In many cases, especially where the illness is life threatening (cancer, for example), breaking bad news is the prerogative of the consultant not the nurses. Thus staff relate to patients within the boundaries of their own role.

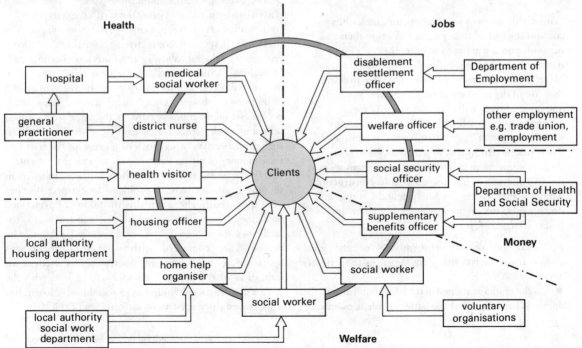

Figure 4.1 Model showing the large number of health and social services available for disabled people and the organisations responsible. (Source: Blaxter, 1978, p.137)

However, whatever the role, it is still work; instead of being dealt with as a person the patient is commonly dealt with as a case.

All these tendencies in their turn produce movements for reform. While some staff support the status quo, others are unhappy with the quality of the service they offer. And, on top of this, there are groups of dissatisfied clients who propose even more radical change. All these points of view can be found in the following two extracts:*

Giving the patient more say in the treatment could be good medicine

The recently set up Patients' Liaison Group, which was formed under the auspices of the Royal College of General Practitioners, has as its aim the promotion of better communications between family doctors in the NHS and their patients ... Failure of communication has been seen to be the root of many doctor patient misunderstandings.

(Margot Lawrence, *Daily Telegraph*, November 9, 1983)

'You decide when to see your doctor and let him confirm the fact of your pregnancy. From then onwards you are going to have to answer a lot of questions and be the subject of a lot of examinations. Never worry about any of these. They are necessary, they are in the interests of your baby and yourself, and none of them will ever hurt you.' These admonitions from a British Medical Association publication [of 1977] ... are intended to console. Their tone is patronizing and their message is clear: doctors know more about having babies than women do. (An alternative, and less charitable, construction would be that women are fundamentally stupid and doctors inherently more intelligent.) (Oakley, in Black, *et al.*, 1984, p.170)

☐ What are the different models of the ideal doctor–patient relationship contained in the extracts above?
■ In the model contained in the BMA publication, the doctor is the expert and the patient's role is essentially

passive. In the RCGP's model, however, patients have a bigger say — the relationship is essentially collaborative. Oakley's comments could be a plea for collaboration or, alternatively, imply yet a third form of the relationship, one in which the conflict of interests and the independent expertise of the patient are emphasised. In this model it is the patient who should dominate while doctors play a purely advisory role.

Despite their differences, those who hold both the collaborative and the conflict models have a good deal in common — both want reform. Since this is so, we will first describe the problems they identify and only then proceed to consider the different solutions proposed.

How far do patients follow medical advice?

If we make the assumption that medical advice is of value, then one test of the effectiveness of many encounters is how far staff persuade patients to follow that advice. The technical term for this is '*compliance*'.

☐ What problems can you see in the use of this term?
■ It seems to imply that patients should be passive and obedient.

This traditional model of patient behaviour informs a good deal of medical research about those patients who, for one reason or another, do not carry out staff's suggestions. Such studies often claim that patients are irresponsible, or even that they have 'uncooperative personalities'. Indeed, patients who do not follow instructions have been termed: 'defaulters', 'disobedient', 'unreliable'; or else they deviate', 'disobey doctors' instructions' or are 'negligent'.*

However, though compliance often carries these prejudicial implications it remains the standard technical term and we shall therefore use it here, though the fault, if such there be, may be as much or more with the staff and their manner of giving instructions, as with the patient.

Having issued this warning, how far is compliance, in the non-pejorative sense, a problem? One aspect that has been quite thoroughly studied is the taking of prescribed medicines. Researchers examine how much and how often medicines have been taken in a specified period. The amounts are compared with what the patient was instructed to take, and any discrepancy is used as an indication of the patient's compliance, or not, with the doctor's instructions. Philip Ley, a social psychologist, has summarised three reviews of such studies (Table 4.4).

---

* The second quotation comes from the article 'Doctor knows best' by Ann Oakley which is to be found in the Course Reader (Part 3, Section 3.9).

* A parallel version of this model of patient behaviour can be found in the Course Reader in the article 'Deaths under 50' by the Medical Services Study Group and the Royal College of Physicians of London (Part 2, Section 2.7).

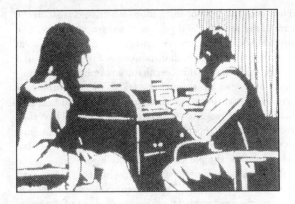 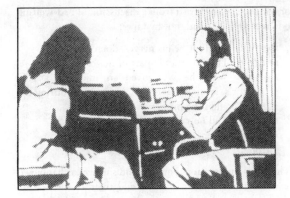

Table 4.4 The percentage of patients who do not comply with doctors' advice to take certain categories of drugs: a summary of three reviews

Type of medication	Ley (1976)	FDA (1929)	Barofsky (1980)
antibiotics	49	48	52
psychiatric	39	42	42
anti-hypertensive	–	43	61
anti-tuberculosis	38	42	43
other medications	48	54	46

(Source: Ley, 1982, Table 2, p.243)

   ☐ How much does the type of medication affect compliance?

   ■ Little — around 40–50 per cent of patients do not comply with medical advice, regardless of the type of medicine.

Indeed, it has been claimed from a study in Australia that around 20 per cent of hospital admissions are due to patients becoming unwell as a result of not complying with their treatment. It should, however, be remembered that a similar proportion of hospital admissions have been attributed to *iatrogenic* causes, in particular, the adverse effects of drugs. Note also that although doctors often complain about patients who do not comply with treatments, it appears that many are unaware of just how common non-compliance actually is. In a general medical clinic in which studies showed that only 50 per cent of patients were complying with medication, 42 per cent of the doctors believed that *all* patients were compliant. Only 11 per cent of the doctors made an accurate estimate of the true proportion (Davis, 1966).

Different conditions require different styles of interaction
Quick-fire questioning and rapid instruction may be fine for some problems but medical conditions vary enormously. They may be life threatening or benign, acute or chronic,

physical or mental; or there may even be doubts (as in pregnancy) as to how far this is a medical condition at all. All these different circumstances require very different types of communication and, equally, very different types of involvement on the part of medical staff and patient.* In chronic conditions such as a colostomy (in one of the nurse–patient extracts) or a thyroid condition (the GP consultation), patients may be largely responsible for day-to-day management. Indeed, some chronic patients become extremely knowledgeable[†] — so much so that staff communication that ignores the patient's expertise will probably fail. So too will that which ignores the patient's emotional state. In her study of surgical nursing Clark concluded:

> Nurse–patient conversations tend to be short, often (but not always) occcur in relation to tasks and, in content, are almost exclusively restricted to technical rather than emotional matters. (Clark, 1981, p.14)

Doctors, too, commonly talk in this fashion. A study of a thousand consultations in children's clinics in Scotland conducted in the early 1970s revealed that although some doctors privately felt that up to half the children they were seeing might have emotional problems which were affecting, even causing, their condition, such matters were never normally discussed. Instead, almost all illness was overtly treated as if it were a purely physical phenomenon — a rule which typically applied even on the very rare occasions when parents themselves raised the matter. Here,

---

*The diagnostic problems involved here are discussed in *Experiencing and Explaining Disease*, Chapter 2, *ibid*.; while later chapters on cancer and mental illness discuss further the delicate matters these involve.

[†]A good example of this is described in the article in the Course Reader 'Coping with migraine' by two migraine sufferers, Sally Macintyre and David Oldman (Part 6, Section 6.2).

for instance, is an extract from a discussion of bed-wetting (one recorded by hand, not by tape):

MOTHER Could it be his nerves, doctor?

DOCTOR That's certainly part of it, yes.

MOTHER Well, he was given an injection at the doctor's. It might be that. He's never wet during the day. Could it be his nerves?

DOCTOR And he's just seven?

MOTHER Seven.

(Strong, 1979, p.53)

Where serious emotional matters did surface, as happened very occasionally, then parents and their children were passed on to other types of staff — to social workers, occupational therapists and child psychiatrists. The paediatricians left emotions to others. So too do many types of doctor, even though some research suggests that psychological problems are extremely frequent in medical practice and closely involved with a wide range of physical conditions. Table 4.5 shows three varying estimates of the prevalence of such matters in general practice.

□ Why do you think doctors often avoid psychological problems?

■ Doctors may feel some or all of the following: dubious about the actual contribution of psychological factors to physical conditions — there is no definite evidence for some of the links that are often made; uneasy about dealing with emotional matters for which they lack any training; busy — emotional issues can take a long time to discuss; helpless — solutions to many of these matters are unavailable; uncertain as to whether the patients themselves actually wish them to be raised — some aspects of psychiatry are commonly criticised as a form of hidden social control.

Thus even the staff of institutions which specialise in the care of the mentally ill do not seem to fare any better. The psychologically oppressive nature of many long-term institutions has been well documented. For example, in a classic study by David Rosenhan, an American psychologist and lawyer, researchers faked the symptoms of serious mental illness. Once admitted to mental hospital, however, the researchers behaved normally. They then recorded what happened when they asked questions such as 'Pardon me, Mr (or Dr or Mrs) X, could you tell me when I will be eligible for grounds privileges?' or '. . . when will I be presented at the staff-meeting?' or '. . . when am I likely to be discharged?' The results are shown in Table 4.6. Perhaps the most important thing to come out of this study was that the fake patients felt powerless, depersonalised and unworthy of account, indeed, at times the researchers felt that they were invisible.

In some other conditions, communication has important physical as well as mental consequences. The major study in this area was conducted by an American researcher, Lawrence Egbert, and his colleagues in the early 1960s. They looked at the effect on patients' recovery from

Table 4.6 Self-initiated contact by fake patients with staff

Responses to contact	Doctors	Nurses and attendants
Moves on, head averted	71	88
Makes eye contact	23	10
Stops and chats	2	2
Stops and talks	4	0.5
Number of respondents	13	47
Number of attempts	185	1 283

(Source: Rosenhan, 1973, p.245)

Table 4.5 Prevalence of psycho-social problems in visits to general practitioners — three estimates

| | Prevalence per 1 000 persons per year in: | | |
	Ommoord (1972)	Netherlands (1967)	England (1971)
Types of reaction (depressive, anxiety-agitated, neurotic, neurasthenic)	173	72	83
Problems of life (sexual, rational, occupational, personality, crises, problems concerning phase of life, others)	183	5	8
Problems concerning young children (sleeping, eating, toilet training, others)	33	–	–
'Psychosomatic' (obesity, migraine, hypertension, coronary ischaemia, asthma, peptic ulcer, urticaria, eczema)	144 .	101	133
'Functional disorders' (cardiophobia, palpitations, spastic colitis, carcinophobia, dysmenorrhoea and premenstrual tension, all cervical and lumbar symptoms, all myalgias, disturbed sleep, fatigue, malaise, hyperventilation, headache)	305	188	152
'True' psychiatry (schizophrenia, paranoid psychosis, oligophrenia, psychotic reaction)	7	5	8

(Source: Lamberts, 1980, p.353)

abdominal surgery when they were given different amounts of information about their treatment. The night before the operation they were visited by the anaesthetist. The patients were randomly divided into two groups, fifty-one in a control group were not told about post-operative pain, and forty-six in a special care group were. Only the special care group were told where they would feel pain, how severe it would be, how long it would last and that they could relieve the pain by using simple relaxation techniques. They were also told that if they could not relieve pain this way, they should request medication. This advice was repeated on the afternoon following the operation. The patients were not told that they were in a study, and the surgeons did not know which patients were receiving special care, nor did the nurses who administered the pain-killing drugs.

When the researchers later examined the drug records, they found that on most days the control group received on average twice as many pain-killers as the special care group. An independent observer, who was not aware of the type of treatment being received, rated special care patients as in better emotional and physical condition than the control group. And the surgeons, who were also unaware of the care each patient received, sent the special care group home an average of 2.7 days earlier than the control group. In summary, therefore, although the management of emotional matters is still highly problematic, research does suggest that in some areas, at least, there are relatively simple methods which can improve matters; methods which are still not, however, used by many staff.

Social class and staff–patient encounters

Another important aspect of staff–patient encounters is the influence of the social characteristics of the patient. Staff and patients are often of different sex and from different classes and ethnic groups, and these differences can plausibly be expected to exert a powerful effect upon the interaction. Unfortunately, little comparative work has been done on the influence of gender or ethnicity, so we shall focus upon social class, which has thus far received the most attention.

While nurses are drawn from all social classes, doctors are not. A survey of all the doctors in England and Wales who were new to general practice in 1969 and 1970 found that 80 per cent of them had social class I or II backgrounds, that is, families where the father was in a professional or managerial occupation;* whereas only about 25 per cent of the general population is in social classes I and II. Consultations between doctors and patients are therefore normally conversations between people of different social

*Methods of categorising social class are described in *Studying Health and Disease*, Chapter 10, *ibid.*

class. There is, however, little suggestion from modern research that the gross form of abuse described at the beginning of this chapter is common nowadays. The working class are no longer simply demonstation material for teaching hospitals. None the less, as Table 4.7 reveals, working-class patients do seem to be treated differently from those in other classes.

Table 4.7 Social class and consultations with general practitioners (92 tape-recorded consultations)

	Middle-class patients	Working-class patients
Average length of conversation time in minutes	6.2	4.7
Average number of problems discussed	4.1	2.8
Average number of symptoms	2.2	3.0

(Source: adapted from Cartwright and O'Brien, 1976, p.89)

☐ What differences can you identify in Table 4.7?
■ On average, middle-class patients had longer consultations, and had more problems discussed, even though working-class patients had more symptoms.

There were other differences too. Upon interview it was found that doctors knew more about the family background of middle-class patients, despite the fact that working-class patients had been with the practice longer — an average of 13.9 years for working-class patients and 10.9 years for middle-class patients. What might explain this? One possible answer is that working-class patients ask fewer questions and therefore receive less information. This theory has been investigated by two social psychologists, David Pendleton and Stephen Bochner, and some of their results are shown in Table 4.8.

Table 4.8 Mean length of consultation and mean number of health-related statements given by the doctor (the tape-recorded conversations were coded into 'units' of information and explanation)

	Social class of patients (female)		
	low	medium	high
Mean length of consultation	5.0	7.0	7.6
Mean number of 'units' of information and explanation volunteered by the doctor, per consultation	2.2	4.0	5.3
Mean number of information and explanation 'units' per consultation response to a question by patient	1.0	2.5	4.6
Total health-related statements per consultation	3.2	6.5	9.9

(Source: Pendleton and Bochner, 1980, p.671)

□ Looking at Table 4.8, to whom do doctors volunteer most information, and what happens when lower-class patients ask questions?

■ Doctors volunteer more to higher social-class patients and give less to lower-class patients even when they ask questions. (So the theory falls down.)

What other explanation of these differences can be produced? One possibility is that rightly or wrongly, doctors' perceptions of the amount of information that people can understand or take in varies with their class: lower-class patients are felt to be less able to cope than higher-class patients. Alternatively, these differences may simply arise out of conscious or unconscious class prejudice on the part of doctors. For all this, working-class patients express more satisfaction with medical consultations than do those from the middle-class, presumably because their expectations are lower, or possibly because they are less confident when interviewed.

Is there sufficient explanation?

Given some of these differences in the treatment of different social classes, it is perhaps not surprising that 23 per cent of the patients in the Cartwright and Anderson study of general practice complained about the lack of full explanation. If patients were given more information about their health and their diseases they might be more willing or able to follow medical advice (always assuming this to be desirable). However, many doctors are bad at explaining things to patients. Indeed, it is often argued, though evidence is still lacking, that many hospital patients pick up important information through cleaners and nursing auxiliaries. Even when information is provided by the doctor, it may not be clear enough for the patient to understand. For example, in the earlier transcript of a GP consultation (page 59), the doctor's explanation of the patient's weight loss is abandoned in mid-sentence. At other times, information may be misunderstood because doctors make mistaken assumptions about their *patients' knowledge*.

One way this has been investigated has been to show patients an outline of the human body, and ask them to locate the position of various organs such as the heart and the kidneys. Some of the results of a survey of almost 1 000 people in the UK are shown in Figure 4.2.

□ How accurate were people's perceptions of the location of body organs?

■ Many were inaccurate: only 50 per cent gave the correct position for kidneys, 49 per cent for the heart, 33 per cent for the stomach, and 31 per cent for the liver.

Given these differences in knowledge between lay people and professionals (though doctors too can get things wrong sometimes), it is hardly surprising that misunderstandings

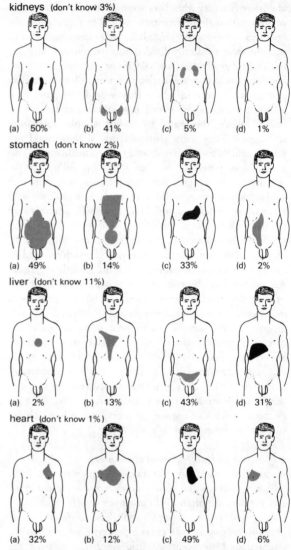

kidneys (don't know 3%)

(a) 50% (b) 41% (c) 5% (d) 1%

stomach (don't know 2%)

(a) 49% (b) 14% (c) 33% (d) 2%

liver (don't know 11%)

(a) 2% (b) 13% (c) 43% (d) 31%

heart (don't know 1%)

(a) 32% (b) 12% (c) 49% (d) 6%

Figure 4.2 Lay people's perceptions of the position of various organs: percentages indicate where people perceived each organ to be located. The correct position is shown in bold. (Source: *Self-health*, March 1984, p.29)

might arise, particularly over what patients actually think. Moreover, even when health professionals do provide clear, accurate information, there is no guarantee that people will remember it. Philip Ley has found that forgetting is related to the amount of information which is given. The more information that is given, the less that is remembered. In one study, patients were given six statements to recall and forgot a third of them soon afterwards. If it is essential that a patient remembers some information, two clear statements seems to be the maximum — though even then one-sixth of people will forget one of them. Forgetting is also related to the type of information. In another study, Ley found that only 44 per cent of people remembered the doctor's instructions about what to do, while only 56 per cent remembered information about their illness — though 87 per cent remembered statements about their diagnosis.

The treatment of the deviant

If social class has strong effects upon the type and amount of information given, other forms of social classification produce even stronger effects upon the interaction. All service occupations such as waiters and hairdressers grade those whom they serve into 'good' and 'bad' types of client; medical staff are no different. Patients considered good may get special favours, those deemed bad may get quite another kind of treatment. The rule applies to all staff: GPs, nurses and porters alike. To see how it works out in one particular instance, you should now read the article by Roger Jeffery in the Course Reader on the behaviour of doctors working in a casualty department.

☐   Why were some patients considered bad?
■   They refused to cooperate; there was little wrong with them; they were thought to be using illness for other ends; or they were held to be responsible for their own illness.
☐   What relationship have these matters got to the sick role?*
■   All break the rules of the conventional sick role.
☐   In what ways do the position and attitudes of casualty staff resemble those of the kitchen staff considered in Chapter 3?
■   Although there is a vast social and economic gulf between them, both are at the bottom of their respective social hierarchies. Moreover, both make systematic distinctions between good and bad work. Treating drunks in casualty is the equivalent of washing lettuces in the kitchen: there's a lot of effort, few rewards and some risks (either the overlooked slug or the drunk who dies on the doorstep after discharge).

Casualty departments, as this and other research has shown, are therefore an exception to the general rule that most staff–patient encounters within the NHS proceed in a relatively polite fashion with little open conflict. All medical staff make a distinction between good and bad patients but here the categories are far more overt and some patients are subjected to open hostility. The same is true of a few other settings and occasions. Unmarried women seeking abortions may sometimes experience similar treatment, and so too may drug addicts seeking treatment. Medicine in prisons and for the armed forces may also sometimes take on these aspects.

A comparison with private practice

So far, almost all the interaction we have examined has occurred within the NHS. How does it compare with that found elsewhere? Addressing the Pilkington Commission on doctors' pay in 1958, a leading consultant, Sir Thomas Holmes Sellors, remarked as follows:

> To put it rather unofficially ... to put it rather crudely, in an [NHS] out-patients session the patient listens to the doctor, whereas in a private practice, the consultant listens to the patient. (Cited in Ferris, 1967, p.34)

If Sellors is right does this mean that the kind of staff-domination uncovered by Byrne and Long's work on GPs and Clark's work on nursing, is peculiar to the NHS? Unfortunately, there has been very little research into the characteristics of private practice. Two small studies of private medical consultation do exist, however. The first two excerpts which follow are from private paediatric clinics in the USA, the remainder from a private oncology (cancer) clinic in London.

(i)
INTERN [a junior doctor who sees the patient before the specialist]   How did you get here?
MOTHER   Well, he's been seeing a psychiatrist and he diagnosed minimal brain dysfunction and prescribed X. But we also want to get Dr Stein's [a neurologist] opinion as we felt we ought not just to have a psychiatric opinion.

(ii)
MOTHER   We liked him [Dr Levy] particularly because he was critical of schools and said, 'Don't believe what they say. That's what got us here.'
DOCTOR   True. It's very important work the Learning Disability Group does in building up consumer appreciation. There's gotta be a dialogue, it's the only way.
(Strong, 1979, pp.78–80)

(iii)
MR J   I'm a member of PPP and so if you send them the account they will pay ... They asked for a report if you can send one.
DOCTOR   What shall I say?
MR J   Whatever you think.
DOCTOR   No, what you say. I'm your agent. I'll write whatever you want.

*The sick role is discussed in *Medical Knowledge: Doubt and Certainty*, Chapters 3 and 8, *ibid.* and in *Experiencing and Explaining Disease*, Chapter 13, *ibid.*

(iv)

DOCTOR   Have you had occasion to see Smith at all?

MRS E   He's very good.

DOCTOR   I thought you were seeing Jones. He thought Smith didn't have anything to contribute.

(v)

MRS B   Now where do we go from here?

DOCTOR   May I ask you something? ...
                    [after a further ten minutes]

MRS B   [standing up] Thank you for your kind attention.

(Silverman, 1984, pp.196, 198, 201)

☐   On this evidence, was Sir Thomas Holmes Sellors right? Are doctors forced to listen more seriously to private patients.

■   It looks like it. In the third extract, the doctor explicitly refers to himself as the patient's agent. In the first, the mother indicates that she is checking out different medical opinions, of which Dr Stein's is merely one. (American patients can refer themselves directly to specialists.) And in the fifth extract it is the patient who steers the course of the interaction and who actually ends the consultation while the doctor is obliged to ask his question in a distinctly subordinate fashion (contrast the way the GP cited earlier asked his questions).

One further feature should be noted. In all these extracts, both parties openly assume that there are good doctors and bad doctors, doctors to see and doctors to avoid. Medical expertise cannot be automatically assumed; it has to be checked. Thus patients let doctors know that they are seeing other doctors and doctors name the other specialists with whom they have discussed particular problems. Some doctors also comment on the competence, or otherwise, of their colleagues. By contrast, in NHS consultations, there is an unspoken but very strongly overt assumption that all doctors are expert and that medical authority cannot be challenged or checked on by the laity. Patients rarely mention other doctors, and doctors avoid passing judgement on the capacity of their colleagues and rarely name those with whom they have consulted.

☐   What might account for the difference between NHS and private practice?

■   In private practice, doctors are selling a named product — themselves. Their authority and their income is based, in part at least, on their personal reputation. Moreover, colleagues are also competitors, while patients want to know who else is worth consulting and who they should avoid — and they are paying for this information.

☐   What would be another explanation for the doctors' subordination, besides the fact that these are fee-for-service consultations?

■   Unlike the NHS encounters cited earlier, some (though not all) of these patients have greater income and status than the doctors.

Reforms and dilemmas

What conclusions can be drawn from all this? British patients seem reasonably content. But despite this, there does seem quite a bit of room for improvement. Medical staff who use an autocratic style may fail to uncover their patients' real worries — or put them off attending consultations altogether. Many doctors and nurses fail to handle their patients' emotional problems or even to communicate basic information, while their ability to get patients to follow advice is strikingly limited. Doctors also have problems communicating with patients of a lower social class than themselves, and there may be far more serious difficulties with patients who have chronic or psychiatric conditions. On the other hand most encounters do seem reasonably polite but, against this, staff can be very rude to patients who don't fit the conventional sick role. Finally, the limited evidence about private practice suggests that, here at last, some patients can enforce a good deal of attention to their wishes.

Problems such as these have produced a great crop of suggestions for reform. One of these is to *change the nature of staff* — either by a different recruitment policy or by increasing their numbers, or else by systematic training in interpersonal skills. All of these present their own problems. Consider for example, skills training. Interaction with patients is videotaped, then played back to staff with systematic analysis of the extent to which they allow patients to speak for themselves. By the late 1970s, the majority of American medical schools had introduced such training, though change in the UK has been slower and mostly confined to general practice and psychiatry. Some nursing schools have also developed such training. These initiatives are still being evaluated, though there is already some evidence to suggest that while such training can indeed modify staff's manner, the change may only last for a short time.

Others, who view the relationship between staff and patients in terms of conflict, have argued that the only solution is to *increase patients' power* significantly. This might be done in two broad ways. The first solution is to increase the public control of the health service. One current experiment is to run a general practice through a lay management committee or, less ambitiously, to develop some form of patient representation. A similar type of proposal is to increase vastly the power of the Community Health Councils, or else to turn health authorities into properly elected bodies. How effective any of these strategies might prove is unknown, and as you have seen in Chapter 3, the trend in the 1980s is to increase central control of the NHS rather than the opposite.

The second approach, though also from a perspective of conflict, is to increase the direct power that individual patients possess. One important way of doing this is to increase patients' knowledge. Education about health and disease might, perhaps, become a central part of the school curriculum or be developed through such means as community-based groups. Another possibility is to modify the law. At present, unlike the USA, it is extremely hard for patients to sue staff. There could be other changes also. At present, though patients have a right both to a second opinion and to change their GP if they wish, in practice these matters are hard to arrange. Perhaps if people were reminded of these rights, say, through an obligatory notice in every ward and consulting room, this too might have an effect? Thinking along these lines, the National Consumer Council has produced the following:

Rights guide issued for NHS patients

The first comprehensive guide to patients' rights, including information on how to complain and how to change your family doctor, was published by the National Consumer Council yesterday — 34 years after the establishment of the National Health Service. Mr John Hatch, the chairman of the NCC working party which produced the guide, said yesterday that patients' ignorance of their rights had contributed to the continuation of practices in the NHS which should have been abolished years ago ... The Department of Health has not commented on the guide. Mr Hatch said ... it was reluctant to become involved in case it upset the medical profession. The British Medical Association, however, gave the guide a good reception ... Around 50,000 copies of the booklet have been printed. The NCC wants to place them in doctors' surgeries and hospital waiting rooms.

(David Hencke, *The Guardian*, July 1, 1984)

Consumerism, the movement to protect the rights of the consumer, can, however, take quite another form. To some critics of the NHS, its failures in customer service are thought to be due principally to the fact that patients cannot exert any direct financial leverage with those who are supposed to serve them. Service, they argue, therefore becomes slack and impersonal, for the customers cannot threaten to take their trade elsewhere as the NHS has a virtual monopoly:

> A government-owned monopoly may not exploit, but the customer has no redress against inefficiency, poor service, high rates and disregard of his or her needs. (Drucker, 1979, p.153)

Since the NHS is free at the point of use the question of high costs does not arise. But there are clearly problems with waiting, impersonality, poor communication and disregard of some of the customers' needs. Would switching to a fee-for-service system improve matters?

☐ What problems might you see in the fee-for-service approach, apart from financial cost and equitable access?

■ There is the key problem of medical expertise. Can even well-educated patients really know what they are buying? And if they do not, how can they really be in control of the transaction? (One might also note that American health care is hardly free from charges of impersonality, poor communication and disregard of customers' needs — it also, of course, has its own form of rationing.)

Consider once again, the first and third extracts from the private practice consultations (pages 67–8). The parents certainly seem to be exercising a good deal of control. But on another interpretation this is purely illusory; instead they are victims of a subtle piece of marketing. The doctor referred to in the first extract (and cited in the second) had been speaking to parent–teacher associations, and telling parents that failure at school might be due, not to childrens' lack of talent, nor to the failings of the teachers or parents, but to a medical condition known as minimal brain dysfunction* — a condition which, luckily for them, he and his fellow neurologists could treat. If true, this is clearly an important service. But many doctors are dubious about its reality. To them and many other commentators, parents' hopes and fears are only too easily exploited by such methods. On this analysis, private practice may certainly produce a more gracious and subordinate manner in medical staff, but that very manner may sometimes be the means through which dubious though profitable therapies are sold to a defenceless public.

---

* This is discussed further in *Experiencing and Explaining Disease*, Chapter 13, *ibid*.

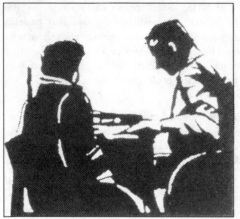

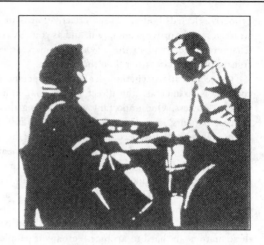

However, as you have seen in Chapter 2, fee-for-service is not the only form of private practice. In Health Maintenance Organisations (HMOs) the customer pays for health care in advance each year, or possibly through government-distributed vouchers. Might not this be *the* solution — a mechanism which avoids the financial costs and potential exploitation of unrestricted private practice while at the same time, through enforcing competition between doctors, also gives patients some control of the personal quality of the service? In practice, however, it is most doubtful whether HMOs do offer these benefits in personal service. The American sociologist Julius Roth, a strong critic of the NHS, has attacked American HMOs precisely because they are too much like the NHS! Or even worse:

> If [people] select a pre-paid plan such as Kaiser Permanente [an HMO], they find themselves restricted to a small number of practitioners, often with no choice at all at the specialist level, no choice of hospital, and no way of obtaining an independent second opinion or alternative service without paying the full cost out of pocket. Even if they are willing and able to pay the costs, they may be treated with considerable suspicion by the outside practitioner or organization to whom they turn, for example ... [being] subjected to a credit examination before being given an appointment. The two organizations whose services they are using may refuse to collaborate by exchanging test results and other information. (Roth, 1979, p.199)

In summary, although there is considerable and widespread interest in ways of improving the service offered to patients,

every method has its drawbacks. Patients' groups may run or advise some practices, but most patients have other things to do and so are not represented. Fee-for-service offers more power to enforce a polite service, but more opportunity for patients to be financially and medically exploited. HMOs may turn out to be as bureaucratic and limited in choice as the NHS, while also creating massive problems of coordination and the possibility of maltreatment. Changes in the law may enable patients to sue more often, but may also lead, as has happened in the USA, to the practice of *defensive medicine*. In this, doctors intervene and investigate patients in every way they can think of in order to avoid the possibility of being sued later on — an expensive and unpleasant business. And as for changes in education — teaching doctors, nurses and receptionists more open-ended methods of communication — just how long would the benefits last once the pupils have left school? Back in their daily jobs staff are faced with the heavy demands that the routine processing of patients creates. Even informing people about their rights may have little effect — most people may still feel it's not worth bothering to object about treatment. Finally, what of the service offered to the mentally ill and the mentally handicapped: how can they get to exert more effective pressure on the way they are treated? Here above all there are formidable difficulties.

None the less, for all these difficulties, pressures to improve the quality of service offered to patients will not go away. Indeed, they seem likely to increase. However, as we have seen, every type of health care system creates its own special problems for the patient. As with the issues discussed in Chapters 2 and 3, customer service faces many dilemmas with few obvious solutions in sight.

Objectives for Chapter 4

When you have read this chapter, you should be able to:

4.1 Describe those aspects of customer service that give rise to dissatisfaction and the effect that poor communication can have on compliance.

4.2 Describe the manner commonly used by many doctors and nursing staff in their interaction with patients and the reasons why that manner is adopted.

4.3 Outline some of the factors that affect the style of staff–patient communication: the type of disease, the social class of the patient, the extent of the patient's knowledge, and the method of payment.

4.4 Comment on the reforms that have been proposed for improving staff–patient encounters: changing the nature of staff, and increasing the power of patients.

Questions for Chapter 4

1 (*Objective 4.1*) Broadly speaking, what are the main aspects of customer service in the NHS that people complain about? Which key aspect do customers *not* complain about?

2 (*Objective 4.2*) The following conversation is between a second-year student nurse and a patient

NURSE   How are you today?
PATIENT   Well, I still feel sick.
NURSE   Sick?
PATIENT   Yes, well you know I'm scared to eat in case I really am sick.

(a) In what way is this extract different from some of the other encounters you have seen in this chapter?

(b) Why don't more staff talk in this fashion?

3 (*Objective 4.3*) The following description is from a study of NHS Drug Treatment Clinics, many of whose patients are heroin addicts. These clinics are the only place where such addicts can receive methadone (a heroin substitute).

> The Clinics are an unusual medical setting in which there is a higher level of overt conflict between patients and staff than is found elsewhere in medicine. (Stimson and Oppenheimer, 1982, p.101)

The Clinics had the following features: staff employed a porter to keep order in the waiting room; they checked the patients' accounts of drug use by carrying out urine tests; they asked patients to enter into treatment and good behaviour contracts; and they penalised patients who did not arrive on time for appointments.

(a) What are the similarities and differences between the treatment of these patients and that meted out to deviant patients in casualty?

(b) In what way does this picture differ from standard medical assumptions about patient compliance?

4 (*Objective 4.4*) To what extent might the privatisation of certain forms of nursing care ensure that the particular style of nursing interaction cited in Question (1) become more widespread in the care of the elderly?

5

Community care: dilemma or prospect?

This chapter is largely concerned with contemporary aspects of community care. Historical accounts of changing attitudes to, and the provision of, institutional and community care appear in *Caring for Health: History and Diversity*, Chapters 2–4 (U205 *Health and Disease* Book VII). Discussion of society's attitude to mental illness and changes in views on the care of the mentally ill appear in *Experiencing and Explaining Disease*, Chapters 6–9 (U205 *Health and Disease* Book VI).

Fears over costs of community care

Taking the old, the mentally ill and mentally handicapped out of institutions, and putting them into the community will not work, say people involved in community health work. They think the proposal is idealistic, impractical and expensive.

Mrs Olive Gibbs, vice-chairman of Oxfordshire County Council said 'On paper this seems absolutely marvellous — old people living in the community with their families. But they don't realise the incredible burden old people, and especially senile old people put on their families.' She said that community care would create an extra burden on the social services department of the county council — and the council did not have the money to cope.

(*Oxford Times*, November 11, 1983)

In the previous three chapters we have considered some of the dilemmas of health care at the levels of central government, districts and the individual patient. While such distinctions help in understanding the underlying issues, they inevitably fail to capture the way the different levels are interrelated and thus affect one another. In addition, we have not so far considered what is perhaps the most important sector of health care — that provided by lay people. Community care, the subject of this chapter, enables us to examine all these matters and also, as the newspaper story illustrates, to reflect on the complex relationship between health and social services.

However, this chapter is not just about dilemmas. The policy of providing more community care is, as the newspaper story reports, seen by many people to be based on an 'absolutely marvellous' ideal. Far from being a dilemma, community care has been seen as a solution. Long-term institutional care has many problems, such as the poor communication between staff and patients discussed in the previous chapter. Community care seems to offer a chance to remedy this. But how far has this policy been realised — and with what effect?

Before considering these questions, we need to consider one other.

☐ What is meant by 'policy'?

■ A conscious decision about the shape of the future. Policies may either seek to change or else to preserve the status quo.*

The development of policy, which can take many years, depends on the accumulation of information and evidence from a variety of sources, which in the UK include research studies, Royal Commissions and official inquiries. Having formulated a policy, the government will sometimes publish it as a *consultative document* (called a *Green Paper*). In the light of the comments and reactions it receives, a *White Paper* may be published, which outlines the government's firm proposals and guidance. Alternatively, the government may simply issue a circular, as you have already seen happened in the case of privatisation. Changes in health care policy do not usually require Acts of Parliament unless they involve alterations to the legal status of official bodies or individuals. Examples of all these various documents appear in this chapter. However, it is important to note that policy pronouncements by central government do not necessarily produce change at district level unless they are supported by some form of compulsion or incentive.

What is community care?

Community care is not easily defined. The term has been used in at least two different ways: as a *prescription* for how people with long-term health and social needs might be cared for, and as a *description* of the actual services and resources involved. In addition, the meaning of the term 'community care' has altered over time. As an explicit objective of government policy, it came to the fore shortly after the Second World War and has largely remained there ever since.

Soon after the formation of the NHS a series of official reports was published which espoused the advantages of providing care for dependent groups such as the mentally ill, the mentally handicapped and the elderly, in places other than the large long-stay hospitals, which were often

*The nature of policy is also discussed in *Caring for Health: History and Diversity*, Chapter 10, *ibid*.

geographically isolated, and which, as you have seen in Chapter 2, were sometimes over a hundred years old and containing upwards of 2 000 patients each (Figure 5.1).

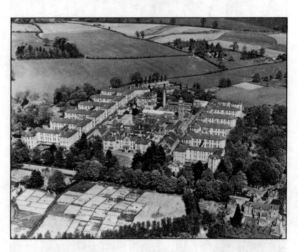

Figure 5.1 Leavesden Hospital for the mentally handicapped. Located away from urban areas, such hospitals were largely self-sufficient. Note the boiler house and water tower.

It is worth noting in passing that such a policy was not new. Similar views were, for example, espoused by St Just in late eighteenth-century France, when he argued for the closure of all hospitals in Paris; while in nineteenth-century Britain, 'outdoor' medical relief was provided under the Poor Law, rather than admitting all the sick to the Poor Law infirmary. A form of community care had indeed been standard for the mentally ill before the great wave of nineteenth-century asylum construction.

Since 1948, community care has been a consistent policy of central government. However, even during this relatively short period 'community care' has been used to mean different things for different groups and at different times. For example, *Health and Welfare*, a government report published in the early 1960s, described the needs of the elderly in the following terms:

Elderly people living at home may need special support to enable them to cope with their infirmities and to prevent their isolation from society. As their capabilities diminish they will more often require such services as home helps, laundry services, meals cooked ready for eating and chiropody [foot care]. Loss of mobility brings the need for friendly visiting, transport to social clubs and occupation centres and arrangements for holidays. When illness is added to other infirmities they need more home nursing, night care and help generally in the home. (Ministry of Health, 1963, p.16)

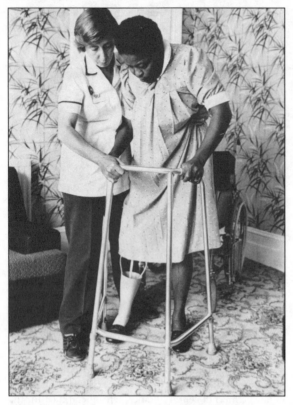

Figure 5.2 Domiciliary physiotherapist helping a woman learn to walk again following amputation of her right leg.

☐ What is the term used to describe the type of services included in this definition of community care and illustrated in Figure 5.2?

■ 'Domiciliary services'.

For the mentally ill and mentally handicapped, however, the same document defined community care services to include provision of residential homes albeit intended that they should be more homely than previous types of institutions (Figure 5.3). Over time, the services and resources involved in achieving the objective of community care have come to be defined in increasingly broader terms. By 1977, in the government's priorities document *The Way Forward*, community care covered:

a whole range of provision including hospitals, hostels, day hospitals, residential homes, day centres and domiciliary support. The term 'community care' embraces primary health care, and all the above services whether provided by health authorities, local authorities, independent contractors, voluntary bodies, community self help or family and friends. (DHSS, 1977, p.8)

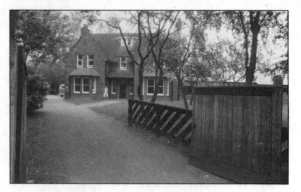

Figure 5.3 Residential hostel for mentally handicapped people. Some, such as this one, are based on existing houses, others are custom built. The key feature is that they are located in residential areas.

The quote also illustrates another important shift of emphasis in official definitions of the services and resources involved in community care. In earlier definitions the focus was on *statutory* provision; that is, provision by public agencies such as the NHS and local authorities. In the 1980s much more attention is being paid to what has been termed the '*mixed economy of welfare*' — that is, to the variety of agencies and individuals providing care: not only statutory services, but also private agencies, voluntary agencies, and families and friends. By including lay care in the definition, the government had belatedly recognised a situation that has always existed — that the overwhelming majority of mentally ill, mentally handicapped and elderly people either live with their families or live alone (Figure 5.4), and are dependent on relatives, friends and neighbours. Another change in emphasis made in *The Way Forward* was a narrowing of the contribution of statutory services. This was made more explicit in *Growing Older*, a White Paper on the elderly published in 1981, which boldly pronounced that:

care *in* the community must increasingly mean care by the community. (DHSS, 1981a, p.3)

This then is what 'community care' has meant over the last few decades. But why has there been such a commitment to providing care in this way, rather than in large institutions?

Why community care?

There have been two persistent beliefs about community care — it is better and it is cheaper than institutional care — beliefs which were neatly encapsulated in the Guillebaud Report:

the development of domiciliary services ... will be a genuine economy measure and also a humanitarian measure, enabling old people to lead the sort of life they prefer. (Cited in Allsop, 1984, p.109)

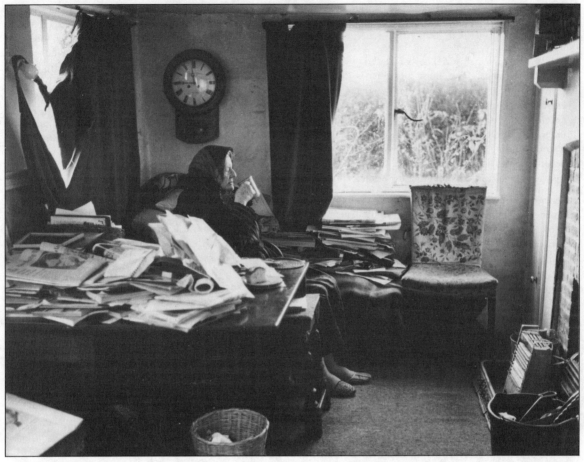

Figure 5.4 Living alone — an elderly woman living alone in a country cottage who had no wish to be moved to 'more suitable' accommodation.

In what way might community care be 'better'? Research carried out during the 1950s and 1960s revealed the degree of *incarceration* and *institutionalisation* of mentally ill and mentally handicapped people in long-stay hospitals. The scale of such provision had increased dramatically during the first half of the twentieth century. Places in mental hospitals, for example, increased from 6 500 places in 1916 to more than 50 000 places in the 1940s, and large numbers of young, mildly retarded people found their way into such care. An American sociologist, Erving Goffman, and a British psychiatrist, Russell Barton, argued that not only were the regimes in these institutions rigidly depersonalising and not conducive to rehabilitation, but that they also exacerbated peoples' disabilities. This was also shown to be true of residential homes for the elderly in a study by Peter Townsend, a sociologist, published as *The Last Refuge* in 1962. More controversially, around the same time a lawyer, Thomas Szasz, and a psychiatrist, Ronald Laing, began to question the very concept of insanity, arguing that public mental health treatment was a way of regulating and controlling the poor and the deprived. In the late 1960s and early 1970s there was also, as was mentioned in Chapter 2, a series of scandals associated with long-stay hospitals. In addition, innovations in medical treatment played their part, with the introduction of new drugs to control the more florid aspects of some mental illnesses thus making care outside of custodial institutions feasible for more patients. Finally, the large remote hospitals were difficult to staff at the time of severe labour shortages in the 1960s, and they were so old that major, costly modification or re-building became necessary.

The belief that community care not only might be better but also cheaper has also been an important influence on its adoption as policy by central government. Such beliefs, however, are based more on anecdotal evidence than on any rigorous consideration of the relative costs and benefits of different forms of care. Many studies of the costs of alternative forms of care have focused only on the costs to public agencies such as the NHS and local authorities, and have ignored the social costs to the person and her or his relatives.

☐ What might such social costs include?

■ Many things. The most obvious is the time provided by any unpaid lay carer, but there may also be extra expenditure on such items as heating, lighting, special diets and laundry, and loss of income for lay carers because of disrupted employment. There may also be housing costs which would only be taken into account if the housing were publicly provided. Costs may also be incurred in adapting the home.

In general, research suggests that *existing* types of care designed to maintain even very incapacitated people in their own homes are cheaper than institutional care. But this may result in existing types of care being inadequate to meet people's needs. There is reason to believe that if adequate support were provided, caring for people in their own homes might be just as expensive as institutional care. Indeed, one interpretation of why governments have supported community care is that it offers the possibility of transferring costs from the public to the private purse and thus reducing public expenditure — in other words, care *by* rather than care *in* the community. Consider now the extent to which such a shift has already taken place.

Community care: assessing progress

Given the different ways in which community care has been defined for different groups at different times, any attempt to assess progress is beset with difficulties. However, if we focus on three aspects of policy — care in large hospitals, in small residential hostels, and services provided to maintain people in their own homes (which would include day centres and day hospitals as well as domiciliary services) — it is possible to get an indication of general trends.

First the large hospitals: *The Hospital Plan* in 1962 envisaged the closure of thirteen psychiatric hospitals, each with over 400 beds, by 1975. In fact, by the beginning of the 1980s only one had been closed. However, the rate of progress has differed between hospitals for the mentally ill and hospitals for the mentally handicapped. The number of hospital beds for the mentally ill had declined in England and Wales from nearly 150 000 in 1955 to an estimated 69 000 in 1983. Figure 5.5 shows the decline in the size of the resident population of psychiatric hospitals since 1954 in England.

☐ What does this suggest about the length of time patients stay in hospital?

■ On average it has fallen, with more admissions occupying fewer beds.

What has been happening in hospitals for the mentally ill is that as the old long-stay patients are discharged or die, they are not being replaced by as many new long-stay patients. However, the same is not true of hospitals for the mentally handicapped where the admission rate of new long-stay residents has meant that the annual decline has remained at only 1 000 places a year and in 1983 there were still around 41 000 places in England and Wales. The failure to reduce the number more quickly is thought to reflect the relative lack of family support for mentally handicapped compared with mentally ill patients. Not only have large institutions for the mentally handicapped remained in existence longer than was planned, but many were still lacking various amenities at the end of the 1970s (Table 5.1).

In the much more severe economic climate of the 1980s there is evidence that health authorities are being put under increasing pressure to close long-stay hospitals more rapidly, a prospect which has given rise to considerable concern not only locally, as the newspaper report at the beginning of the chapter illustrated, but also centrally. During 1984, for example, the *Social Services Committee* in the House of Commons carried out an inquiry into community care. This committee, established in 1977, is one of a series of all-party sub-committees that monitors a particular area of government activity. The Social Services Committee is appointed 'to examine the expenditure, administration, and policy of DHSS, associated public

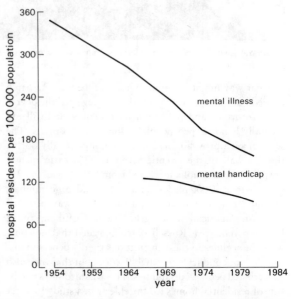

Figure 5.5 Residents of psychiatric hospitals in England expressed as the number of residents per 100 000 total population, 1954–1981. (Source: *Facilities and Services of Mental Illness and Mental Handicap Hospitals in England 1972*, HMSO, 1974; *1980–1*, HMSO, 1984)

Table 5.1 Numbers of mental handicap hospitals (over 200 beds) in England below minimum tolerable standards in various amenities, 1972–79

Amenity	Number of hospitals in:		
	1972	1975	1979
Medical staff	11	3	6
Nurses on wards	31	18	6
Ward orderlies and domestics	67	49	58
Night space	16	12	8
Day space	10	11	4
Patients' personal cupboards	6	9	9
Patients' personal clothing	8	9	7
Large dormitories	25	13	10

(Source: CIPFA, 1985, Table 5, p.74)

bodies [e.g. the NHS] and similar matters within the responsibilities of the Secretary of State for Northern Ireland'. These sub-committees' powers to call civil servants and government ministers to give evidence and to answer questions about government action makes them potentially very influential.

Warning of 'care on the cheap'

A programme to move nearly 100,000 vulnerable mentally handicapped and ill people from hospitals into the community on the cheap could be disastrous the all-party Commons Social Services Committee said yesterday...

It warns Mr. Norman Fowler the Social Services Secretary: 'Any fool can close a long-stay hospital: it takes more time and trouble to do it properly and compassionately. The minister must ensure that mental illness and mental handicap provision is not reduced without demonstrably adequate alternative services being provided before hand'.

(*The Guardian*, March 1, 1985)

☐ What particular aspect of community care policy was the social services committee concerned about?

■ The inadequate provision of alternative facilities *before* hospital care is reduced.

This brings us to the second aspect of the policy — the development of alternative residential facilities to the large institutions. It was planned that facilities for mental illness would include psychiatric units for acute admissions in district general hospitals in addition to small residential units spread throughout the district. The former have been slow to develop while the latter have often failed to materialise altogether. However, plans to provide hostels for the mentally handicapped made some progress during the 1970s and 1980s. For example, places in local authority hostels increased from 3 000 to 10 000 during the 1970s.

Finally, what progress has been made in developing services for the vast majority of dependent people who live in their own homes? At the beginning of the 1970s the DHSS provided guidelines on the level of provision that public agencies should aim to achieve by the early 1980s. These official *targets* were thought to be inadequate by some people. In 1962, Peter Townsend argued that the target for the provision of home helps (Figure 5.6) should be twenty per 1 000 population by 1973 whereas the DHSS target in 1972 was only twelve. However, not even the lower target of the DHSS had been achieved by 1978/9 (Table 5.2).

Table 5.2 Progress towards achieving DHSS guidelines in relation to selected services

	Places per 1 000 population	
	DHSS target (established 1972)	Provision 1978/79
Day care		
Elderly over 65	4.0	1.1
Mental illness	0.6	0.1
Mental handicap	1.5	0.8
Domiciliary Services		
Home helps to over 65s	12 wte*	6.3 wte*
Meals on wheels	200/week	112/week

* wte = whole time equivalent
(Source: Goldberg and Hatch, 1981, p.6)

More recently, the DHSS has moved away from the setting of targets, partly because of doubts over their relevance and partly because 'they no longer looked achievable on a reasonable time scale'. As the Minister for Health told the Social Services Committee in 1984: 'I am not persuaded there is any satisfactory way of drawing up useful national guidelines' (Social Services Committee, 1985, p.cvii).

☐ How does this view compare with developments in the role of central government in managing the NHS discussed in Chapter 3?

■ There is a tendency to increase the degree of central government control through such means as accountability reviews of the performance of health authorities.

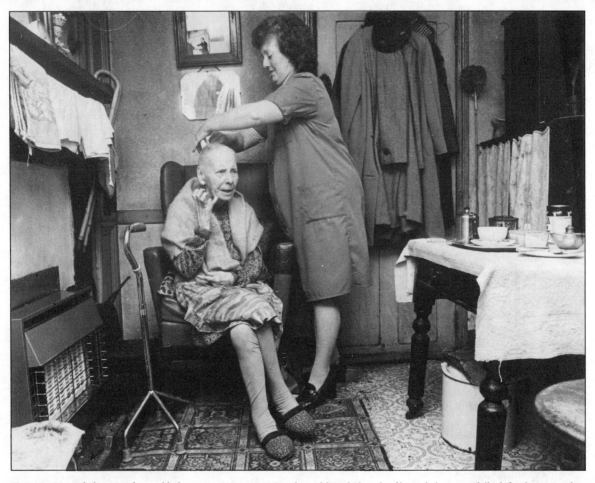

Figure 5.6 Home help caring for an elderly woman in Battersea, London. Although the role of home helps is carefully defined, most perform many additional tasks for elderly people in their homes.

This contradiction between the Minister's view and the trend in NHS management was not lost on the Social Services Committee:

> The Minister recently intervened actively to pressurise authorities to make specific closure plans for their large mental hospitals. Local government finance ... is now founded on a complex series of detailed norms and indicators. In other words, there does not seem to be in general any reticence in principle about detailed central intervention. (Social Services Committee, 1985, p.cvii)

In addition, since the late 1970s local authority expenditure has been significantly curtailed by central government, which has restricted both the rate support grants (funds from central government to local authorities) and the level of rates that local authorities are able to levy. This has adversely affected the level of provision of many community care services (Table 5.3).

As with the provision of health care, considerable geographical variation exists between local authorities in the level of provision of social services (Figure 5.7).

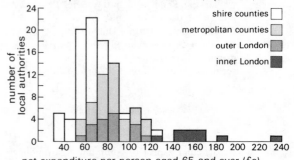

Figure 5.7 Levels of expenditure per person aged 65 and over by Local Authorities in England and Wales, 1980–1981. (Source: Department of Environment, 1983, Exhibit 3.1)

Table 5.3 Some trends in community care services, 1979–1981

Residential	1979/80 compared to 1978/79 (%)	1980/81 compared to 1979/80 (%)
Elderly	−0.7	−2.4
Mentally ill	+8.7	−8.0
Mentally handicapped adults	+10.3	−0.8
Mentally handicapped children	+4.8	+9.1
Physically handicapped	+2.7	−6.7
Domiciliary services		
Home helps		
number (WTE)	−2.4	+3.5
cases	+4.4	−6.1
hours service	+0.5	+0.7
hours service per case	−2.7	+7.2
Meals on wheels	+5.9	−3.3
Telephones		
number of installations assisted	−20.7	−33.8
number of rentals assisted	+15.1	−11.4
Aids	−5.1	−4.6
Adaptations	−21.1	−0.6
Holidays	−0.7	−21.3

(Source: Social Services Committee, 1982, p.80)

□ Looking at Figure 5.7, what geographical pattern is there in local authority expenditure?

■ Shire counties spend the least and inner London authorities the most — around two to three times as much.

□ What may account for these differences?

■ The level of need *per capita* is almost certainly higher in the inner cities than in the shire counties. In addition, those in political control of the latter tend to spend less on all local authority services, not just social services, than local government in urban areas.

The effect of different levels of expenditure on available services can be seen in Figure 5.8 which shows that there was almost a ten-fold difference in the rate of provision of home helps between local authorities.

The failure both to provide sufficient care in the community for people in need and sufficient support for lay people providing unpaid care can have profound effects. A DHSS research report published in 1981 acknowledged that the reality of community care may be rather different from the theory for many people discharged from psychiatric hospitals:

studies ... suggest that the majority live at home on continuing medication but with little community

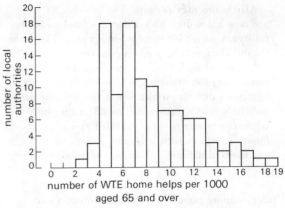

Figure 5.8 Number of WTE home helps per 1 000 people aged 65 years and over by Local Authorities in England and Wales, 1980–1981.
(Source: Department of Environment, 1983, Exhibit 3.9)

support other than that of their general practitioner and often the community psychiatric nurse, and that whilst most are free of psychiatric symptoms and are glad to be home, both they and their families may lead somewhat deprived lives. (DHSS, 1981b, p.36)

What does 'somewhat deprived' actually mean in practice? The following example provides an answer:

The Homers live in a council maisonette in an inner city area. They have two children, Alan who is in the sixth form at a local comprehensive and Alex who attends a special school and is severely subnormal, hyperkinetic [markedly and persistently overactive] and epileptic. Mrs Homer has managed to care for Alex for many years with no outside help. He requires constant attention and almost total nursing care in routines such as washing, dressing and toileting. Recently, he has achieved a degree of bladder control, but as he frequently has epileptic fits, it is still necessary to change his clothing at least once a day.

The fits continue during the night and as there is a danger that he might injure himself, Mr and Mrs Homer and Alan maintain an all-night vigil, taking four-hourly turns to watch over him.

When Mrs Homer becomes too tired to carry on, her husband takes days off work to relieve her. In this way he uses up his annual leave and the family have not had a holiday since Alex was born. The long nights take their toll and Mr Homer is very worried that he may soon be sacked as his attendance at work is unreliable and he feels ... he does not give satisfactory service ... His wife has taken a part-time job since Alex started school and she feels that it is keeping her sane. But she too fears that she may lose the lifeline of an outside interest.

Alan has recently performed badly in his 'O' levels and now has to drop back a year at school ... but he resists any suggestion that his brother should leave the family. The family have reached the end of their tether. In writing for help on their behalf the consultant paediatrician said: 'This continues to be an immensely difficult problem where medical help has been only marginal and sometimes damaging and where community facilities provided have really been limited to school, with little more than good intentions in addition'. (Cited, in Finlayson, 1983, p.204)

Understanding policy failure in community care

Both the cold statistics and the personal experience of many individuals testify to the considerable gap between the political rhetoric and the reality of community care (Table 5.4). While many factors have contributed to this policy failure, a *lack of resources* combined with *managerial difficulties* are the most important.

Table 5.4 Community care — targets and achievements, 1970/71 to 1980/81

	Target change (numbers)	Achieved change (numbers)	Shortfall (%)
Hospital beds (all ages)			
England	− 27 500	− 10 400	62
Wales	− 800	− 250	69
Scotland	− 1 400	− 1 100	21
Local Authority homes and hostels (all ages)			
England	27 615	7 927	71
Wales	1 672	447	73
Scotland	2 141	689	68
Day care (adults)			
England	47 508	21 735	54
Wales	3 135	1 801	42
Scotland	4 937	2 022	59

(Source: CIPFA, 1985, Table 2, p.71)

Why has there been a lack of resources? First, the groups for which community care is primarily designed are relatively powerless within society. Second, demographic changes have led to an increased need for services at a time when central government has been attempting to reduce public expenditure. And third, the transfer of people to community care has been expected to take place using existing resources.

☐ Why does this present problems?

■ Existing resources are tied up in hospital care. The health authorities are faced with a 'Catch 22' — they cannot release resources from the hospitals until patients have been transferred to community care, but the transfer cannot take place until resources are available to provide the necessary services in the community.

Even some extra resources in the form of bridging loans to 'pump-prime' may not be sufficient to get things moving, as it is not possible to close hospitals or make savings until a substantial proportion of the patients have been transferred.

☐ Can you suggest why this is so?

■ While there are still patients in a hospital, even if only a few, it is necessary to continue to provide certain essential services such as heating. There is also a minimum level of staffing that cannot be further reduced until the whole hospital is closed. Finally, and of greatest importance to building new community hostels, it is not possible to sell the hospital and grounds until the last patient has gone.

Another way of looking at this issue is to compare the *average cost* of a patient's care in hospital with what is called the '*marginal cost*'. For example, the average cost per case could be calculated as the total cost of running the hospital divided by the number of cases treated. But the marginal cost per case would be the *extra* amount that it would cost the hospital to increase its number of cases by one.

To illustrate the distinction, assume that the average catering cost per patient is £5 a day. It would not necessarily cost the hospital an extra £5 to feed one more patient — it might only cost £2 (the marginal cost). The reason the marginal cost might be less than the average cost is because it is not necessary to employ more catering staff or build more kitchens to feed one more person, indeed, the only extra cost would probably be the ingredients of the meals. The converse of this situation is that *reducing* by one the number of patients being fed each day would not reduce costs by £5; again, the staff, kitchens, and so on represent relatively fixed costs, and so only marginal savings could be expected. The marginal cost of a hospital patient, and therefore the marginal savings, depends on the type of hospital and patient involved. In the case of patients affected by community care policies, marginal savings are probably between a half and a third of the average cost. Bridging finance is therefore vitally important to allow alternative services and eventual closure and sale of hospital and land before sufficient savings are accrued from the transfer of patients. One problem facing health authorities has been that bridging finance has not been widely available.

Consider now the managerial difficulties that health authorities have faced. These arise from the DHA's relationship with various groups: NHS occupational groups, the public and local authorities. As you have seen in Chapter 3, local health service policy can be strongly influenced by individual employees and occupational groups, particularly, though not exclusively, doctors. For example, if consultants dislike particular policies, they have considerable power to delay change. There has certainly been some resistance from the medical profession towards the proposals to shift resources from hospital to community care. In addition, other staff groups working in large old hospitals have been resistant to change work routines that have become familiar over the years. Health and local authorities have also met resistance from another important group, members of the public, who are anxious about the implications of community care for themselves.

Mental anguish

People living in a smart street have reached for the panic button because their new neighbours are mentally handicapped. They fear for children at a nearby primary school, and are worried that the value of their homes will drop. One resident said 'We feel these people shouldn't be here'.

(*Kettering Evening Telegraph*, June 6, 1981)

Finally, managerial problems have arisen between DHAs and local authorities. Community care may mean very different things to these two agencies. For local authorities it may mean reducing the number of places it maintains in old people's homes and increasing day care facilities and domiciliary services. However, such a reduction in the availability of residential accommodation decreases the opportunity for the DHA to discharge patients from hospital.

One of the most difficult aspects of the joint planning of services, as you have seen in Chapter 3, concerns finance. The bulk of current expenditure in respect of mental illness and mental handicap is on hospital in-patients-funds that come from central government finance for the NHS. Yet community care involves replacing hospital care with services provided by local authorities: personal social services, education and housing. Extra services provided by local authorities will put an additional burden on the ratepayers. There is thus a financial incentive for local authorities to do nothing. Joint finance, introduced in 1976, has undoubtedly acted as a small impetus for change in services for priority groups. But the total funds available — an estimated £105 million in 1985/6 — are far too small to achieve a major transfer of responsibility from the NHS

to local authorities, representing as they do only around 3 per cent of personal social service expenditure and less than 1 per cent of NHS expenditure. In 1982, in an attempt to accelerate change, the government permitted DHAs to pay local authorities or voluntary bodies on a *long-term* basis, as long as the latter accepted particular patients or residents from NHS care. At the time of writing it is not clear what effect this change will have on promoting community care.

The future of community care

While the impact of medical innovations, such as the replacement of joints and the development of more effective drugs, might be expected to prevent some disability, estimates suggest that there will nevertheless be an annual increase of around 1 per cent in the numbers of severely disabled people: that is about 5 000 a year. The problems of a growing number of dependent people may be exacerbated if the current high divorce rates continue or increase and the average family size decreases, resulting in fewer lay people to care for elderly relatives. Additionally, as women are the major providers of lay care, their increasing involvement in paid employment can be expected to have an impact on their ability to provide such care* (Figures 5.9 and 5.10).

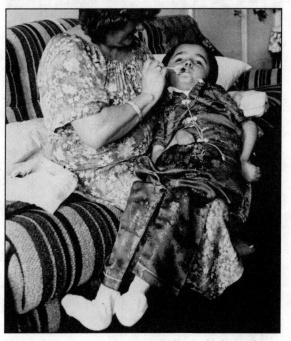

Figure 5.9 Lay care — mother caring for her disabled son at home.

*These issues are all discussed in greater detail in The Open University (1985) *Birth to Old Age: Health in Transition*, Chapters 4 and 12, The Open University Press (U205 *Health and Disease*, Book V).

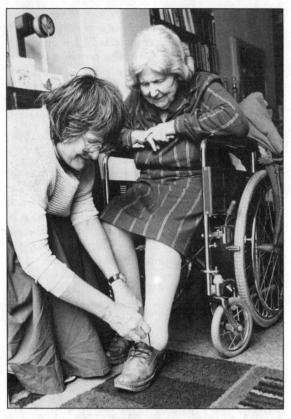

Figure 5.10 Lay care — a daughter looking after her elderly, disabled mother at home.

Lay carers play a crucial role in helping to make community care effective (and efficient) and the high social, emotional and financial costs that such care can involve will have to be increasingly recognised by the statutory agencies. Without support it is inevitable that many families will be placed under great stress and many may break down. There are also many people for whom the community, in the sense of family or friends, does not exist and for them care *by* the community will prove to be an isolated and desperate experience. The Social Services Committee noted that:

> there are hundreds if not thousands of mentally ill people living unsupported in the community, many of them former hospital patients. Large numbers are sleeping rough in archways and under railway bridges ... Many more are in hostels for single homeless. These are the often invisible victims of past and present deficiencies in community care. (Social Services Committee, 1985, p.lxxxiv)

Too little attention has also been paid to the views of those in need. Even where considerable support is provided,

dependent people often have little say in the form it will take. There is considerable resistance, for example, to providing cash grants to allow people to purchase the kind of care they prefer, though some experiments in this sphere are proving successful.

There are two further issues involved in the future pursuit of community care. First, the past concentration on the interface between health and social services has obscured the importance of other services, especially those of social security, housing and employment, and indeed the influence of economic and social policy in general on the capacity to care of individuals and communities. To a large extent the success of the community care policy will depend on the extent to which the wider social and economic environment allows caring relationships to be developed.

Second, there is a danger that any policy of community care will further increase the moral pressure on women to care. Some commentators have argued that further policies must avoid putting women under a greater obligation to care than men. So, for example, the right to compassionate leave from employment should be equally available to men and women. However, others have argued that the gender divisions which exist in health care in general and community care in particular will not be removed without fundamental social changes such as improvements in the position of women in the labour market. These are, however, issues which transcend the immediate concerns of implementing a policy of community care in the 1980s.

Finally, throughout this chapter we have been concerned less with the pros and cons of the *idea* of community care than with its implementation. As the newspaper cutting at the beginning of this chapter indicates, the prevailing view of the idea appears to be that 'on paper this seems absolutely marvellous'. But is it? A review of changing ideas towards the institutional care of the mentally disordered by Patricia Allderidge provokes a thought on which to end:

> when in 1907 Henry Maudsley finally set in motion the foundation of a *small* specialist mental hospital, in direct reaction against the massive county asylums, he was in fact recycling a model which had previously been used at the end of the fourteenth century, in 1713, and several times in the second half of the eighteenth; and which had already been proposed this time round in 1867 and had been circulating in one form or another ever since. (Allderidge, 1979, p.333)

Thus, although the idea of community care seems broadly accepted at present, this may change. The following account was written in 1985 by someone working in a large hospital about to be closed.

> The size of the long-stay patient population, now about 850, actually creates valuable opportunities for

a variety of facilities; occupational and industrial therapy (considered to be the best in the world); special units for music, art and pottery, psychotherapy, and social skills; the provision of different diets and religious services; patient clubs and a cafeteria; a gymnasium with remedial gymnast; hairdressers and a boutique; and the specialist services, such as dentistry and physiotherapy, that patients fail to utilise out of hospital. All these amenities are provided in extensive and attractive grounds and constitute, despite the connotation of 'the total institution', an ongoing community. Such provisions for rehabilitation and organised outings, such as swimming, are made possible by the sheer size of the hospital. (Weller, 1985, p.570)

Is this a straw in the wind, suggesting the idea that large institutions are the best way to create a community of care? Perhaps not, but it serves as a reminder that no policy should be considered as the final word on an issue. The policy of community care also illustrates the difficulties that central government can face in trying to implement a change in direction. Finally, it demonstrates how a well-intentioned strategy which is intended to improve people's lives can, as in the case of the Homer family, turn out very different in practice. While policy formulation is essential to the resolution of many of the dilemmas facing health care, it must also be remembered that new policies themselves can produce their own new dilemmas.

Objectives of Chapter 5

When you have read this chapter you should be able to:

5.1 Discuss some of the different ways in which community care has been defined and the factors that have contributed to support for such a policy.

5.2 Comment on the extent to which community care, as an alternative to institutional care, has been successfully established and discuss some of the factors which have constrained policy implementation in this field.

Questions for Chapter 5

1 (*Objective 5.1*) Community care can be used either prescriptively or descriptively. Describe (i) the prescriptive and (ii) the descriptive ways in which the term 'community care' has been used, and (iii) the main factors that have led to support for community care.

2 (*Objective 5.2*) What have been the main reasons for the relatively slow decline in the size of the residential population of hospitals for the mentally handicapped in England (shown in Figure 5.4)?

6

The way of the new

In the previous chapter you have seen how the problems of caring for the old, the mentally ill and the mentally handicapped are being approached by changing the way services are provided. In other words, the current response to that particular dilemma is to seek new ways of organising health care. In a similar manner, attempts are being made to reduce the high costs of acute hospital care by the introduction of day surgery, in which people are admitted to hospital for only a few hours rather than several days. This is another example of what is referred to as *process innovation*. In many ways these types of innovation attract less attention, particularly from the mass media, than *product innovations*.

> ## Hospital buys big banger to shatter kidney stones
> A radically new form of treatment to remove kidney stones from the body without a surgical operation is to be introduced in Britain. A private London hospital is paying more than £1 million for a German-made lithotripter machine. At present there are only seven such machines in the world, four in Germany and three in America.
>
> (David Fletcher, *Daily Telegraph*, June 5, 1984)

It may appear that product innovations, such as 'big bangers' have little in common with new ways of organising services. In fact, the two are often closely connected. For example, although the introduction of day surgery has largely resulted from the need to reduce health care costs, it has only been possible because of the development of new anaesthetics from which patients recover in a matter of minutes or hours. This chapter is concerned with the ways in which both product and process innovations arise, the factors that determine whether or not they are adopted by the NHS, and if adopted the way innovations spread or diffuse.

One way of viewing the history of an innovation is to consider its career: its creation through *research and development*; its *adoption* by, and *diffusion* through, a health care system; and finally its *abandonment* in the face of new, alternative developments. In this chapter we shall concentrate on the first two phases. The third phase, abandonment, usually occurs when a replacement becomes available which has been shown to be, or is believed to be, more effective, efficient or humane — aspects that we will consider in the next chapter.

Research and development
There is a myth that innovations arise by accident. One of the best known surrounds the series of events that led to the discovery of the antibiotic, penicillin. The myth is that one day in the 1920s Alexander Fleming left a dish of growing bacteria by his laboratory window in Paddington, London. By chance some spores of a fungus that produces the substance penicillin floated in and when he examined the dish he found that where the fungus had landed, the bacteria had been killed. The era of antibiotics had dawned.

Needless to say, this myth ignores several key features of the story. The first is that the whole of Fleming's research had been devoted to the search to find an effective antibiotic ever since he had become aware, during the First World War, of the vast number of wounded soldiers who died not from their immediate wounds, but from ensuing bacterial infections. He was therefore well prepared to respond to what he found in his dish of bacteria. The second is that his discovery remained a laboratory curiosity, because the technology to grow the fungus in bulk and harvest the penicillin it produced did not exist. It was not until the Second World War made the question urgent once again that Fleming's laboratory curiosity was rediscovered by a team in Oxford. The resources of the American pharmaceutical industry were brought into play, and penicillin rapidly became a medically useful substance.

This story illustrates the two models that are often proposed to explain how innovations come about. The first sees new ideas as arising out of developments in what is called *basic* or *pure science* — that is, scientific research carried out without practical aims in view other than obtaining knowledge about the world. This model assumes that such research then leads to other more *applied* developments — that is, developments which exploit new techniques or ideas to generate new products and processes to solve health care problems. This is known as the *science-push* model. The second model suggests that those engaged in health care — whether as clinicians, managers or manufacturers of equipment and drugs — identify needs which then result in the necessary research being commissioned. This is the so-called *market-pull* model.

In practice, neither model offers an entirely adequate explanation. On the one hand the market often doesn't know that it *has* a need until pure science has developed new knowledge. For example, no one envisaged the possibility of looking inside the living human body without having to cut it open until the discovery of X-rays at the beginning of this century suddenly opened up that prospect. On the other hand, even scientists engaged in pure research don't search *entirely* at random for problems to solve, if only because scientific research is expensive, and they are dependent on funding bodies which have some interest in the possible application of the findings of pure research. In practice, most innovations are the product both of science-push and market-pull, though one or the other may predominate.

At first sight it may appear that research which results in product innovations, such as the development of antibiotics, can have little in common with that which results in process innovations. Product innovation is largely the result of investigation of the natural world whereas new ideas in the organisation of health care largely result from study of the social world. In addition, while pursuit of the latter is still accessible to lay people, natural science research is now almost exclusively the province of professionals. However, these differences are a matter of degree. While it is possible for lay people to make some contribution to the study of the social world, much research in this area requires high levels of funding and the application of sophisticated analytical methods, similar to those used in the natural sciences.

One final general comment on the uses of natural and social science research in the field of health care: developments often involve the application of both. Pharmaceutical companies use market research to inves-tigate the need for and acceptability of products before applying pharmacological research in developing a new drug. Conversely, social science research may be dependent on developments in the natural sciences, such as the development of microchips in computers.

Despite all these similarities and contrasts between methods, the key aspect of research that affects both natural and social science alike is that of the need for high levels of funding. Not only does this limit the amount of research that can be undertaken but it also has important consequences in the determination of subjects for study. We therefore need to consider two interrelated questions. Who funds research? And how are the topics for research chosen?

☐ There are three principal sources of funds for research in the UK. What do you think they may be?

■ 1 The state — through the universities, the research councils, and government departments such as the DHSS and the Ministry of Defence.
2 Industry — in particular the pharmaceutical and electronics companies.
3 Charities and trusts.

The precise sums involved are difficult to calculate for several reasons. These include both the difficulty of defining which areas of research are primarily related to health, and determining the proportions of expenditure devoted to research by such bodies as universities, charities and trusts. However, it is possible to estimate the approximate scale of the contribution to health research (Figure 6.1). Figures of this magnitude acquire more meaning when compared with expenditure on other areas of research, in other countries, and with amounts spent in the past.

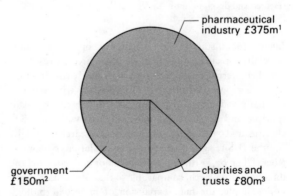

Figure 6.1 Estimates of Research and Development Funding in the Health Field, 1983–1984.
(Sources: (1) Office of Health Economics, 1985b, Table 18, p.24; (2) MRC, DHSS, NHS plus estimates of other sources; (3) projection from 1976 and 1980 levels of funding).

Somewhere between 10 and 25 per cent of the total national research budget (which was about £8 000 million or almost 2.5 per cent of Britain's GNP in 1984) is spent on basic science, health and welfare, while 75 to 90 per cent goes on military and industrial research. The growth of this huge enterprise is essentially a post-1939 phenomenon. In the 1930s, spending on research was perhaps as little as 0.1 per cent of the GNP, and it was scarcely a matter of government concern; a much higher proportion of the research funds then came from charities or industry. The Second World War changed all that; research spending increased considerably during the war, then doubled as a percentage of GNP every 7–10 years from 1945 until the mid 1970s, with the state becoming more and more important as the major source of funds. Since the 1970s spending on research has barely kept pace with inflation and the contribution of government, as opposed to industry, has fallen back slightly.

How does the UK compare with other countries? The total research budget represents a similar proportion of GNP as that spent by other EEC countries and by the USA. In addition, the major involvement of the state is matched in all other industrial countries. On the other hand the choice of priorities — between say military and civil research — differs from country to country (Figure 6.2).

by public money and thus more dependent on grants for research funding; and the different tax systems for charities set up by commercial companies.

Having seen, in broad terms, who funds research in the UK we need to turn our attention to the way this money is spent. For not only do the sizes of the contributions from each of the three main sources differ (Figure 6.1) but so do the types and subjects of the research they support.

The state

In the UK, the state funds research through a number of channels. Figure 6.3 shows how the government distributed its £3 656 million share of the research and development budget in 1984.

Research on health, disease and health care is funded through the DHSS, the NHS, the universities and the research councils. Most of the research supported by these funds is done in universities, the rest in hospitals and specialised research institutes. While the whole of the allocation to the DHSS and the Medical Research Council (MRC) is spent on health research, it is not possible to tell from Figure 6.3 how much of the Economic and Social Research Council (ESRC) allocation went towards

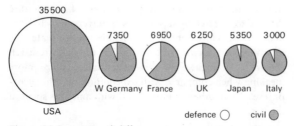

Figure 6.2 International differences in government spending on research and development in the civil and defence sectors. (Source: Connor, 1984, p.4)

Japan, for instance, has specifically opted for commercially-directed rather than military-directed research. Another international difference is the relative contribution of industry and charities. By comparison with the US, Germany and Japan, British industry invests much less in research and development, and compared with the USA, charities and trusts play a smaller role in research in the UK. In the USA, giant charitable foundations such as Rockefeller or Ford can exert a major influence on the direction of research, comparable to that of the state itself. For example, the huge expansion of molecular biology from the 1940s to the 1960s owes much to the Rockefeller Foundation. This feature of the research enterprise in the US arises for two reasons: the weaker position of the universities, which are proportionally less well supported

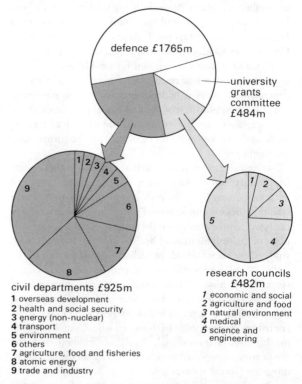

civil departments £925m
1 overseas development
2 health and social security
3 energy (non-nuclear)
4 transport
5 environment
6 others
7 agriculture, food and fisheries
8 atomic energy
9 trade and industry

research councils £482m
1 economic and social
2 agriculture and food
3 natural environment
4 medical
5 science and engineering

Figure 6.3 Spending by British government on research and development, 1983–1984. (Source: *Annual Review of Government Funded Research and Development*, HMSO, 1984, Table 2.1)

research in the health field. What is clear however is that while the provision of services consumed about 10 per cent of the total public expenditure, it received less than 5 per cent of the government's research budget. By contrast, defence, which also consumed around 10 per cent of public expenditure received 53 per cent of the research budget.

Although both the DHSS (£27 million) and NHS (about £5 million) provide funds for research, the main sources are the research councils (at least £113 million). This reflects a longstanding principle that research should be commissioned independently of the government department which has a direct interest in the outcome. In 1916, a government report on the machinery of government (the Haldane Report) proposed this arrangement for state funding of civil science and it has persisted, with modifications, ever since. Even before the Haldane Report, a Medical Research Committee had been established, funded on the principle of one penny per person per year insured under Lloyd George's National Insurance Act of 1911. This was the first and only example in the history of British research policy where an attempt was made to quantify the support given to a particular research area on the basis of *need*, as assessed by the scientists and researchers. After 1916, the Medical Research Committee was reconstituted as the Medical Research Council (MRC).

The MRC uses its funds both to finance research projects in universities and to support a number of major biomedical research institutions (such as the National Institute for Medical Research in Mill Hill, London; the Clinical Research Centre in Harrow; and the Molecular Biology Laboratory in Cambridge). In addition it supports some projects in community medicine, psychology, and medical sociology. Increasingly these find themselves in competition for a share of a static or even shrinking budget — occasionally resulting in dramatic closures of research projects:

> **Medical research funds to be cut by 21% next month**
>
> Leading medical scientists have been told privately that their funds will be cut ... Projects at risk include cancer research at Cambridge, test tube work at Edinburgh, and research into blood diseases at Oxford.
>
> (Andrew Veitch, *The Guardian*, March 14, 1984)

The MRC determines its own directions and priorities for research. Although it coordinates its activities with those of the other research councils, it jealously guards its own autonomy.

☐ This arrangement in which the MRC, rather than the government, DHSS or NHS, is the main funding body has been criticised by some people. Can you suggest why?

■ This arrangement assumes that the scientists and researchers at the MRC know best what research should be done. People have questioned this and suggested that the DHSS and NHS are in a better position to judge the needs and priorities for research in the field of health as they have a responsibility for providing health services.

In 1970 a committee of inquiry under Lord Rothschild attempted to produce a major alteration in the Haldane principle when they proposed that funds should be diverted from the MRC to the DHSS. The DHSS, acting as a *customer*, should then specify what research it needed and researchers in universities and research institutes acting as *contractors*, should carry it out. In practice the MRC and major scientific establishment figures resisted strongly what seemed like an attack on their autonomy, and within a few years the policy was reversed. Meanwhile, similar criticism was being made of the other research council which has an involvement in the health field. The ESRC (formerly the Social Science Research Council (SSRC)) responded by introducing more lay people into its decision-making committees. What effect this will have on the nature and topics of research that are funded is still not clear.

Although all these funding bodies are dominated by scientists and experts, there are some distinct differences between them as regards the type of research they fund. The MRC tends to fund *biomedical research*. If asked to identify its greatest successes, the MRC would undoubtedly point to the large number of Nobel laureates whose work has been done under its auspices, notably the groups which first identified the structure of DNA, sequenced a protein and cracked the genetic code. These have indeed been amongst the most exciting advances in biology in the last thirty years.

In contrast, the DHSS and the NHS (both at regional and district level) are on the whole more interested in funding *health services research* — the evaluation of the effectiveness, efficiency and humanity of existing health services. The DHSS funds several research units concerned with such topics as health services management and perinatal epidemiology.

Although most state-funded research takes a biomedical approach, there is, however, some support for social research, through the MRC, DHSS and ESRC. However, social research is very much the poor cousin of biomedical research. The dominance of the latter is not peculiar to state-funded research but is a feature both of industrial and charitable support also.

Industry

Clearly many different types of industrial product are relevant to health, some directly, others less so. The design of hospital beds directly affects the comfort and to some degree the speed of recovery of patients, and the work of nurses and other staff. The development of automated laboratory equipment by scientific instrument manufacturers has transformed both the work of hospital pathology laboratories and the techniques of medical diagnosis. The revolution in information technology has put the microchip at the heart of many new instruments and the computer increasingly at the centre of the modern hospital's record systems. For several reasons product innovation in the context of health care calls to mind the pharmaceutical industry. First, it is big business — in 1982, 383 million prescriptions were dispensed through the NHS at a cost of £1 500 million. Second, unlike many other health care innovations which emerge from universities or government institutions, new drugs come almost exclusively from the drug companies. And third, the pharmaceutical industry has attracted a great deal of attention as regards its pricing and advertising policies. For these reasons, we will concentrate on the role of the pharmaceutical companies (Figure 6.4).

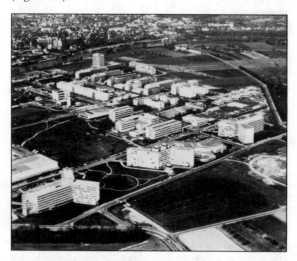

Figure 6.4 A modern pharmaceutical factory.

□ What is the overall goal of the pharmaceutical industry?

■ Pharmaceutical companies, like other companies in the private sector, can only continue to exist by making profits, if not in the short term then over a reasonably foreseeable period. Profitability has to be their underlying objective.

To pursue this objective, the pharmaceutical industry has to be able both to produce and to market products which provide it with an adequate return on capital invested. The products that are produced and marketed are, relatively speaking, a means to an end, not an end in themselves.

Given that there are a lot of drugs already available, why should the pharmaceutical industry do research at all? The answer to this question lies partly in the nature of the laws regulating the production and marketing of drugs. Any new drug is *patented* by the company which produces it. This means that only that company, or its licensees, have the rights of production and marketing for a period of seventeen years. In other words, the company is granted a monopoly by the Patents Office for a particular product and can in principle fix the price at which it will sell it. Whereas the chemical constituents of the drug may cost only a few pence to produce, the pharmaceutical company can sell it for many times that figure. For example, the chemical substance frusemide (used as a diuretic to decrease the retention of fluid by the body in conditions such as heart failure) costs £5 a thousand tables. As *Lasix*, a brand of frusemide marketed by Hoechst, it costs £60 a thousand. Similarly, the tranquillizer benzodiazepine costs about £20 a kilo to manufacture; Roche of Switzerland sell their brand, *Valium*, to their sister company for marketing in the UK at £922 a kilo.

The purpose of patent laws, like copyright laws, is to try to ensure that innovators are rewarded, which might not occur if everything were left to market forces. But in the pharmaceutical industry, patent laws have had a profound effect on research: if other companies wish to share in the market for a particular type of drug that is protected by patent, then the only alternative to waiting for the patent to lapse, is to engage in an intense research effort to produce another drug that is as similar to the patented drug as possible but doesn't infringe the law. The result of this is that any successful new drug on the market is usually followed by several similar products, often referred to as 'me-too' drugs, manufactured by competitors. For example, *Valium*, one of the most commercially successful drugs of all time, gave rise to a galaxy of similar tranquillisers, none of which was very different in effectiveness. A variant of this type of research strategy is the development of new *combinations* of existing drugs. Many of these are very familiar from TV commercials — for instance, headache treatments that contain various combinations of analgesics (pain-killers), muscle relaxants, and even anti-depressants.

Pharmaceutical companies, rather than universities or other academic institutions, have been responsible for developing most of the important new drugs since the war, including tranquillisers, oral contraceptives, most anaesthetics, anti-malarials and anti-histamines. But they may also contract work out to specialist research institutes or to universities (some £17 million worth in 1982/83). Recently, this has been true of one particular area of research — the development of *genetic engineering* techniques as a major source of fundamentally new drugs. These techniques offer new and cheap ways of producing, on a large scale, substances ranging from hormones such as insulin to a potential anti-viral agent, interferon. A novel aspect of these developments has been the rise of the new growth industry of biotechnology during the late 1970s and the 1980s in which university researchers have spawned independent companies with names like Biogen, Genetech, Celltech and Cetus, to exploit the new methods. The big drug companies have been quick to buy in. Sometimes they have negotiated deals on industrial products: the insulin producer, Eli Lilly, now produces human insulin with a method developed by Genetech.

Pharmaceutical companies also make wholesale deals with universities and hospitals, funding new research institutes within them. For example, the German company, Hoechst, contracted a $50 million deal with the Massachusetts General Hospital in the USA for biotechnological research. The effects that these powerful industrial links may have on the universities and the question of commercial ownership rather than free publication of the scientific research that results from such marriages of convenience raise questions about control of research and scientific ethics which have seriously concerned many people in recent years.

However, not all drug company research is of this path-breaking kind. There is, in addition, the careful synthesis and screening of many hundreds of thousands of different types of chemical compounds for possible therapeutic effects. Before a new drug can be brought onto the market, it first has to be shown, almost always by animal experimentation, to have some type of desired biological effect. Detailed studies then have to be carried out on its effects within the animal, its toxicity and so forth.* Finally, it has to go through a period of clinical trials to assess its value by comparison with existing drugs and procedures. Of the many hundreds and thousands of substances studied by this type of molecular roulette, only a tiny proportion ever finds its way onto the market.

Since the thalidomide tragedy of the 1960s, the regulations controlling the licensing of new drugs have been tightened up by the Food and Drug Administration (FDA) in the USA and the Committee on Safety of Medicines (CSM) in the UK. The CSM is also responsible for monitoring the effects of drugs once they are on the market and in use. This is known as 'post-market

surveillance' and is discussed further in Chapter 7. The drug companies have argued that the very long time taken to get any new drug onto the market (ten years) leaves very little time to recoup their research expenditure before their patent protection (seventeen years) runs out, thus reducing the financial incentives to innovate. It has also been argued that the benefits of getting an effective drug onto the market more quickly than at present are lost, and that this must be set against the protection that regulations give against unsafe drugs.

However, critics of the industry claim the regulations are still too lax. They believe that the terms of reference of the CSM, which only require them to consider whether or not a drug is safe and more effective than a placebo, are inadequate. In addition, argue the critics, a medical need for a new drug should be proven. This may be compared with the system in Norway, where an application for a new drug is accepted only if a need can be medically demonstrated. But, as you have seen in Chapter 2, defining 'need' is not straightforward. A few years ago the World Health Organization determined that of the 60 000 or so drugs available on the world market, a basic list of a mere 220 was all that were really needed.

Drug companies these days tend to be multinational industries, and of the twenty-five largest only three are British — ICI, Beechams and Glaxo — and none of these is in the top twenty. They operate a pricing structure for their products which is geared to what the local market can bear rather than the actual production costs of the substances themselves. At present, overseas-based drug companies meet three-quarters of the NHS drug requirements.

Within Britain, prices for drugs are fixed by an agreement between the industry and the government on the basis that the prices charged to the NHS are no higher than those charged for export, which in turn is based on a formula of 25 per cent return on capital. In 1983, this formula produced at least £300 million profit for suppliers to the NHS. In 1979, gross profits on NHS sales were 21 per cent, with some companies showing as much as 30 per cent — a figure which may be compared with pre-tax returns for the chemical industry as a whole for that year of 18.2 per cent (Shulman and Rentoul, 1984). On this basis, only advertising and oil are more profitable than drug manufacture. The drug companies response to these arguments is that its pricing policy has to take into account the fact that of the many thousands of compounds they research as possible drugs, only a handful ever reach the market; the prices charged for these must be such as to cover the costs of the research and development for those compounds that never reach the market.

How successful is the industry at producing new drugs? It is probably true to say, as the industry's representatives

---

*This is discussed further in *Studying Health and Disease*, Chapter 3, *ibid*.

often do, that only the commercial and competitive environment of private industry is able to generate so many new products. They tend to point out that fewer new drugs are developed in the Eastern Bloc. What is open to question of course is how many of the new products developed by the industry are really necessary and beneficial?

Charities and trusts

Charities and trusts are legally recognised, non-profit making institutions compelled by their charters to disburse money for defined goals which may be concerned with education, welfare or research. But charities are also big business. It has been estimated that the total income of the 135 000 registered charities in the UK in 1982/83 was over £7 000 million (Posnett, 1984). It is reckoned that approximately £475 million, or 6.5 per cent of the income was for charities involved in the health field.

Charities can be thought of in three main categories based on their major source of income. The first are those which rely mostly on *voluntary donations* (shown in Figure 6.5) and tend to be involved with some particular client group (such as the physically disabled) or some disease or diseases, such as cancer. The second category, usually referred to as *trusts* or *foundations*, relies primarily on investment income, and tends to support a wide range of activities. The final category depends on *fees* and *charges*

for services provided, such as independent schools (including Eton!), housing associations and nursing homes.

Charities concerned with health raise over half their income from donations (55 per cent), the remainder coming from fees and charges (23 per cent), investment income (13 per cent) and statutory grants, such as those from government (6 per cent). Indeed, health charities dominate the market for voluntary donations.

☐ Looking at Figure 6.5, what proportion of the top 200 charities in terms of voluntary income, are related to medicine and health?
■ 33 per cent (67 out of 200).

It would appear, therefore, that health-related charities are very popular with the public, compared, for instance, with charities for the arts or youth organisations. Why should this be so? Some clue as to why people donate money to health charities is provided by looking at which subjects the public support.

☐ Looking at Figure 6.5, which three health subjects attracted the most money?
■ Cancer, physical disability and blindness.

It has been suggested that the favouring of these particular topics reflects the concerns and fears of donors, who tend

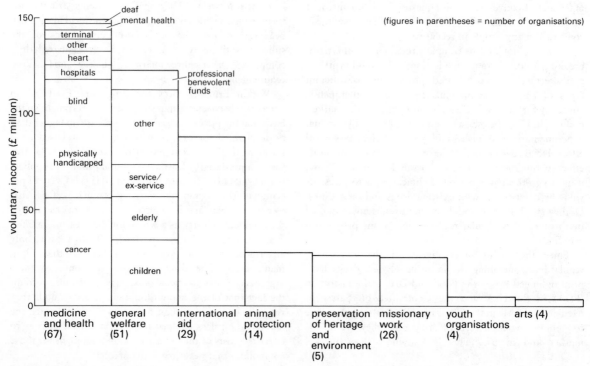

Figure 6.5 Charities attracting the largest voluntary donations, 1983–1984. Based on the 200 charities with the largest voluntary incomes. (Source: McQuillan, 1984, p.94)

in the main to be elderly or approaching old age. If this is so, then it is interesting that charities concerned with ageing, rather than any particular disease, get relatively little support.

The proportion of income that health charities spend on research varies dramatically. One trust, the Wellcome, where funds come from a parent drug company, Burroughs Wellcome, now spends more on supporting university-based biomedical research than any other body in the UK outside the MRC, as well as funding its own research institute. Other influential trusts and foundations include Ciba — again funded from the drug company of the same name — Nuffield, whose money originally came from the car industry, and Leverhulme, set up by Unilever.

In addition to these trusts, some charities that depend largely on voluntary donations devote much of their income to research. These include two of the largest and oldest fund-raising charities, the Imperial Cancer Research Fund (ICRF) and the Cancer Research Campaign (CRC). The former was established at the turn of the century, and the latter was an offshoot in 1923 in an attempt to provide even more support for research. In 1982/83 their combined income was over £43 million. Much of their money comes from legacies left by people dying from cancer (over £25 million). The scale of their operation can be judged from the fact that their combined assets amounted to £84 million, providing them with nearly £7 million in investment income alone. The CRC has over 1000 local committees of supporters throughout the UK and hundreds more local honorary organisers. Their advertising budget and style makes them able to compete with major private industries (Figure 6.6).

While the aim of the CRC is 'to attack and defeat the disease of cancer' through biomedical research, other health charities are concerned with innovation in the field of health care delivery and organisation. There are many examples of charities pioneering new developments in the face of conservative statutory authorities — the Family Planning Association, the Samaritans, the National Marriage Guidance Council, and the Women's National Cancer Control Campaign (which pioneered screening for cervical cancer). Some of these initiatives were later adopted by the statutory authorities, while others still await official recognition.

Apart from support for biomedical research and health care innovation, some charities have been most active and effective in the field of public policy. One such example is the Spastics Society. Although most of their £24 million income in 1982/83 was spent on providing special schools and centres (only 1.3 per cent on research), their major impact has been influencing government policy in obstetric and paediatric care. Their 'Save a baby campaign' in the 1970s carried the message to the public and to the

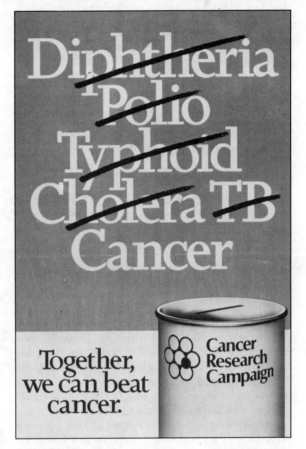

Figure 6.6 Cancer Research Campaign poster. Charities use commercial advertising agencies to promote their causes. The campaign that this poster was part of what was mounted in spring 1984 and included 500 giant sites as well as smaller sites donated free by the poster advertising industry. In addition, the CRC used press advertisements in mass circulation daily newspapers and weekly magazines.

government that the prevention of cerebral palsy (brain damage resulting in spasticity) lay in better provision of intensive facilities in hospitals such as the monitoring of *all* births and more special care baby units.* Despite the fact that such developments are either of unproven value or only have a marginal effect on the incidence of cerebral palsy, the campaign was successful in encouraging the government and the Social Services Committee in their policy objective of all births taking place in hospital with much greater use of medical technology such as foetal heart monitors.*

While the Spastics Society spends most of its income on providing facilities for spastics, other charities are explicitly

*The use of these techniques is discussed in *Birth to Old Age, ibid.*

concerned with the study of policy. They are mostly trusts which are not dependent on public support — the Rowntree Trust with its interest in social research, Nuffield and Leverhulme concerned with policy in social and health affairs, and the King Edward Hospital Fund involved in monitoring statutory services.

The technological imperative

At the beginning of the chapter a distinction was drawn between product and process innovation.

> ☐ Which of these two forms of innovation seems to be the priority for most of the biomedical and phar- maceutical research, and which seems to attract most interest and attention among health care providers and users?
> ■ Product innovation.

Most of the incentives in health research and medical practice are strongly biased towards product innovations: Nobel prizes, professional status, research awards, the kudos of pure science, all tend towards expanding the frontiers of what can be done, rather than doing in a different way what is already being done. In consequence, it is normally taken for granted that health care innovation is an outside force inexorably marching forward and inevitably resulting in higher costs (referred to as the 'technological imperative'): the DHSS, for example, assumes 'that additional expenditure on the hospital and community health services nationally of half per cent a year is necessary as a contribution to the costs of this constant process of medical innovation' (DHSS, 1983a, p.17). But the scope for process innovation in health care is just as wide as anywhere else: innovation could be cost-reducing rather than cost-increasing.

> ☐ An example of a process innovation was mentioned earlier in the chapter. Can you recall what it was?
> ■ Day surgery, which can make use of a new technology — short-duration anaesthetics — to give a different way of providing surgery at less cost.

Let us now consider how the adoption of innovations does or does not take place in the NHS, and in particular, the differences between process and product innovations.

Adoption and diffusion

How does change come about in the NHS? Why is it that different people working in the same organisation can feel either frustrated at their inability to bring about change or disturbed by the pace of change and the way nothing seems to be left well alone? By considering three particular examples of change, we hope to show the wide range of factors that determine whether the adoption and diffusion of an innovation is a success or a failure. Two of the

examples are of product innovation: in vitro fertilisation techniques and CT scanners; while the third is a process innovation: changing patient waking times in hospital. However, before discussing these examples let us consider some of the factors that we might expect to influence adoption and diffusion. A major study carried out by Barbara Stocking, a health policy analyst, suggested there are three main aspects to consider: the characteristics of the innovation, the influence of the environment, and the role of individuals or specific groups.

The characteristics of the innovation include such aspects as how compatible it is with existing work arrangements; how complex a change will be necessary if it is adopted; whether or not it is possible for people to see it in use or try it out in advance of deciding whether or not to adopt it; and what advantage it will confer over existing technology or organisation.

Stocking saw the influence of the environment taking several forms: society's attitude and expectation, the prevailing philosophy about how health care should be organised, the physical environment of health service buildings, and the amount of marketing. An obvious example of the last is the marketing of drugs carried out by the pharmaceutical industry. In 1981/2 they spent £120 million on promoting their drugs, which as a proportion of turnover was three times as much as the average for the rest of British industry. Advertising ranges from pages in the professional journals, through direct mail shots, to visits by sales representatives (there was one drug sales represen- tative for every eight GPs in the UK in 1982). Each GP received about 50 kilograms of advertising material a month, including about forty free medical magazines (Shulman and Rentoul, 1984).

The third and final influence, that of individuals or groups, is perhaps the most important. Stocking identified the crucial role that some individuals played in initiating change, that others contributed as promoters of innova- tions, and yet others as disseminators.

As you read through the three case studies, try to identify the factors that were most influential in leading to the adoption of each innovation and, in addition, try to decide which model of research — science-push or market- pull — best fits each example.

In vitro fertilisation (IVF)

First frozen embryo birth

The birth in Australia of the first baby from a frozen embryo, announ- ced yesterday, could be matched in Britain within two years. The embryo had been frozen for eight weeks at −196°C. Although an important advance, the birth is also likely to provoke a fresh debate on the ethical and legal implications.

(Thomas Prentice, *The Times*, April 12, 1984)

Only six years after the British research team of Dr Robert Edwards and Mr Patrick Steptoe had announced that they had succeeded in producing the world's first 'test-tube' baby, news of the first frozen embryo baby was reported. Not only does this illustrate the speed with which product innovation takes place, but also its international dimension.

☐ What other aspect of innovation does the newspaper report illustrate?
■ The ethical and legal implications of some product innovations.

IVF techniques are but the most recent in a long line of efforts to treat infertility and thus relieve the distress it causes. A substantial number of women who want babies cannot conceive them by the normal procedures of human fertilisation. In some cases this is because the woman does not produce ova, or there are obstructions in the Fallopian tubes so ova cannot reach the uterus. For other women their sexual partner may be impotent, or have a low sperm count, or his sperm may not be fertile. IVF also offers the chance of pregnancy to women who want to have a baby without sexual involvement with a male.

If a woman *can* produce her own ova, these can be collected by means of a relatively simple surgical procedure and fertilised *in vitro* (in a glass dish) either by her partner's or a donor's sperm, and then reimplanted in her uterus.

Not surprisingly, the first success with IVF, the birth of Louise Brown in 1978, had a dramatic effect on infertile couples. After years of despair their hopes were raised by reports of the possibilities that lay ahead. The effect was to create, more or less over night, a demand for IVF:

Thousands queue for £1,000 'test tube' babies

Thousands of women desperate to have babies are on the waiting list for treatment when Britain's first 'test-tube baby clinic' opens in the autumn.

(*Daily Telegraph*, July 14, 1980)

Such euphoria and optimism frequently accompanies product innovations; but very often the initial enthusiasm of the innovators can have unintended repercussions for those very people who stand to benefit most. By 1982 the reality of IVF was becoming clear.

'False hope' charge over fertility claim

The head of Britain's largest infertility clinic yesterday spoke of the misery suffered by thousands of would-be mothers as a results of the public enthusiasm for test-tube babies. Reports of a one-in-four success rate were out of all proportion to the published results, said Mr Robert Winston.

'Virtually every infertile patient now has the fantasy that if she is able to save up the money and get herself into the hands of somebody practising *in vitro* fertilisation, that she is going to have a baby', he said.

(Andrew Veitch, *The Guardian*, October 14, 1982)

By 1982 it appeared that the success rate of IVF was nearer 10 per cent than 25 per cent, although technical developments may improve on this in the future. The story of IVF demonstrates some other aspects of product innovation. One is the unexpected side issues that often arise. In the case of IVF it has been the production of 'spare' embryos, an inevitable consequence of the technique. The doctors and biologists involved in developing IVF never considered the fate, at least not in public debate, of the extra embryos they would produce. Having produced them, the doctors have found themselves under pressure from geneticists and developmental biologists, anxious to acquire the spare embryos for research purposes. But this presents ethical problems about the 'rights' of embryos.

In 1984 a British Government Committee of Inquiry into some of the ethical and legal implications of IVF and related techniques, chaired by the philosopher Mary Warnock, proposed an absolute upper limit for research on embryos of fourteen days post-fertilisation. This is the time at which, during normal embryonic development, the neural tube begins to form.* At this point, the committee concluded somewhat arbitrarily, the embryo begins to develop into a 'person' and must be legally protected against research manipulation.

*The development of embryos is discussed in The Open University (1985) *The Biology of Health and Disease*, Chapter 4, The Open University Press (U205 *Health and Disease*, Book IV).

These recommendations and proposals are still being discussed as this book is being written. Meanwhile, public feeling is running high. A private member's bill to ban all embryo experimentation and to control very tightly the availability of IVF has come before Parliament.

Two million sign call for ban on human embryo tests

More than two million people have signed a petition calling for a legal ban on experiments on human embryos, LIFE, the anti-abortion organisation, announced yesterday.
(David Fletcher, *Daily Telegraph*, February 27, 1985)

In contrast, some feminists see the techniques as being developed by male scientists and doctors without concern for a woman's right to control her own body. Some were also critical of the Warnock Committee for not paying attention to some groups of women who wished to submit evidence to the Committee.

While the Warnock Committee report represents a comprehensive attempt to deal with some of the issues involved in IVF (as well as other related techniques), it leaves other issues unresolved and even undiscussed. To begin with, the issues are presented in strictly ethical terms. The question of ensuring pregnancies for those who are infertile is part of a larger question of ensuring that all those who want children can have healthy living babies. This raises the question of whether priority should be given to research into treating infertility or to reducing the marked disparities in perinatal mortality rates that exist in the UK between social classes.*

The question of priority is tied up with that of who should provide IVF — the state or the free market? In 1985 IVF is not yet available on the NHS, only by private payment. Some gynaecologists predict that the techniques could eventually be developed by the NHS at a cost of about £200 per woman, as opposed to the £2 000 being charged privately in 1985. This will raise the question of whether or not the 'right to have a baby' should be part of NHS provision, or should only be available to those who can afford it.

IVF illustrates another dilemma that product innovations often raise — how can the concerns and fears of the public about possible abuse of the innovation be allayed? If the government were to accept the recommendations of

the Warnock Committee then they would have to set up a licensing authority to approve both places where IVF is carried out and those in which experimentation on human embryos are conducted. The proposed authority would have substantial lay representation to reassure the public about the activities of the scientific community.

☐ What problems would a lay person have on such a committee, assuming the other members were scientists and doctors?
■ Inevitably much of the committee's business would be of a highly technical nature which a lay person may have difficulty in understanding.

In other words, a lay representative may face the same sorts of problems that lay members of health authorities face when confronted with clinicians and professional managers. In this respect, the management of product innovations presents the same opportunities and dilemmas as the established aspects of health care.

CT scanners

Faced with a patient complaining of a range of symptoms, the doctor's initial task is that of diagnosis. Diagnostic techniques often depend on being able to measure and monitor aspects of the patient's biochemistry, physiology and, in general, internal state. Playing an increasing part in monitoring these internal states are *non-invasive methods* — methods that avoid incising or piercing the body in any way. The oldest of these methods involves X-rays, but more and more procedures involving ultrasound, radio-isotopes and fibre-optics have appeared over recent years.* Often the machinery to visualise what is going on internally can be linked to computers to enhance the quality of the picture or improve the analysis of the data. While the new instruments may dramatically improve information and diagnosis, they are also very costly and the extra information they provide may be of greater value to research than to the patient being examined. So what are the arguments in favour of introducing the new machinery, and how far should scarce resources be invested in it? We will consider the use of one particular innovation, the CT scanner.

A CT (computer tomography) scanner is essentially an X-ray machine linked to a computer (Figure 6.7). The X-rays are used to take pictures at various levels of the body from many different angles, and the computer then analyses the data to give a series of cross-sectional pictures of, for example, brain, spine or liver. The CT scanner is a major improvement on X-rays because it allows soft body tissues as well as bones to be seen, enabling, for example, brain tumours to be identified (Figure 6.8).

---

*These inequalities are discussed in *The Health of Nations*, Chapter 9, *ibid*.

*Some of these methods are discussed in *Studying Health and Disease*, Chapter 3, *ibid*.

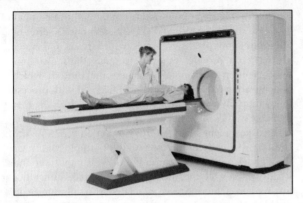

Figure 6.7 CT scanner: the patient is slid through the opening in the X-ray machine so that serial sections can be taken.

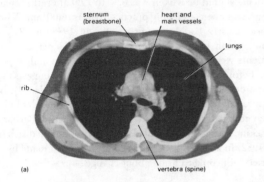

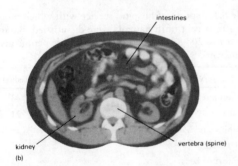

Figure 6.8 CT scans showing views through (a) the thorax and (b) abdomen.

CT scanners were pioneered in the UK. Their development resulted from combining concepts and strands of knowledge from several disciplines: basic research in physics and engineering; image enhancement techniques from the experience of military and space researchers interested in extracting the maximum possible information from pictures; and biological knowledge about the biochemistry and physiology of the body. As the medical potential of the technology became apparent so the

development of new generations of machines began to be separated out from the general development of image anaylsis devices for other, non-medical, purposes.

Originally slow and unable to handle the whole body, the first CT machines were only capable of scanning the head. However, as technology improved it became possible to picture any area of the body. As a result, CT scans have replaced a number of diagnostic procedures that are either less accurate, create discomfort for the patient or carry significant risks. However, despite these advantages there is no convincing evidence that the use of whole body scanners improves patients' survival.

Despite having pioneered the techniques, the adoption and diffusion of scanners in Britain has been relatively slow. By 1980 there were about three times as many head scanners and ten times as many body scanners per head of the population in the USA compared with the UK. In all, the US does more than five times as many scans, adjusted for population size, than in the UK. While this difference may partly reflect a greater degree of scepticism on the part of British doctors, another factor is probably of more importance.

☐ What do you think is the main reason for these differences?

■ Cost — not merely capital cost, but running cost. (In 1980 a CT scanner cost about £700 000 and up to £300 000 a year to run; each individual scan was costing about £100.)

The consequence of this is that in deciding on the purchase of a scanner it is not enough only to take into account the capital cost — planners have also to consider the revenue costs of staff, overheads, and maintenance which a machine requires. A substantial proportion of the machines available in British hospitals have been bought by charities — sometimes big national foundations, and sometimes as the result of more locally based appeals, as you saw in Chapter 3. In 1980, about half the thirty-five body scanners in use or on order were paid for, fully or partially by donated funds. But meeting operating expenses is a much less attractive proposition for a public appeal than buying the machine in the first place. The operating costs must therefore normally be met from a health authority's own funds. In a time of scarce resources, this cost has to be assessed against other demands, and in some instances the offer of a 'free' scanner purchased with donations has had to be refused by health authorities unable to afford the running costs.

What should determine how many scanners are available? Aaron and Schwartz, whose work was referred to in Chapter 2, report that some radiologists in the USA suggest that eventually every hospital with 200 or more beds and a diverse caseload could justify having a CT scanner. On this basis there could eventually be more than 3 000 scanners in the USA, and, pro rata, some 600 in the UK. The annual running costs alone could amount to some £200 million (at 1980 prices).

☐ Where might the pressure for the introduction of the new machines come from?

■ You might have thought of several different sources — patients or relatives of patients who have read of the new methods and assert their right to them under the NHS; doctors who believe the machines will enhance the service they can offer, and reduce the use of alternative invasive techniques such as surgical operations, or who are concerned that *not* to have access to such equipment will lower their status with colleagues in better equipped hospitals; instrument manufacturers who stand to make substantial profits from the sale of new equipment; the health authorities who wish their hospitals to be fully up-to-date; the media, local or national, which may mount campaigns for particular equipment to be installed; and, of course, local and national politicians.

Apart from the additional cost, there are other potential disadvantages in introducing the new machines. One is that a health authority has to commit revenue funds which are then tied up for the length of the life of the equipment. It is not generally possible to make small reductions of funding without the whole enterprise having to stop. A second disadvantage is that resources have to be *centralised* in one particular hospital, hence contributing to the overall trend of closing small dispersed facilities, such as local general practitioner hospitals, and concentrating most services on one central site.

A third quite separate class of problem is the pace with which technology develops. Machines become obsolete within a very few years of installation. Indeed, CT scanners themselves have been virtually outdated during the early 1980s by the development of a new class of scanner whose imaging properties depend not on X-rays but on other properties of atoms: nuclear magnetic resonance and positron emission (NMR and PET scanners). NMR scanners can in effect look through bone, at tissues that are inaccessible to CT scanners, while PET scanners are about 1 000 times more sensitive than CT scanners in detecting the tracer chemicals that are used to locate abnormal tissues and cells. However, the new machines cost much more than CT scanners and involve much heavier running costs. Just those pressures which led to demands for CT scanners are likely to lead to demands for the installation of more of the new generation of scanners, with consequent greater costs, and greater centralisation.

Patient waking times in hospitals

The case studies on IVF and CT scanners raise a series of questions about priorities, provision of services and ethics arising from product innovations. Our third example, which concerns attempts to change the time at which patients are woken in hospital, is concerned with process innovation. By comparison with the issues which the first two case studies raise, the time at which patients should be woken may seem relatively trivial. Yet in terms of the comfort of hundreds of thousands of people who pass through hospitals each year in the UK it is important and it illustrates well the, perhaps unsuspected, difficulties involved in achieving even a relatively small change in established practice.

In 1961 a report prepared by a nursing committee in the Ministry of Health recommended that the earliest that patients should be woken was 6.30 to 7.00 am rather than what was then common practice, before 6.00 am. This report clearly had little impact, for in 1979 the Royal Commission on the NHS reported that 44 per cent of patients were still being woken before 6.00 am and 76 per cent before 6.30 am. It also found that early waking was the commonest cause of patient dissatisfaction (Table 6.1). In an attempt to understand why later waking times had not been adopted by hospitals and health authorities, Barbara Stocking undertook a detailed study in four health districts in 1982. In all four districts, attempts had been made by a variety of people to bring about change.

Table 6.1 Aspects of hospital service with which more than 10 per cent of in-patients were dissatisfied. Based on a survey of 700 adults. Percentages exclude people giving 'no answer'.

Aspect of service	dissatisfied (%)
woken too early	43
food	21
washing and bathing facilities	19
toilet facilities	15
comfort of beds	13
noise during daytime	12
privacy during examination and treatment	11
Based on 797 people (all ages)	
information about progress	31
difficulty understanding doctors (apart from using medical terms)	15
notice of discharge	12

(Source: Royal Commission on the NHS, 1978, p.125)

☐ Who do you think might have tried to promote change in the waking time?

■ You may have suggested patients, who perhaps have most to gain; the Community Health Council, whose job is to represent the interests of patients; and NHS staff, partly out of concern for patients, but also if a change would benefit their own work. The latter might be true for night nurses.

There were in fact examples of all these categories having tried to promote change. In addition, some nurse managers, administrators, a university department of nursing, and the chairperson of the district's hospital consultants had also tried. Despite the considerable amount of effort by these people they had met with only limited success. They had met a wide range of obstacles including inadequate nurse staffing levels, the clinical management of patients, knock-on effects on other staff, patient expectation, and ward design.

While most nurses were keen, at least in principle, to change the waking time, in practice they were reluctant to do so, because of *nursing staff shortages* (particularly on long-stay wards) and the implications that change would have for the balance of work between day and night staff. One reason given to justify early waking on long-stay wards was the fact that patients were put to bed early by the day staff before they went off duty. This was necessary because there were insufficient night staff to cope. In addition, it was found that the night staff, who tended to have been employed longer than the day staff, were more resistant to change of any sort.

Another reason for early waking was to enable various *clinical procedures* to be carried out, such as preparation for operations, routine observations of temperature, pulse, blood pressure and so forth, and early treatments to be administered. While not all patients had to be woken for these activities, the design of 'Nightingale' wards (Figure 6.9) meant that it was impossible for staff to avoid disturbing all the patients' sleep. In addition, some consultants demanded that the ward should be ready for their arrival for a ward round at about 9.00 am. They insisted on all domestic and catering activities being completed so their round would not be disturbed.

Objections to organisational change were not confined to the clinical staff — doctors and nurses — but extended to ancillary staff as well. In one hospital, the catering service pointed out that as later waking would mean patients going to bed later, the evening meal would have to be served later (in one long-stay hospital it was served at 4.15 pm!). If it was to be served later, then staff shifts would have to be altered and catering costs would rise as a result.

Staff not only pointed out their own objections to change, but also sought to show that the patients wouldn't welcome a later waking-time. Reasons cited by staff included the patients' desire to go to bed early and get up early, as this was seen as a traditional pattern of behaviour in the district the hospital served. Staff in a psychogeriatric hospital believed that the patients were insufficiently clear about what was going on to worry anyway. In another hospital the staff felt the benefits of later waking were

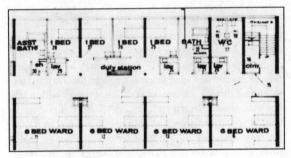

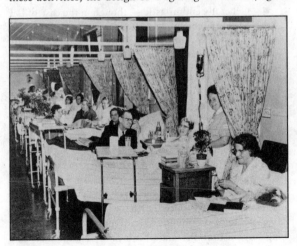

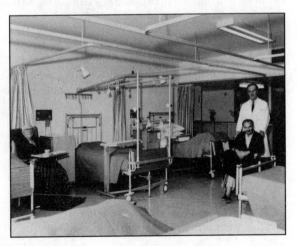

Figure 6.9 Hospital ward design. The large 'Nightingale' wards (a) containing 20–30 beds have been replaced by wards sub-divided into single, two, four and six-bedded rooms (b).

outweighed by the costs to patients of having to have bed baths in the afternoon rather than in the early morning.

Given that several obstacles exist in each hospital, it may seem improbable that any progress could be made in the adoption of a process innovation such as changing the waking time. However, in practice some hospitals have made some progress. Several factors seemed to encourage adoption: if another more major change was taking place, such as the opening of a new hospital; if the nurse managers were interested and committed to the change; and if medical staff were prepared to review the necessity of routine early-morning observations of patients and the need for the ward to be specially prepared for their round. Pilot studies or trials of the new arrangements appeared to meet with little or no success in changing attitudes, and in one hospital attempts at persuasion by managers was abandoned as a failure and replaced with an authoritarian style of management. The latter successfully altered the waking time, but possibly at the cost of antagonising staff. This highlights an important aspect of such organisational change — the need to balance the costs and benefits both for staff and patients.

As Stocking concluded, change may be beneficial to patients in terms of giving them more rest in hospital or, on long stay wards, in providing a more home-like environment. Usually it only causes problems to staff. They may get their rewards in seeing that it benefits patients or in pride at running a more up-to-date hospital, but these gains may be bought at a high price in terms of the disruption of routines, threats to working relationships within the hospital, and a heavier workload. If flexibility for the individual patient is the aim, it may begin to feel as if there are no routines at all. Yet people need routines to reduce stress. For these reasons changing waking times is perhaps one of the most difficult changes to bring about in the NHS.

Conclusions

Let us now consider the three innovations just described plus that of community care discussed in the preceding chapter. It is clear from these accounts that adoption of the two product innovations has been much more successful than that of the two process innovations. Why has that been so? The first point to note is a difference in the models of research and development that lay behind the innovations.

☐ How do product and process innovations differ in this respect?

■ Product innovations tend to result from science-push whereas process ones arise from market-pull.

This distinction is not absolute — as you have seen in Chapter 5, some of the impetus for community care arose

from the development of new drugs for the care of the mentally ill.

☐ Turning to the characteristics of each of the four innovations, are there any differences between them that could account for the variation in their adoption?

■ Some characteristics of IVF and CT scanners definitely helped their adoption: they both offered some medical advantages to patients over the existing technology; both could be seen and tested by potential adopters (the manufacturers of CT scanners actually took a machine around the country on a lorry to display in hospital car parks); and, on the whole, their adoption was compatible with existing work arrangements (although the adoption of CT scanners sometimes led to disputes both between hospitals and radiologists as to their siting and who was to be in charge).

In contrast, several characteristics of the two process innovations jeopardised their chances of success: neither was compatible with existing work arrangements; both involved fairly complex changes; neither could be easily tested in advance (though they could be observed in other places); and neither produced much direct advantage for the staff.

It is worth noting in passing that when a product innovation also requires major changes in processes for its adoption, such as the introduction of computers for record keeping, it can run into the same problems that process innovations meet.

Let us now turn to what Stocking describes as environmental factors: society's attitudes and expectations, and aspects of the physical environment?

☐ What has been society's attitude to IVF and to CT scanners?

■ Generally enthusiastic — though in the case of IVF this has been tempered with anxiety and concern about the long-term consequences of interference with embryos and 'nature'.

As you have seen from the newspaper reports, product innovations tend to get exaggerated claims made about them, thus raising people's expectations higher than is justified. The introduction of CT scanners was accompanied by wild claims that it was the long-awaited cure for cancer. In contrast, the issue of patient waking time has created little or no media interest. While surveys suggest that such issues have a good deal of support from patients while they are in hospital, there is little active support or interest from people once they have been discharged. The same is true of community care. Reports of conditions in long-stay institutions and the lack of community care services are generally deplored by the public. Television documentaries may lead to official inquiries but are unlikely to produce a sustained demand from the public for change and improvements. It often appears to be the case of 'out of sight, out of mind'. However, it is important also to recognise the serious obstacles to change that the physical environment poses for process innovations: the difficulties of building hostels as an alternative to large institutions; and the design of 'Nightingale' wards which mean 'one awake, all awake'.

Finally, let us consider the role of individuals and groups in initiating change.

□ Broadly speaking, how do those most intimately involved with the four innovations discussed differ as regards their status and power?

■ There is a striking difference. IVF and CT scanners were both initiated and supported by powerful groups of doctors working in high status acute specialities and based in the most prestigious regional and teaching centres. In addition, CT scanners were backed up by manufacturers who invested much time and money in promotion and marketing.

In contrast, patient waking time and community care have the support of relatively powerless groups: nurses, doctors working in low-status specialities and therapists. In addition, these groups are not united — some of the most effective opposition to change was mounted by members of the same groups. And in comparison with the product innovations, the hospitals involved with community care are isolated and far removed from the traditional centres of power in the NHS.

It is apparent from these four examples that the adoption of product innovations has been considerably more successful than that of process innovations. In many ways, the promoters of the latter have a much harder task than those involved with new products. They have to convince a wide range of people, with different and sometimes conflicting interests, that change is desirable. That in turn requires the use of evaluative techniques to explore the alternatives and demonstrate the advantages of the proposed innovation. The ways in which that can be done are the subject of the next chapter.

Objectives for Chapter 9

When you have studied this chapter you should be able to:

6.1 Distinguish between science-push and market-pull models of innovation.

6.2 Describe the differences between the three main sources of research funding in terms of the size of their contributions, their research interests and their motivation.

6.3 Explain, using examples from the case studies, why product innovations tend to be adopted more readily than process innovations.

Questions for Chapter 6

1 (*Objective 6.1*) The 'Big Banger' machine for treating people with kidney stones, referred to at the beginning of this chapter, uses sharply-focused sound waves to shatter stones inside the patient's kidneys. The alternative treatment requires a surgical operation. Which model of research, science-push or market-pull, do you think lies behind this innovation?

2 (*Objective 6.2*) Broadly speaking, what are the main research interests of (i) the MRC, (ii) the DHSS, (iii) the pharmaceutical industry, and (iv) charities?

3 (*Objective 6.3*) What factors do you think would (i) assist, and (ii) discourage, the widespread introduction of 'Big Banger' machines in the NHS?

7

Evaluation and monitoring

This chapter includes discussions of several methods (randomised controlled trials, qualitative and quantitative social research) which were described in Book I, *Studying Health and Disease*. During this chapter you will be asked to read three articles contained in the Course Reader: 'Effectiveness and efficiency' by Archie Cochrane (Part 3, Section 3.2), 'The economics of treating varicose veins' by David Piauchaud and Jean Weddell (Part 3, Section 3.5) and extracts from 'Ethical dilemmas in evaluation' (Part 3, Section 3.6).

For any disease there are usually several possible treatments. For any service there are many ways in which it may be organised. And for any health issue there is a range of policies that might be adopted. How then are decisions to be taken and choices made between alternative treatments, different organisational arrangements and competing strategic policies? The plethora of questions that need answering forms a daunting list but they can be boiled down to the following four key questions. Do health services provide *effective* forms of care? Are services organised in the most *efficient* manner possible? Are services *equitably* distributed so that everyone has an equal opportunity of receiving care? And finally, are the people who use the services treated with *humanity*?

These questions cannot be resolved without methods of systematic *evaluation*: the process of relating results to objectives. For example, assessing the proportion of people with pneumonia who recover after receiving an antibiotic, or the cost of producing meals for hospital patients by one method rather than another. The crucial feature is that explicit objectives are set and outcomes are measured. Thus the setting of clear objectives is of central importance to evaluation.

Although attempts at evaluation have been made since at least the seventeenth century,* there has been a major expansion and investment in such studies since 1945. Many new, elaborate techniques have been developed in the fields of epidemiology, social and economic research, management studies and operational research. (The last mentioned approach was developed during the Second World War to describe the increasingly scientific methods adopted in the planning of military operations.) The wide range of methods that have been developed reflect not only the range of questions that need answering, but also the range of activities that require evaluation. This extends from evaluating a single encounter or a single drug to that of a

---

*Historical examples of evaluation appear in *Caring for Health: History and Diversity*, ibid.

complete policy — from a surgical operation to the use of psychotherapy, and from the organisation of hospital catering arrangements to capital spending on kidney transplant facilities.

There are several ways in which the various methods of evaluation can be categorised. One crucial distinction is that between an *experimental* and *non-experimental design*.* Experimental methods are the more powerful, but they are also more difficult to use. A proper experiment demands that researchers have some systematic control over their subject matter so that they can vary its operation under different experimental conditions. Where the topic is the effectiveness of a drug, this is relatively easy. But consider instead the question of whether the NHS has been effective in reducing inequalities in the mortality rates of different social classes.† Experiment is impossible here, so what methods can be adopted instead? One method is to examine the mortality rates for all classes over time. It can be observed that the rates for classes I and II have fallen faster than those of classes IV and V. In other words, there has been a relative widening of the gap between higher and lower classes.

□ So has the NHS been effective in reducing inequalities in mortality rates between social classes?

■ There is insufficient evidence to answer. In fact, there are three equally plausible answers: (i) the NHS has failed to reduce inequalities; (ii) the NHS has partially succeeded — the gap may have been even greater without the NHS; and (iii) the NHS had no effect on changes in mortality rates.

□ How might you try to assess which explanation, if any, is correct?

■ You might compare the UK experience with that of another country which has not had a state-run health system. However, other countries will inevitably differ in other ways apart from the type of health care system.

Generally speaking, evaluation attempts to impose as great a degree of experimental control as possible. In the case of biomedical aspects of health care, experimental designs are usually possible, whereas psychosocial aspects often, though not always, require the use of non-experimental approaches. Examples described in this chapter are drawn from across this spectrum.

The first crucial division is between experimental and non-experimental research, but a second is that between *evaluation* and *monitoring*. Once the value of an activity has been demonstrated and generally accepted as

worthwhile, there is no need for further evaluation to be carried out. There is, however, a need for continuous monitoring to assess first whether or not the activity is being implemented and second, even if it is, that it is achieving the results expected from the initial evaluation studies. Despite the distinction between evaluation and monitoring, it is not always possible, in practice, to separate the two activities. For example, when assessing the impact of a policy it may be necessary to both evaluate and monitor it while it is being implemented. This has largely been true of the community care policy and the various recent reorganisations of NHS management.

Finally, it is important to appreciate that despite the major expansion in evaluation and monitoring that has taken place over the past forty years, the proportion of current health care practices that has been adequately studied remains small. There are a number of reasons for this. Not only may studies meet such obvious obstacles as lack of funding, but there can also be opposition from groups with an interest in preserving the status quo. In the case of the medical profession such an interest group has the power to prevent evaluation. For example, the value of a surgical operation can only be studied with the active cooperation of surgeons. And even when measures have been evaluated, interest groups have to be persuaded to change their own practices — something that can take many years to accomplish. The factors that may either promote or discourage such changes are considered in the context of each of the approaches discussed.

We shall first consider the four main aspects of evaluation — medical effectiveness, economic efficiency, equitable provision and humanity. Although we shall consider each one separately, those responsible for making decisions about health care provision have to take all four simultaneously into account for they are interdependent. Each aspect has to be balanced against the other three. Consider, for example, a very expensive drug to treat cancer. Suppose that 2 per cent of patients benefit from the drug, but not the other 98 per cent, and that it is impossible to predict who will benefit in advance. Moreover, the drug also causes severe adverse effects such as hair loss and vomiting. For a few people the drug is definitely effective, but has to be judged against both its poor efficiency (the small benefit would be bought at a high cost) and the high degree of patient dissatisfaction resulting from the adverse effects it produces. Broadly speaking all decisions about providing health care should involve weighing up the effectiveness, efficiency, equality and humanity of a measure. While evaluation may be able to measure each of these, the final decision as to what action to take is political; that is, it depends on the relative importance that the decision-makers put on each aspect.

---

*This distinction is discussed further in *Studying Health and Disease*, ibid.

†Social class differences in mortality rates are considered in *The Health of Nations*, Chapter 8, *ibid*.

Effectiveness

As already mentioned, the effectiveness of remarkably few health care activities has been scientifically evaluated. Some notable exceptions include the eighteenth-century work of Lind in demonstrating the antiscorbutic qualities of lime juice;* and in the 1830s Louis' evaluation of blood-letting and homeopathy,† both of which were shown to be ineffective. Clearly some medical procedures do not require this type of approach as their value is plain to see. Immobilising a fractured bone in plaster to reduce pain and accelerate healing, the use of penicillin to combat some bacterial infections, and the surgical removal of the appendix in cases of appendicitis are just three examples of procedures that do not require experimentation to establish their value.

There are, however, many other aspects of medicine that require, but have never been subjected to, evaluation by an experimental method. The method best suited to this task is known as the *randomised controlled trial* (RCT).‡ Its strength lies in its conceptual simplicity. Consider the following example:

Value of vitamins in preventing birth defects to be tested

Sixteen hospitals are to conduct trials to test the value in pregnancy of vitamin supplements for preventing spina bifida and anencephaly (absence of brain) births, or malformations known as neural tube defects (NTDs).

Volunteers are mothers with a history indicating that they might be at risk. Some will be given a multi-vitamin preparation in addition to their normal diet.

(Pearce Wright, *The Times*, June 8, 1984)

In this study, which commenced in 1984, one group of pregnant women (cases) are given multi-vitamin tablets, while a second group (controls) are given a pharmacologically inert tablet, called a 'placebo'. A key feature of an RCT is that people are allocated to the two groups at random.

☐   Why is randomisation so important?

*Lind's work on scurvy is discussed further in *The Health of Nations*, Chapter 12, *ibid*.
†Louis' work is discussed in *Medical Knowledge: Doubt and Certainty*, Chapter 2, *ibid*.
‡Further details of the design of RCTs appears in *Studying Health and Disease*, *ibid*.

■   If a sufficiently large number of people are allocated at random it is reasonable to assume that overall the two groups are similar apart from whether they receive the drug or the placebo. Thus any difference in outcome between the two groups can be attributed to a difference in the effectiveness of the drug they received rather than to any difference between the individuals taking part.

Given the simplicity and power of RCTs in assessing effectiveness, why have relatively few aspects of health care been subjected to such scrutiny? There have been a number of reasons, some of which are discussed in an article by Archie Cochrane which appears in the Course Reader. The author is an epidemiologist whose book *Effectiveness and Efficiency*, published in 1971, has had an international influence. The article of the same name, which you should now read, is taken from his book.

☐   Cochrane cites several reasons why more aspects of health care have not been subjected to RCTs. What reasons are they?
■   1 Ethical objections are sometimes raised.
2 There is a lack of objective outcomes for assessing the effectiveness of many health care activities.
3 Resistance by authoritarian social systems, which feel threatened by RCTs.

A fourth obstacle, that Cochrane does not mention in this particular extract from his book, is the cost involved and the long duration necessary for many RCTs. Let us consider each of these four main obstacles in turn.

☐   In what way may *ethical* considerations prevent an RCT being conducted?
■   Many doctors believe that it is unethical to withhold a treatment that has become established clinical practice simply because its effectiveness has never been demonstrated.

However, as Cochrane points out, it is equally unethical to continue using a procedure that is of uncertain value. Despite his view, the opinion of most doctors is that to do nothing is unethical if a treatment exists that is *believed* to be beneficial. Such ethical disagreement is particularly apparent when investigators wish to use a placebo for comparison rather than some other form of treatment, as in the study of vitamins and NTDs referred to in the newspaper story. The ethical debate that took place prior to the setting up of the RCT can be seen in the collection of articles and letters that appears in the Course Reader — 'Ethical dilemmas in evaluation'. Of these you should read *The Lancet* editorial of May 1980, the letter from Peadar Kirke, and *The Guardian* articles and letter of December 1982.*

*If you have time you may wish to read all the material in this collection.

□ On what grounds did some people oppose the RCT?

■ On the grounds that 'to deprive women of a totally harmless vitamin cocktail seems unethical', to quote John Lorber, a professor of paediatrics. In other words, even though the benefits of vitamins are not proven, the possibility of some benefits makes it unethical to withhold them.

□ On what grounds did people support the RCT?

■ On the grounds that the benefits of vitamins were not proven and there was a possibility that vitamins could cause harm to some fetuses. To prescribe vitamins without first carrying out an RCT would, in the view of one correspondent, be 'sanctioning what amounts to a situation of uncontrolled experimentation on mothers and babies'.

A second obstacle to RCTs is the assertion that some therapies cannot be evaluated by this means because the benefits can only be judged subjectively, and not measured objectively. Cochrane gives the example of psychiatry. This view has considerable support within psychiatry. The psychiatrist, Anthony Storr, maintained in his book, pointedly titled *The Art of Psychotherapy* (1979), that psychotherapy cannot be a scientific enterprise, for the therapist forms part of a reciprocal relationship with the patient and 'cannot maintain the type of detachment which characterises the scientist conducting a chemical experiment'. He adds that 'the changes which occur as a result of successful psychotherapy do not lend themselves to precise description or measurement'. How true is this?

While such measurements do present difficulties, there have in recent years been several attempts to develop measures of a person's quality of life — known as *health status indicators*.* One such example was that developed by Rachel Rosser and Vincent Watts to measure changes in patients undergoing psychiatric treatment. The indicator recognised eight levels of disability plus four levels of distress (Table 7.1)

□ Do you think that an indicator combining disability and distress is a meaningful indicator of a person's health status?

■ It may be, but equally there may be other dimensions — such as the duration of ill health — which should be included.

Rosser and Watts got psychiatrists to assign patients to different points on the scales of disability and distress, though equally they might have got patients to do it themselves. The use and limitations of their approach can best be seen by considering an example. Let us assume that

*These are also discussed in *Experiencing and Explaining Disease, ibid.*

Table 7.1 Health status indicators — measures of disability and distress

Disability
This describes the extent to which a patient is unable to pursue the activities of a normal person at the time at which the classification is made.

1 No disability.
2 Slight social disability.
3 Severe social disability and/or slight impairment of performance at work. Able to do all housework except very heavy tasks.
4 Choice of work or performance at work severely limited. Housewives and old people able to do light housework only, but able to go out shopping.
5 Unable to undertake any paid employment. Unable to continue any education. Old people confined to home except for escorted outings and short walks and unable to do shopping. Housewives only able to perform a few simple tasks.
6 Confined to chair or to wheelchair or able to move around in the home only with support from an assistant.
7 Confined to bed.
8 Unconscious.

Distress
This describes patients pain, mental suffering in relation to disablement, anxiety and depression.

1 No mental distress.
2 Mild mental distress.
3 Moderate mental distress.
4 Severe mental distress.

(Source: Rosser and Watts, 1972, pp.363–364)

there are three individuals (A, B and C) whose health status has been assessed as follows:

	Distress	Disability
Patient A	3	3
Patient B	3	5
Patient C	2	4

The position of A is shown in Figure 7.1 with a reading of

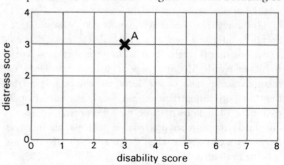

Figure 7.1 Graph of distress and disability as measured by the indicators shown in Table 7.1.

3 on distress and 3 on disability. Plot the position of B and C.

□ Is the health status of A better or worse than that of B and C?

■ Assuming of course that we have a valid measure of health, then A's status can be said to be better than B, because although they are experiencing the same amount of distress, B is experiencing more disability. As regards A and C, A is experiencing more distress than C but less disability. It is not clear whether the health status of A is better or worse than C.

The only way in which the relative status of A and C can be resolved is by deciding which aspect of ill-health — distress or disability — is worse. Such a decision is inevitably a social judgement. Someone has to say which dimension — distress or disability — is to be given greater weight. Just who should make such social judgements is a matter of debate. It could be health professionals, patients, or other members of the public. And it is possible that each group would decide differently from the others. This is just one further aspect of the difficulties of measuring health status.

The third obstacle to RCTs that Cochrane cites is *authoritarianism*. Whether or not his explanation of the influence of Catholicism and communism is true, it is certainly the case that as with all scientific inquiry, RCTs actively promote uncertainty. Does psychotherapy do any good? How effective is community care? Will pregnant women or just the manufacturers of the products benefit from vitamin supplements? Iain Chalmers, an epidemiologist, has pointed out how a lack of evaluation led well-intentioned doctors and nurses in the past to starve, purge, and cool newborn babies in the hope of preventing the development of various complications and to use excessive concentrations of oxygen in the case of premature babies, which occasionally led to blindness.

Attempts to obstruct scientific studies of effectiveness have taken several forms. One has been to insist that all participants in an RCT are *fully* informed about the method of randomisation and the known risks and benefits of alternative treatments. While most people would agree that fully-informed consent is essential, it is ironic that it is something that is rarely obtained in normal clinical work. In other words, doctors impose stricter standards on themselves and their colleagues when conducting a trial than they do during their routine work: they accept that treatment of unknown value may be prescribed to ill-informed patients when no trial is in progress, but insist on *fully*-informed consent when the treatment's effectiveness is being evaluated.

The fourth reason for few RCTs having been performed is that they are an expensive form of evaluation, partly because it may be necessary to follow the participants for many years to establish the outcome. For example, a major study in the 1970s of the effectiveness of coronary artery bypass grafts (a surgical operation to improve the blood supply to the heart muscle) took about ten years to complete and cost $24 million.*

Despite this series of potential obstacles, an increasing number of RCTs are being performed. With this growth in the number of trials, a new, key actor has emerged in the world of health care — the statistician. As studies have become larger and more complex, statisticians have assumed greater importance. It is they who are centrally involved in both designing the studies and analysing the results. In a light-hearted review of these changes, two American statisticians, A.A. Rimm and M. Bortin, have summarised the views of the three protagonists involved in RCTs — the patient, the physician and the statistician (Figure 7.2).

Efficiency

As with the evaluation of medical effectiveness, the amount of health care activity that has been subjected to formal economic evaluation remains small. It is increasing rapidly, however, and in some instances — for example, major capital expenditure decisions in the NHS — it is now obligatory to conduct an economic appraisal before any final decision is taken.

Why is it necessary to consider economic efficiency, and what techniques exist to examine it? A basic tenet of modern economics is that we live in a world of relative *scarcity*, in which *choices* have to be made in allocating resources. Using resources in any activity that produces benefits inevitably involves *not* using those resources in some alternative way that would also produce benefits. Logically, therefore, we must consider the costs of building hospitals, or prescribing drugs or implementing health and safety regulations, in terms of the benefits that have been foregone elsewhere. This concept is known as the *opportunity cost*. If we are to compare the costs and benefits of different ways of spending scarce health care funds, then we need to be able to measure both costs and benefits in such a way that they can be weighed one against the other. We can explore the problems of doing so a stage at a time.

One of the most frequently encountered decisions in health care is choosing between different forms of treatment. One aid in making this decision, as you have just seen, is to conduct an RCT into the effectiveness of the different treatments. One such RCT conducted in the late 1960s investigated two methods of treating varicose veins and concluded that in terms of effectiveness there was

---

*Coronary artery surgery is discussed further in Chapter 11.

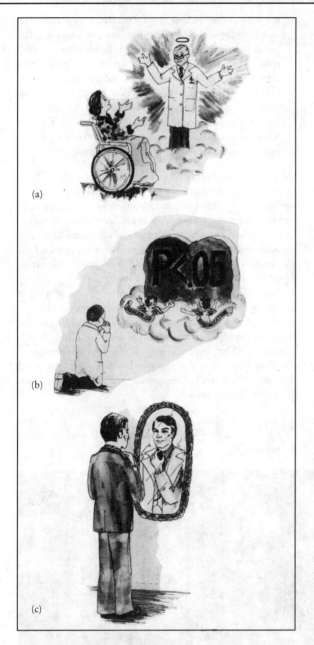

Figure 7.2 Three perceptions of God: (a) the patient's, (b) the physician's and (c) the biostatistician's.
(Source: Rimm and Bortin, 1978, p.61)

nothing to choose between them. For evaluating efficiency this is an ideal situation, for if the effectiveness (or benefit) of each method is the same then all that has to be measured and compared are the costs: whichever costs less would be more *cost-effective* in these circumstances. This is what two researchers, David Piauchaud and Jean Weddell, did, as you

can see in their report of the study which appears in the Course Reader (Part 3, Section 3.5). You should read it now.

□ How did they assess the effectiveness of the two treatments, and what were their findings?

■ They assessed effectiveness in terms of need for further medical care, and found that the difference in the proportion of each group not requiring further treatment was statistically insignificant — 86 per cent in the surgery group, 78 per cent in the injection-compression group.

□ In discussing the results of their cost analysis, the authors report that injection-compression treatment cost around £10 per case, whereas surgical treatment cost £44 per case. What costs do they not include in these figures?

■ They do not include the costs to the patients themselves, only those incurred by the health service.

□ Would adding in these costs have altered their finding that injection-compression was the most cost-effective treatment?

■ No. As they show, the cost to patients receiving surgical treatment was greater by £89 for those in employment, and by seventy hours for those not in formal employment. The differences reinforced rather than countered their finding.

Cost-effectiveness studies have a wide range of applications in health care. They avoid the difficulties of trying to convert benefits (such as having no need for further treatment) into money values. But they are crucially dependent on the certainty that the benefits of alternative treatments really are similar.

□ What does the postscript to the Piauchaud and Weddell article reveal?

■ That five years after treatment there *was* a difference in outcome between the two groups. The probability of not requiring further treatment was significantly greater for those treated surgically, thus undermining the conclusions from the findings in the original paper based on results after three years.

The second limitation of *cost-effectiveness studies* is that they can only show the least-cost way of doing something. This leaves open the possibility that the benefits, may in fact be less than the costs: in other words, none of the options may be worth doing. These problems return us to the difficulties of measuring benefits, difficulties addressed in another main form of economic appraisal, *cost-benefit analysis*. The basic notion of cost-benefit analysis can be stated simply: in deciding whether or not to build a hospital, or a motorway, or hire more nurses, or improve a health authority's sterile supply services, all the gains (benefits) and all the losses (costs) should be identified and measured. If the benefits exceed the costs, the project is worthwhile (although some other project might be even more worthwhile, so benefits exceeding costs is a necessary but not sufficient condition); if the costs exceed the benefits it is not worthwhile. The technique has been adopted in many countries and for many purposes, from the dam-building of the Tennessee Valley Authority to the Jubilee-line extension of the London Underground, and a steadily increasing number of cost-benefit studies have been attempted in the field of health care, though far fewer than the technique's advocates would wish.

Central to this form of evaluation is the notion that it is possible to measure costs and benefits in such a way that they can be compared, and the only candidate for a common yardstick is money. But how feasible is this? In health care, for example, the benefits of a particular project or activity ideally should be measured in terms of the impact on health (taken to include mortality, morbidity, or disability). How can a monetary value be attached to these measures in order to make a comparison between benefits and costs?

One way of tackling this problem is to assume that the value of individuals' lives can be approximated by their productive contribution to society, calculated on the basis of their earnings. Thus, for instance, the benefit of providing a new health care facility that reduced disability could be expressed in terms of the additional earnings that could be expected by individuals whose disabilities were reduced.

□ What difficulties can you detect in this approach (one was raised by Piauchaud and Weddell)?

■ First, many people make a productive contribution to society but receive no earnings: women working in the home are the obvious example. Second, earnings may reflect a whole series of things apart from productive contribution: discrimination by gender or ethnicity, for example. Third, the method takes no account of the views of the individual involved. Fourth, appeal to everyday experience shows that we still attach value to individuals who have no productive contribution left to make: people who have retired, for instance.

Despite these and other difficulties, this approach has been in use at least since the work of William Petty, a seventeenth-century English economist. Loss of prospective earnings frequently figures in court compensation settlements. A good example of the method's application is to be found down the middle of the UK's motorways (Figure 7.3). Researchers at the government's Transport and Road Research Laboratory calculated the cost of accidents arising from vehicles crossing the central reservation when barriers were absent: these costs included not only those of accident services, health services and damage to vehicles, but also the lost earnings due to death or injury of the casualties. The benefits of installing barriers could therefore be measured as the avoidance of these costs, and the costs simply reflect how much it cost to erect a given length of crash barrier.

□ To conduct a cost-benefit analysis of erecting barriers, what additional piece of evaluation is required?

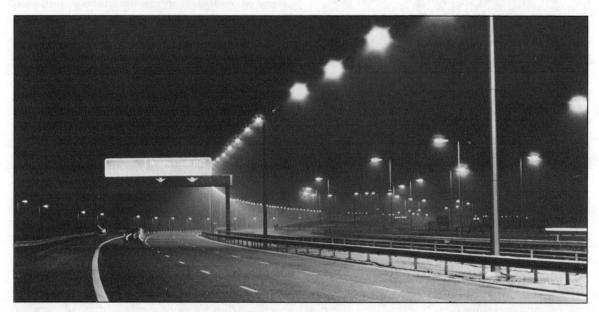

Figure 7.3 Motorway barriers along the central reservation to prevent vehicles crossing over into oncoming traffic.

■ An evaluation of the *effectiveness* of crash barriers in preventing accidents.

This was done by what amounted to a controlled trial — comparing the accident records of two stretches of the M1, only one of which had a barrier. The results showed that on stretches of six-lane motorway where the average daily traffic volume was 30 000 vehicles, the benefits of erecting barriers exceeded the costs by a ratio of 4.2 to 1. What effect did this finding have?

Partly as a result of this study, but also because of pressure from the media and the public, the Minister stated in 1971 that a programme to erect barriers on about 1 000 miles of motorway would be begun. Thus the cost-benefit analysis study in this case not only provided guidance on *whether* or not barriers should be erected, but also, because of the differential levels of benefit with different traffic volumes, *where* barriers should be erected and hence *how many* miles of barrier were desirable. (Mooney, *et al.* 1980, p.101)

The most recent attempt to find a measure of benefit that avoids the problems associated with a person's productive capacity is something called the Quality Adjusted Life Year (QALY), a measure initially developed by an American, M.C. Weinstein. The measure attempts to combine the quality of any change in life expectancy attributable to treatment (life-years) with the quality of life, for there may be a choice between a few extra years of high-quality life expectancy or a larger number of extra years of low-quality life expectancy. One way of doing this, demonstrated by British health economist Alan Williams and his colleagues,

was by getting a panel of seventy people to offer judgements on how they would trade off quality and quantity. Using this method, a collective view emerged that one high-quality life year was equivalent to 1.5 medium-quality life years, two low-quality life years, etc. Thence, by considering each QALY as a 'unit of health', the benefits of different treatments could be expressed in these standard units, and compared with the cost of producing these units in different ways. Thus, preliminary calculations suggest that to obtain one QALY by heart transplant costs £5 000, by kidney transplant £3 000, by replacing a hip £750, and by implanting a cardiac pacemaker £700. Of course, just as many objections and difficulties surround the measurement of benefits by reference to productive capacity, so the application of cost-benefit analysis using QALYs engenders many mixed reactions. A key word to note in all this is '*guidance*': cost-benefit analysis, unlike RCTs, doesn't claim to make decisions about crash barriers, or hip surgery, or pacemaker implantations; or at least it shouldn't, and its more reputable practitioners don't. And although criticised by some as 'techno-bureaucratic obscurantism masquerading as scientific decision-making', in reality the key thing is not so much the results that it suggests as the questions it poses. If the assumptions of scarcity and choice are accepted, then these questions about costs and benefits do not disappear because the technique is rejected.

Cost-benefit analysis, therefore, claims to make explicit what would otherwise occur anyway, and in doing so to increase rationality in decision-making. In making these claims it can appeal to some interesting evidence. Table 7.2, for example, shows four situations in which decisions were made that had an effect on lives. Implicitly, each decision

Table 7.2 The monetary value of life implied by four public policy decisions

Comment	Decision	Implied value of life
1 In 1968 it was estimated that if maternal oestriol concentrations were screened the cost per still-birth averted would be £50. Up until this date the screening procedure was not widely used, implying that the value of life was less than £50.		£50 maximum
2 In 1971 the government decided not to proceed with the child-proofing of drug containers. Allowing for the cost of drug-proofing and savings to the NHS from a reduced number of admissions, it was calculated that a child's life was implicitly valued at under £16 000.	Not to introduce child-proof drug containers	£16 000 maximum
3 In 1969 the fitting of cabs to farm tractors, to reduce the mortality risk for drivers, was made compulsory. The cost per annum was estimated at £4 million (£40 for each of 100 000 tractors). About 40 lives would be saved a year; the implied value of life was thus £100,000.	Legislation on tractor cabs	£100 000 minimum
4 After the partial collapse of the Ronan Point high-rise flats, killing five residents, the report of the inquiry recommended changes in building standards of such blocks. From estimates of the change in risk and the costs involved, the implied value of life was £20 million.	Change in building regulations	£20 million minimum

(Source: Card and Mooney, 1977, p.6)

placed a monetary value on each life saved or lost, and those values varied enormously, from less than £50 to more than £20 million. Such examples of 'life-or-death' decisions could be multiplied: they arise in the design of cars, trains, aircraft and roads, in workplace safety regulations, food and drink standards, gas and electricity supply. Far from being priceless, life seems frequently to be saved or lost according to monetary sums implicitly attached to it. Of course, it is quite possible that the same decisions would have been made even if the implicit valuations of life incorporated in them had been known at the time. But advocates of cost-benefit analysis and other forms of economic evaluation are committed to the possibility of improvement. In the words of Alan Williams:

> ...I am anxious to ensure that we know how little we know when we do what we have to do. Let me quote again here my favourite story about Maurice Chevalier, which I regard as very apt to the cost-benefit approach to life generally. When asked by someone how he viewed the prospect of old age, he is alleged to have replied: 'Well, there is quite a lot wrong with it, but it's not so bad when you consider the alternative'. (Williams, 1974, p.256)

Equality

One of the founding aims of the NHS was that of equality of *access* to health care on the basis of people's needs. To what extent has this been achieved? To answer this question it is necessary to measure both the need for health care and the use made of health services by different social groups. While measurement of the latter is reasonably straightforward, assessment of need is, as you have seen in Chapter 2, notoriously difficult.

☐ In what three ways may 'need' be defined?
■ 1 *Felt need* is an individual's perception of their own need.
2 *Expressed need* is the need for care that a person presents to health professionals (this is also referred to as 'demand').
3 *Need as defined by health professionals* (regardless of whether or not the person recognises they have a need).

Although inequalities in health service use based on age, gender, ethnicity and social class all occur, we shall concentrate on the last of these, not because it is more important but because it is here that research has concentrated. Relatively little comparative work has yet been done on gender and ethnicity, for example.*

*Some background material is summarised in *The Health of Nations*, Chapter 9, *ibid*.

One of the earliest studies was carried out by a community physician, John Brotherston, who compared the ratio between the use and felt need of different social classes. He contrasted the number of general practitioner consultations (use) with the number of days on which people felt that their normal activities were restricted because of ill-health (need) (Figure 7.4).

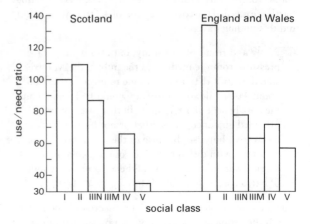

Figure 7.4 Use/need ratio by social class in Scotland, and in England and Wales, 1972.
(Source: Brotherston, 1976, Table X)

☐ Which social classes used more services than would have been expected on the basis of their felt need?
■ Higher social classes (I, II, IIIN).

In contrast, members of lower social classes used fewer services than expected. We will consider possible explanations for these differences in a moment. This approach was taken further by an economist, Julian Le Grand, who included not only GP consultations but the use of all types of hospital services as well. Using a sample of 5 000 people, he calculated their total use of health services (measured in expenditure terms) and then apportioned the amounts used by different socio-economic groups (a method of social stratification similar to social classes). These proportions were then compared to the proportions of felt need reported by the groups (Table 7.3).

☐ On the basis of felt need which socio-economic groups use the most services and which the least? Look at the right-hand column.
■ SEGs I and II use the most, and SEGs V and VI the least.
☐ How much greater is the use of services by SEGs I and II than would be expected if everyone used the same amount as SEGs V and VI?
■ 41 per cent — the ratio for SEGs I and II is 1.41 compared with 1.00 for SEGs V and VI.

Table 7.3 The distribution of public expenditure on health care in England and Wales, 1972

Socio-economic group (SEG)	Percentage of total reporting either limiting long-standing illness or acute sickness	Percentage of health care expenditure	Ratio of expenditure per person reporting ill to that for SEGs V and VI
I and II: Professionals, employers and managers	13.9	16.8	1.41
II: Intermediate and junior non-manual	19.7	22.5	1.33
IV: Skilled manual	34.5	33.4	1.13
V and VI: Semi- and unskilled manual	31.9	27.3	1.00

(Source: Le Grand, 1978, Table 2, p.131)

These data should only be taken as indicative rather than definitive, given the fairly crude methods used both to measure health service usage and to assess felt need. However, while the exact figures may be inaccurate, the overall pattern that emerges is one in which lower-class people do not use as much formal health care to meet their felt needs as do higher-class people. Why might this be so? Does it reflect a failure on the part of the NHS to provide as many services and to respond to the felt needs of lower-class people? Or is it either that these felt needs are not expressed as readily, or not expressed as effectively, by lower as compared with higher-class people? If it is the case that lower-class people do not express their needs as much as others, does this reflect their doubt about the value of health care; their lack of satisfaction with previous encounters with health professionals; or their being unable to afford health care, such as may arise if they are unable to get time off work without losing pay?

One of the first people to suggest an explanation was a social policy analyst, Richard Titmuss. He argued that:

> Higher income groups know how to make use of the service; they tend to receive more specialist attention; occupy more of the beds in better equipped and staffed hospitals; receive more elective (non-emergency) surgery ... than low-income groups — particularly the unskilled. (Titmuss, 1968; cited in Hart, 1971, p.405)

In other words, Titmuss considered that differences in service use reflected differences both in the expressed need for health care between social groups and in the provision of NHS facilities when care was sought. In 1971, Julian Tudor Hart, a general practitioner working in a small South Wales community, argued strongly in support of the latter explanation:

> In areas with most sickness and death, general practitioners have more work, larger lists, less hospital support, and inherit more clinically ineffective traditions of consultations, than in the healthiest areas; and hospital doctors shoulder heavier case-loads with less staff and equipment, more obsolete buildings, and suffer recurrent crises in the availability of beds and replacement staff. These trends can be summed up as the inverse care law: that the availability of good medical care tends to vary inversely with the need of the population served. (Hart, 1971, p.412)

Hart argued that what he termed the '*inverse care law*' had originated before the inception of the NHS when the provision of primary health care services were largely subject to market forces which drew doctors towards wealthier, middle-class areas. Although he recognised that inequalities in access to care had lessened since 1948, he claimed that the inverse care law could have been modified even more if the original objectives of the NHS had been adhered to more rigorously. In Hart's view, equality of use can be achieved by ensuring that everybody has equal access to health services providing good medical care. His view, however, ignores the other main explanation for inequality in service usage — differences in the expresssed needs of different social groups.

There are two main theories to explain why lower social classes express less need for health services. The first is that they have lower expectations about health than do higher social classes. For example, two sociologists, Mildred Blaxter and Elizabeth Paterson (1982), found that working-class women in Aberdeen accepted as normal quite considerable levels of symptoms. Children suffering from recurrent ear infections and coughs were viewed as essentially healthy. Such attitudes were combined with an air of fatalism as to the cause of many diseases and the sense of inability of being able to do anything to alter the course of many illnesses.

The second explanation stresses the different costs and benefits of health care to different social groups. Time is the key cost: working-class people are less likely to have a telephone and to own cars. The impact this can have has been shown in a study by another two sociologists,

Bronwen Earthrowl and Margaret Stacey,* who examined the visits that parents made when their children were in hospital. The financial costs and the practical difficulties of travelling were much greater for working-class than for middle-class parents.

There are then several competing explanations of the differences in use of health services by social classes. Which is correct? Or do they all have a part to play? Mildred Blaxter has suggested that:

There are many problems associated with the disentangling of factors of health service provision from those of differential utilisation, of utilisation from need, and of need from perception of the meaning of symptoms and the salience of health events to the individual — a sequence which comes full circle, since the final factor may depend to some extent on the first. (Blaxter, 1983, p.1145)

If these diverse factors are to be disentangled, it will require the combination of several different perspectives — including epidemiology, sociology, psychology, statistics and economics — jointly engaged in multi-disciplinary research.

Humanity

The final aspect of health care evaluation to consider is that of humanity. Imagine a health service which treated everyone — whoever they were — in the same way, which was run extraordinarily efficiently and which provided only the most effective treatments. Would even that be quite enough? Wouldn't most of us want something else as well — to be treated, not as objects, but as people. In other words, rational health services need to recognise people's own rationality, as well as their emotions, their everyday needs, the complexity of their lives and the importance of human dignity. The need for *humanity* in health care, and the occasional lack of it, was a central theme in Chapter 4. Despite this universal demand there is sometimes very little agreement over just what is meant by 'humanity'. Is it more humane to tell people they are dying than to conceal it from them? Should staff work *with* the disabled or *for* them? Differences in ideas as to what is and what is not humane need not, however, prevent evaluation: all that is necessary is that the criteria which are used be made explicit.

There are three key areas in which debates about humanity occur. The first most obvious one, and that which provokes the most bitter debate, concerns the value and definition of life itself: how much is a human life worth? You have already seen an economistic attempt to answer this. The second key area concerns the demand that patients

health services recognise that most people have a life beyond and outside the health service. Similar to some other organisations, health services have a tendency to be greedy, demanding that patients rearrange their lives to fit with the staff's schedules.

☐ What examples can you think of in this area?

■ There are many, such as in maternity hospitals where labour may be induced to fit in with the work patterns of staff;* the long campaign to increase visiting hours in hospital; and the concern that medical care be available on a twenty-four hour basis and that doctors be prepared to make home visits.

The third key area concerns the demand that patients should be treated as persons, not as mere objects for processing (no matter how effectively, efficiently and equitably). Health services should not only make adequate recognition of patient's emotions but also treat them as reasoning beings with a right and a capacity to exercise rational choice over the course of their own lives.

☐ Bearing in mind the discussion in Chapters 3 and 4, what implications does this have for health services?

■ It means that patients be treated courteously, listened to, allowed time to answer, given key information, presented with options, allowed to make or take part in decisions, and given the right to complain and to get recompense when wronged. And it also means that lay people be given a say in the shaping of the service.

Here, then, is a rich crop of topics for evaluation. How should it be done and who should do it? Certainly, there is a central role for lay people — those who use the service. But, having said that, there is also an important role for more systematic evauation. How should this be done? What sorts of methods should be used: quantitative or qualitative?† Let us first consider quantitative studies.

☐ What were the main findings of the surveys of patient satisfaction cited earlier in Chapters 4 and 6?

■ The main complaints were about being kept waiting, the quality of hospital food, being woken too early and the failure to explain things adequately. But, overall, patients expressed very high levels of satisfaction with the care provided by nurses, hospital doctors and GPs — indeed, over 90 per cent expressed confidence in all three.

Surveys of patient and public satisfaction are amongst the

---

*An edited version of this study, 'Social class and children in hospital' appears in the Course Reader, Part 6, Section 6.7.

*These issues are discussed in *Birth to Old Age: Health in Transition*, Chapter 6, *ibid*.

†Qualitative and quantitative methods are discussed more fully in *Studying Health and Disease*, Chapters 9 and 10, *ibid*.

most popular methods of evaluating the humanity of health services. They enable the rapid assessment of the opinions of very large numbers of people. However, despite these major advantages, there are also problems.

☐ If you are interested in people's perceptions of the care that they receive, what two drawbacks can you see in relying solely on questionnaires?

■ First, if we want to get the opinions of the elderly, mentally infirm or mentally handicapped, surveys may be of little use. Second, assessing the humanity of a service and describing the way one was treated is a highly complex matter which may be difficult both to define and to quantify.

There is, therefore, a major role for qualitative studies of people's perceptions of the humanity of the health service — from novels, autobiographies and informal interviews. However, such qualitative approaches face a major difficulty — people's satisfaction may simply reflect very low levels of expectation rather than any great humanity in the service. This last point was put more generally by the nineteenth-century philosopher and economist John Stuart Mill. What would happen, he said, if we asked slaves whether they were happy and they all replied that they were? Would we then conclude that slavery was a good thing? Or might we not argue instead, that since many might not know what freedom was like, they were not in the best position to assess their situation? An alternative qualitative approach that avoids these particular problems is that based on observation or the analysis of records. Some, termed *ethnographies*, use the methods of anthropology: living among the people being studied to see how life looks from that point of view. In some instances, the researcher actually lives the same life as those who are studied (known as 'participant observation'), in others he or she simply spends time with them (known as 'non-participant observation').

☐ Which of these methods were used in the studies by Paterson and Jeffery discussed earlier?

■ Paterson used participant observation — she herself actually worked as a kitchen-maid. Jeffery was a non-participant observer in the casualty department. (But note also that in both of these studies, there was also a large amount of informal interviewing.)

☐ Overall, the evaluation of the humanity of health care would appear to be beset with methodological obstacles. What possible dangers can you see in such evaluation?

■ It may give the providers and managers of health services the grounds for preferring their own perceptions and beliefs, dismissing those of the people they are studying. Alternatively, it may mean that humanity is not taken into account when services are being planned or assessed.

All too often in health service planning and management, the importance of humanity is underestimated — pre-eminence is given to efficiency, and increasingly the question of effectiveness is being considered. But humanity and, indeed, equality are rarely given sufficient attention. The importance of such aspects was elegantly demonstrated in a study of patients recovering from a cholecystectomy (removal of the gall bladder). Roger Ulrich, a geographer, compared a group of patients who had a view of trees outside their hospital window with a group who looked out on to a blank wall. It was found that those with a view of trees recovered significantly faster and required less analgesics (pain-killers). It appeared that the view of trees was more humanly satisfying. In other words, just as the effectiveness of a procedure will affect both its efficiency and its acceptability to patients, so aspects of the humanity of health care may influence efficiency and effectiveness. This underlines how closely interrelated all aspects of care are, and how important it is that all are considered when care is being evaluated.

Monitoring

Establishing the value of some aspect of health care does not guarantee that either an individual or society at large will benefit from its use. To take two simple examples: a drug might be shown to be effective in a carefully designed study, but in general use it might be prescribed too frequently or not frequently enough; day surgery, in which patients go into hospital for their operation but do not stay overnight, might be a safe, more efficient way to provide a service, but that does not guarantee it will be widely adopted by health authorities. Thus evaluation is not sufficient. It is also necessary to *monitor* health services to see whether or not they are providing the best possible services within their limited resources. In view of the large number of methods that exist for monitoring health services, our account can only indicate the diversity of approaches that have been used. Let us start by considering a specific area of the monitoring of effectiveness — the safety of new drugs.

Drug suspended after reports of 61 deaths

The DHSS has suspended the anti-arthritis drug Opren after 3500 reports of adverse effects, including 61 deaths ... More than 500,000 patients have been prescribed Opren in the past year.

(Pat Healy, *The Times*, August 5, 1982)

In 1980 a new drug known as benoxaprofen (Opren) was launched in a blaze of publicity. Clinical trials on over 3 000 patients had shown that it was a highly effective drug for alleviating the pain and discomfort of arthritis. Two years later the government suspended the drug company's licence to market Opren after reports of serious adverse effects, including sixty-one deaths. How did this happen? How had clinical trials failed to detect these disastrous effects? What had been evaluated as being a highly effective drug turned out in practice to have unacceptable adverse effects. Should Opren never have been granted a product licence by the government's expert advisory group, the Committee on Safety of Medicines? Unfortunately there is no way that anyone can know, prior to mass use whether or not a new drug will cause serious adverse effects if these only affect a very small proportion of users, such as less than one in 1 000. Even rigorous clinical trials of effectiveness may not bring rare adverse effects to light. Similarly, any adverse effects of taking drugs for long periods can, by definition, only be detected after people have been prescribed the drugs for a long time. Thus, what is technically known as the *post-marketing surveillance* of drugs, is an essential form of monitoring.

In practice, most monitoring of effectiveness is based on a *comparison* of performance, such as between doctors, hospitals (Table 7.4), health districts, or countries. For example, the perinatal mortality rates (PNMR) of different countries are often compared to provide some indication of their relative performance.

□   What is absolutely crucial when making comparisons?

■   Ensuring that like is being compared with like.

In the case of PNMRs, international comparisons have frequently been made which suggest the UK has a higher rate than France. However, the French rate does not include liveborn babies who die before their births have been formally registered. As registration need not take

Table 7.4 Survival of kidney transplant patients in eight different hospitals in the UK and Ireland

Hospitals	Patients surviving two years (%)
A	96
B	82
C	98
D	94
E	88
F	90
G	84
H	94

(Source: Taylor, Ting and Briggs, 1985, p.801)

place until the third day after birth, some perinatal deaths are excluded from the statistics. Caution must therefore be exercised when considering comparative data.

Given the difficulties involved in monitoring the effectiveness of one aspect of health care, such as perinatal services, there are clearly going to be far more problems in assessing a complete health service. A recent attempt to compare the effectiveness of NHS areas was made by a group of researchers at St Thomas's Department of Community Medicine. They compared the effectiveness of the ninety-eight area health authorities that existed in England and Wales between 1974 and 1982. They calculated mortality ratios — standardised not only for age and sex, but also for some social conditions — for fourteen causes of death in people under the age of sixty-five years which they considered were preventable with effective medical treatment. These included cancer of the cervix, asthma, anaemia, and pneumonia. The SMRs for each condition were compared, and each area was ranked from 1 (lowest mortality group) to 6 (highest mortality group). The ranking for all fourteen conditions were added to give an overall rank for each area. The best and worst areas are shown in Table 7.5.

As with all forms of monitoring, this particular

Table 7.5 Ranking of health areas on basis of mortality rates for 14 conditions amenable to medical treatment (standardised for age, sex and social factors).

	Health area	Overall rank
Best ten	N. Tyneside	26
	Oxfordshire	28
	Sheffield	29
	Gloucestershire	30
	Newcastle-upon-Tyne	31
	Bromley	31
	Avon	32
	Suffolk	33
	Cumbria	33
	Hampshire	35
Worst ten	Bradford	50
	Birmingham	50
	Staffordshire	51
	Cleveland	52
	Warwickshire	52
	Lancashire	53
	Wolverhampton	54
	Sandwell	58
	Bolton	58
	Walsall	62

(Source: Charlton, *et al.*, 1983, Table IV, p.694)

approach has methodological limitations. For example, it only considers fourteen causes of death which together account for only a few per cent of all deaths. While it takes some differences in social conditions between the areas into account, a doubt inevitably remains as to whether this was sufficient for the researchers to conclude that any remaining differences in mortality ratios were due to differences in health care provision. Nevertheless, despite these methodological doubts, this form of monitoring can serve as a useful indication of possible shortcomings in health services and might lead to improvements in care.

At the opposite extreme from comparing complete areas is the intensive investigation of individual adverse events: the *disaster approach*. An example is included in the Course Reader (Part 2, Section 2.7): the Royal College of Physicians' Medical Services study of deaths in people under fifty years of age. Another example is the DHSS *Report of Confidential Enquiries into Maternal Deaths* (during pregnancy and childbirth). The latter, in its report for 1976–1978, estimated that 59 per cent of maternal deaths included one or more factors that potentially could have been avoided. Unlike comparisons between countries or areas, the disaster approach identifies the individuals involved in providing care. Not only that, but such an approach means that their performance is exposed to the scrutiny of outsiders. Such *external* monitoring is not welcomed by most health care staff. If there has to be monitoring, then most staff would prefer it to be carried out *internally* — an activity known as *peer review*. As you may imagine, this is found much less threatening than external reviews. However, while peer review is attractive to those involved, its findings may remain secret from other staff (such as doctors in other specialities), the managers of the service, and, perhaps most significantly, patients and the public. Some people have therefore called for a more public method of monitoring:

Audit of operations urged by surgeon

Some surgeons have death rates among patients which are two or three times greater than others and there is a need for a careful audit of all operations carried out in Britain, according to Mr Brendan Devlin, consultant surgeon at Stockton-on-Tees. He calls for an audit of all operations which, he says, would not be an enormous drain on the NHS because much of the material is already collected but is not organised.

(Penny Chorlton, *The Guardian*, April 15, 1981)

Indeed, the almost complete lack of any form of audit in the UK reflects the clinical autonomy of doctors which was discussed in Chapter 3. Beyond the few extreme instances of personal incompetence or negligence (discussed in a moment), there is no statutory or compulsory monitoring carried out. There is also little in the way of continuing education for most health professionals. With the rate of innovation in health care ever increasing, it is now possible for a newly-qualified doctor to lose touch with the latest ideas within a few years. If health services are to benefit from advances and improvements in the effectiveness of care, they are going to be forced into investing much more in *continuing education* in the future. In turn, it may be that the NHS will expect, and perhaps even demand, evidence from its staff that they are maintaining their competence and keeping up to date.

While some doubt remains about the extent to which central government will impose systems for monitoring effectiveness in the future, there is no such uncertainty as regards their intention in the monitoring of efficiency.

My job is to give you all the facilities, resources, apparatus and help I can, and then to leave you alone as professional men and women to use your skill and judgement without hindrance. (Aneurin Bevan in 1948; cited in Watkin, 1975, p.139)

... We believe we must improve the efficiency and effectiveness of the service even further ... We have developed a regional review system to give leadership and a clearer sense of policy direction to the service. We have set up a management inquiry. We are introducing performance indicators, manpower planning and control, and policy scrutinies. We are introducing new approaches to supplies and purchasing methods and introducing information technology to the service. (Norman Fowler, Secretary of State for Social Services, DHSS, 1983a, p.ii)

How closely monitored is the efficiency with which the NHS uses its resources? Have the improvements been as dramatic as the contrast between the two quotes above could suggest? To begin to answer these questions we need to start in the centre with the machinery of government and the DHSS.

Broadly speaking, there are three ways in which Parliament can monitor the efficiency with which resources are used by the NHS. The first is the accountability of the Secretary of State and the Ministers who have to accept responsibility for the legal and efficient running of the NHS down to its most detailed aspects. The other two monitoring procedures both concern Parliamentary scrutiny of how effectively the government is fulfilling its responsibilities: the first is the Social Services Committee (which has been discussed in Chapter 5), and the second is the *Public Accounts Committee* (PAC), which monitors the efficiency of all public expenditure. It comprises fifteen MPs, reflecting the strength of different political parties, and is always chaired by a member of the opposition. Its strength lies in the fact that it has the backing of the Comptroller and Auditor General and his staff of 500–600 in the National Audit Office.

The £60m hospital rip-off

Fraud involving private patients' fees could be losing Health Service hospitals up to £60 million a year it was claimed last night. A shock report by the public's spending watchdog showed that checks in 37 health authorities revealed losses of £10 million a year in fees from private patients treated with NHS equipment and manpower.
(Chris Hampson, *The Daily Mirror*,
April 27, 1985)

As a result of their examination in 1981, the PAC recommended a tightening of central control of the NHS to achieve a more thorough monitoring of efficiency. This was to be accomplished in part:

by a flow of information about the activities of the districts which will enable the regions, and in turn DHSS, to monitor performance effectively and to take necessary action to remedy any serious deficiencies, or inefficiency, which may develop. (Public Accounts Committee, 1980/81, p.xvii)

In response, the DHSS developed a new monitoring system based on *performance indicators*, unveiled in 1983. These performance indicators have attracted much attention; as one of the introductory quotes indicates, they have been cited by the Secretary of State as an example of the government's determination to improve NHS efficiency. What are they, and what in fact is their purpose?

Ideally, the way to measure the efficient performance of a hospital, or district, or region, would be to compare resources used against the output achieved.

☐   In health care, why is this a problem?
■   As we discussed earlier in the chapter, it is extraordinarily difficult to find a way of measuring effectiveness — the impact of health care on health status.

Because of these difficulties, the performance indicators only attempt to assess performance in terms of resources

used. The regions and all 192 districts are issued with a list of around seventy different indicators, showing how they compare with one another. The measures fall into five different groups, covering clinical activity, financial performance, staffing, estate management, and ambulance and support services. Performance indicators for clinical activity include such measures as the average length of stay of patients in hospital, the proportion of patients treated on a day-care basis, and the length of waiting lists (Figure 7.5).

Performance indicators present a fundamental problem: how are the figures to be interpreted? If the number of in-patients in relation to population is higher in Region A than Region B, does this mean that Region A is good/efficient, and Region B bad/inefficient, or vice versa? This is a problem that those who developed the indicators are well aware of, and is the reason why they provide no guidance at all on how the figures should be interpreted.

In the face of such conceptual and technical difficulties, should it therefore be concluded that performance indicators promise much more than they deliver and should be abandoned? There is certainly good reason to use them with caution and to be wary of extravagant claims on their behalf, but a number of reasons have been suggested for their retention and further development. First:

despite the inadequacies of both the concept of indicators and the data that help to generate them, we quite often find that the variation is absolutely enormous. Threefold variation in staffing rates in mental handicap hospitals that cannot possibly be explained by differences in dependency levels ought to leave us aghast. (Yates, 1983, p.111)

You have already seen similarly striking differences in the provision of services by local authorities (Figure 5.8). Performance indicators help to pose and focus questions that are worth investigating. Second, it has been argued that they help to create an 'organisational culture' in the NHS:

henceforth all DHAs, not just those with 'progressive' administrators and clinicians, will be obliged at least to go through the motions of comparing their local measures with those of other districts, both within their region and nationally. Reasons will have to be given for indicators or groups of indicators with 'unusual' values. (Pollitt, 1985, p.7)

However, valuable as it may be to encourage a national perspective among the regions and districts of what is, after all, a *national* health service, this is some way removed from the starting point of a mechanism to monitor health service efficiency. Apart from the obstacles that have already been noted, two concluding difficulties should be acknowledged. First, the 'top–down' approach to

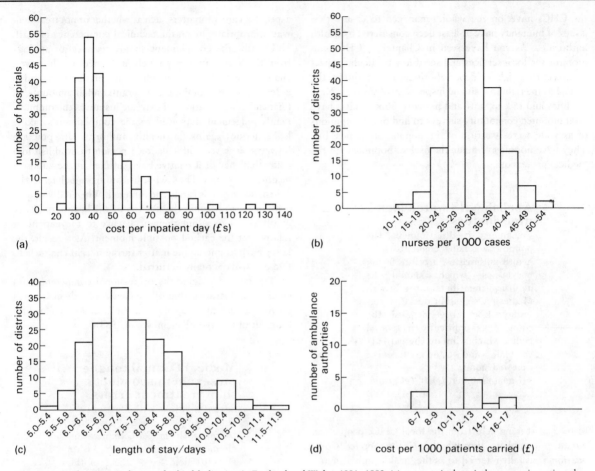

Figure 7.5 Performance indicators for health districts in England and Wales, 1981–1982: (a) community hospital costs per in-patient day; (b) number of nurses per 1 000 in-patient cases; (c) length of stay in general surgery; and (d) cost of ambulance services per 1 000 patients carried.
(Source: DHSS, 1983b, pp54, 94, 144, 167)

monitoring does not come to grips with the fact that it is clinicians at the 'sharp end' of the health service who inevitably set in motion a whole series of resource consequences each time they make a clinical decision. What is required, according to this argument, is some mechanism for making clinicians more accountable for the resource consequences of their action through incorporating them more directly in monitoring procedures. We have already mentioned peer review in the context of effectiveness — maybe this should be extended into the realms of efficiency?

Second, although central government may encourage Parliamentary scrutiny of the efficiency with which its policies towards health care or other programmes are carried out, it is likely to be hostile to scrutiny of the policies themselves: no government likes to be told by all-party committees that it is pursuing inefficient or foolish ideas. The short history of Programme Analysis and Review

(PAR), introduced in 1970 as just such a Parliamentary monitoring mechanism, is a case in point. Viewed as a threat, regarded with suspicion, and encountering secrecy and obstruction by departments, it was abandoned in 1979. As one senior civil servant remarked, 'Socrates was the first person to do a PAR. He went round Athens asking fundamental questions. Socrates was put to death. I do not want to do another PAR' (cited in Heclo and Wildavsky, 1974). Monitoring efficiency involves a great deal more than the right technique.

And what of monitoring humanity, the poor cousin of effectiveness and efficiency? Although its importance was recognised in the reorganisation of the health service in 1974 by the establishment of bodies with the specific purpose of monitoring consumer satisfaction — the Community Health Councils (in England) — these bodies were given little power to influence decisions. Despite this the CHCs have, on the whole, managed to ensure that issues of humanity have at least been considered by health authorities. As you have seen in Chapter 3, CHCs can monitor the local services and see if any particular aspect is subject to a high incidence of criticism. In addition, the CHC has the right to visit and inspect any of the local NHS facilities and talk to staff and patients. Some CHCs have even mounted community surveys to find out the opinions of as wide a cross-section of the population as possible. They have not always made themselves popular with the medical profession:

Abolish NHS watchdogs, urge doctors

Community Health Councils, the public's watchdog committees on health authorities, are interfering busybodies which should be abolished immediately, the British Medical Association declared yesterday. Doctors condemned the councils as politically motivated bodies which whip up the patients complaints and waste a great deal of time and money.

(David Fletcher, *Daily Telegraph*, July 11, 1980)

Instead of seeking help from the local CHC, people can pursue a complaint through the *Health Service Commissioner*, usually referred to as the 'health ombudsman'.

Ombudsman criticises surgeons

A consultant orthopaedic surgeon who failed to explain details of a child's operation to its parents, is criticised by the Health Services Ombudsman today. In a report ... Mr Cecil Clothier says that he found some justification for complaint in 36 out of 50 investigations.

(David Fletcher, *Daily Telegraph*, November 11, 1981)

The health ombudsman investigates some 400 complaints each year, and normally finds about 40 per cent to be justified. These cover all aspects of health services — medical, nursing, administration and ancillary services — and concern such issues as delays in receiving treatment and poor quality care. The ombudsman is not, however, qualified or allowed to pass judgement on the clinical aspects of care, or matters such as whether or not treatment was appropriate, or on the technical competence of staff.

Usually, the complainant simply receives an apology from the health authority involved. Sometimes, however, changes are made to the health services in question, and in a few cases the ombudsman grants small amounts of financial compensation. In extreme instances the ombudsman's judgement may lead to the complainant's taking legal action against a health authority. In practice, however, it is very difficult for a person to establish in a court that they or a relative have suffered at the hands of health service staff. Thus, while litigation is much feared by British doctors, it is rarely encountered. When it does occur it often arises because the doctors or the health authority involved fail to admit their negligence to the patient or relatives at the earliest possible moment. As a result, the latter have to pursue the matter through legal channels to find out what actually occurred.

The task of judging the professional competence and conduct of doctors is that of the General Medical Council (GMC), a body made up almost entirely of doctors (eighty-four out of ninety-one members in 1983).*

Medical Council tougher on sexual misconduct than treatment errors

Sexual relations with a patient are more likely to get a doctor into trouble with the GMC than wrong diagnosis or treatment. Or, as Mr David Tench, legal officer of the Consumers' Association says: 'A doctor is in real trouble if he puts his hand on the knee of a female patient; but if he kills her by wrong diagnosis, in terms of professional misconduct he could well be in the clear'.

(Peter Evans, *The Times*, March 6, 1984)

All doctors have, by law, to be registered with the GMC if they wish to practise in the UK. The GMC has a responsibility to the public to maintain doctors' standards of conduct and training. The proportion of doctors who are brought before the Professional Conduct Committees has been about 0.025 per cent each year since 1960, i.e. it is a very rare event. Of the thirty-six doctors referred in 1983, disregard for professional responsibilities to patients (such as GPs failing to visit patients at home) and dishonesty

*The establishment of the GMC is discussed in *Caring for Health: History and Diversity*, ibid.

(such as frauds with the NHS) accounted for about half the cases. This, however, is not reflected in the media coverage of such legal hearings, which tend to concentrate on the 'sex stories' — five of the thirty-six in 1983. Margaret Stacey, a sociologist who was a lay member of the GMC disciplinary committee in 1983, commented thus on her experience:

> On that committee too I realised that some of the public notions of what the GMC is or is not derive from highly selective reporting by the press. It saddened me to see the public gallery, crowded with press reporters for cases relating to alleged sexual misconduct, empty as soon as that case was disposed of. One time I remember the subsequent case was about a doctor's alleged failure to attend a child in a proper manner; the gallery was nearly empty. (Stacey, 1983, p.22)

Despite the existence of many official means of monitoring, there is an important role for non-statutory bodies. These *pressure groups* range from those concerned about defending the NHS against financial cuts to those with an interest in specific health issues. Examples of the latter include MIND (concerned with the care of the mentally ill) and MENCAP (who lobby to get improvements in the care of the mentally handicapped). Such organisations may also be involved in other activities as well. Their effectiveness varies. MIND was very influential in the drawing up of the 1983 Mental Health Act, and as you have seen in Chapter 6, the Spastics Society strongly influenced the Social Services Committee in their 1980 report on perinatal care, which, in turn, has had a considerable influence on government policy.

The contribution of pressure groups illustrates the diverse ways in which health services can be, and are, monitored. As you have seen, these range from large, expensive, computer-based systems for the post-marketing surveillance of drugs, to individual complaints investigated by the health ombudsman. The powers of these monitoring bodies also vary — the GMC can ban a doctor from practising in the UK, whereas comparisons of mortality rates between areas simply raise further questions for investigation. And finally, there is a diversity in the extent to which monitoring is open to public scrutiny: the disaster approach maintains a high level of confidentiality, whereas pressure groups actively seek publicity. Such diversity reflects the complex range of activities that health services perform and the need to consider their effectiveness and efficiency, equality and humanity.

Objectives of Chapter 7

When you have read this chapter you should be able to:

7.1 Explain how the effectiveness of many aspects of health care have not been scientifically evaluated because of ethical objections; because of the lack of objective measures of outcome; because of authoritarianism; and because of cost.

7.2 Describe some of the difficulties in evaluating the economic efficiency of health care and the ways and extent to which cost-effectiveness and cost-benefit analyses overcome such obstacles.

7.3 Describe how comparisons of the use/need ratios of different social classes reveal inequalities in health care, and the suggested explanations for these differences.

7.4 Explain why the systematic evaluation of the humanity of health care has proved so difficult.

7.5 Describe the diverse ways in which health services are monitored.

Questions for Chapter 7

1 (*Objective 7.1*) What do you think the major obstacles would be in evaluating the effectiveness of community care for mentally handicapped people by means of an RCT?

2 (*Objective 7.2*) A surgeon plans to start sending many of his patients home from hospital three days sooner than has been his practice previously.

(i) Would such a change increase the efficiency of the health service?

(ii) What type of study would you use to investigate this further?

(iii) Such a change would release some funds for an alternative use. How might you decide on the most efficient use of such savings? What is the major practical difficulty of such an approach?

3 (*Objective 7.3*) The proportions of women of different social classes staying in a maternity hospital five days or more after delivery are shown in Figure 7.6. What explanations can you suggest for these findings?

4 (*Objective 7.4*) A survey of hospital in-patients (Table 6.1) found that 31 per cent were dissatisfied with the information they received about their progress. What methods might you use to investigate this aspect of care further?

5 (*Objective 7.5*) The prescribing habits of individual GPs are monitored by a government agency. This has revealed that some GPs prescribe much more than others. Which GPs should be sanctioned — the high or the low prescribers? What does this example reveal about monitoring?

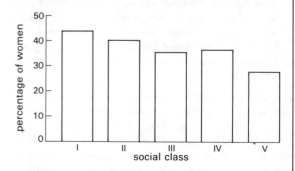

Figure 7.6 Proportions of women of different social classes staying five days or longer after childbirth.
(Source: John Radcliffe Maternity Hospital, Oxford, 1983 — unpublished data)

8
Screening

This chapter contains some worked numerical examples. If you have difficulty following the calculations don't worry, as long as you understand the broad principles involved. The biological and medical aspects of the diseases included in this chapter are discussed in Book IV, *The Biology of Health and Disease*.

Cancer screening 'saves lives'
Early detection of breast cancer can reduce the risk of death from the disease by almost a third, a new survey claims … Dr Wright, of the BUPA medical centre, said: 'The only hope for improving the attack for breast cancer victims lies in early detection and simple local surgery'.

(Annabel Ferriman, *The Times*, October 10, 1980)

Faced with medical and surgical treatments which are limited in their effectiveness, screening appears to offer considerable hope in dealing with some diseases, such as breast cancer. By routinely examining apparently healthy people, screening aims to detect either those who are likely to develop a particular disease or those in whom the disease is already present, but not yet producing symptoms.

This approach is not new. Ever since people became aware that most diseases include a *pre-symptomatic stage*, there have been attempts to find ways of intervening to prevent the development of the symptomatic stage. This practice is so common it often goes unnoticed — the standard history-taking and physical examination people receive in medical consultations* involves a search both for suspected and unsuspected conditions. Everyone has heard of someone who has gone into hospital for one reason and come out with a disease they had never suspected they had. In a sense, this is a form of individual screening. Our concern here, however, is with *population screening* — the mass examination of a whole population, or selected sub-groups.

An early effort to inspect a seemingly healthy population for evidence of hidden disease was made in the late nineteenth century on school children, and centred around examination for contagious diseases.† In the early

*The clinical method is discussed in *Studying Health and Disease*, Chapter 2, *ibid*.

†Surveillance in childhood is discussed further in *Birth to Old Age: Health in Transition, ibid*.

decades of this century the scope for screening expanded to include not only physical impairments in children, but diseases in adults as well. The use of mobile X-ray machines to examine people for tuberculosis was one of the earliest major screening programmes (Figure 8.1).

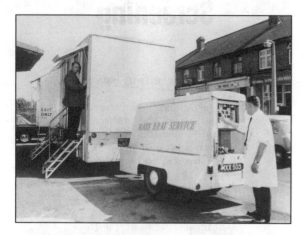

Figure 8.1 Mobile X-ray vans for screening people for signs of respiratory tuberculosis. The screening of civilians in the UK started in the mid-1940s. Between 1943 and 1950, six million people were screened. This revealed unsuspected tuberculosis in over 22 000 people. With the decline in the incidence of the disease it eventually became inappropriate to continue screening people. From the 1960s onwards mass radiography was gradually abandoned.

Much of the attraction of screening arises from some notable successes, such as the virtual elimination of infant deaths from haemolytic disease.* During the 1940s it had been discovered that the underlying cause of this condition was that the mother's and the baby's blood group differed. By screening women during pregnancy it was possible to identify those pregnancies which were at risk, and, as a result to institute measures that would protect the baby from harm. When a screening programme for the disease was established in the early 1950s haemolytic disease was still responsible for over 500 infant deaths a year in England and Wales. By 1973 the number of deaths had fallen to around 100 a year, and by 1983 to a mere twenty-two.

Given the spectacular success of that and other screening programmes, why was it that in 1980 screening for breast cancer was not available as part of a national programme? The simple answer is that the decision whether or not to establish a screening programme depends not only on the availability of a test but also on several other factors — the

*A disease in which the mother forms antibodies against her baby's red blood cells. When these antibodies cross the placenta and enter the baby's blood they cause the baby's red cells to collapse (haemolyse). The commonest form of this disease is rhesus incompatibility.

effect that earlier treatment has on the prognosis of the disease, the relative costs and benefits of the programme, and the acceptability of screening to the population at risk. We will consider each of these aspects in more detail. As you will see, when these wider aspects are taken into account, the question of whether or not to establish a screening programme can become extremely difficult to answer. In 1980, screening for breast cancer was not as obvious a solution as the quoted doctor from BUPA claimed.

The nature of the screening test

For examining large numbers of people, it is essential that any screening test is simple, quick and cheap. At the same time, the test must satisfy three other criteria. First, it must be relatively *safe*. While this has not been a problem for most screening programmes, there have been some notable exceptions. The original mammograms (X-rays of the breasts to detect lumps) in the 1960s delivered a dose of radiation high enough actually to *cause* cancer in a very small number of women; and the use of amniocentesis (removing some of the fluid surrounding a fetus by means of a needle via the mother's abdomen) for detecting fetal abnormalities occasionally results in premature labour.

Second, the test must be *repeatable*, such that if the test were repeated the same result would be obtained. Lack of repeatability can arise in at least two ways. It may be that the property being measured, such as a person's blood pressure, is not constant, but varies with time and place. This is one reason why services such as those offered in the USA (Figure 8.2) in which a blood pressure measurement may be obtained casually in a supermarket car park, are of doubtful value. Account also has to be taken of *observer variation*. In some tests, not only will two or more observers fail to agree on the measurement, but the same observer may get different results on subsequent occasions. These difficulties arise with tests in which the measurement involves some personal judgement, such as examining an X-ray or taking a blood-pressure reading. The impact of observer variation can be seen in a study carried out by an American epidemiologist, Abraham Lilienfield, of the interpretation of chest X-rays by nine radiologists (Lilienfield and Kordan, 1966). He found that on about 10–20 per cent of occasions any two of the radiologists disagreed on what an X-ray showed. When the radiologists were given, without their knowledge, the same X-rays to interpret again, their level of disagreement with their own first examination was also about 10–20 per cent. While the nature of the test may make it impossible to eliminate completely the possibility of observer variation, it can usually be reduced by ensuring all observers use the same criteria when judging the result.

The third aspect to consider is the *validity* of a test: the extent to which the test is actually measuring what it

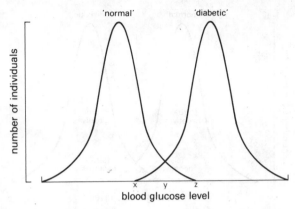

Figure 8.3 Blood glucose levels of two populations: 'normals' and 'diabetics'.

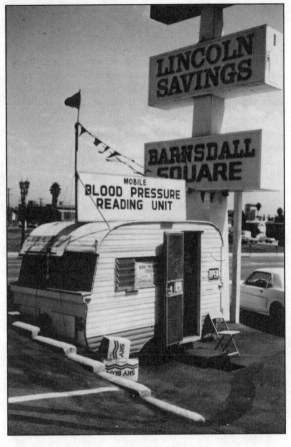

Figure 8.2 Blood pressure caravan parked outside a supermarket in Los Angeles, 1979.

purports to measure. For example, does mammography show up *all* lumps that exist in a breast, *and* do all the shadows on a mammogram represent true lumps? As screening tests must be simple, quick and cheap, some degree of validity is inevitably sacrificed. Some loss of validity for this reason is usually acceptable, as the alternative of *either* no screening *or* the use of a very expensive test may be even less acceptable. This, however, is not the only problem regarding validity. There is also the difficulty that can arise in defining whether or not someone has a disease. This can best be explained by considering an example.

People with diabetes have raised levels of glucose (a type of sugar) in their blood.* Checking the blood glucose level could therefore be a useful screening test for detecting people with diabetes long before they suffer any irreparable harm. This would be the case if there was a blood glucose

*Screening for diabetes is also discussed in *Studying Health and Disease*, ibid.

level above which everyone had diabetes, and below which no one had the disease. Unfortunately this is not so. Figure 8.3 shows the distribution of blood glucose levels for two groups of people — those in whom doctors have diagnosed diabetes on the basis of more sophisticated tests and those who were not thought to have the disease, labelled 'normal'.

□ Suppose you had a blood glucose level of *y* units — would you be a diabetic?

■ You might be, though equally you might not. A level of *y* units is compatible with either diagnosis.

□ At what blood glucose level should a screening test be set to distinguish diabetics from normals? What would be the result of setting the level at (1) *x*, (2) *y*, and (3) *z*?

■ 1 At *x* units, everyone with diabetes would be correctly identified, but in addition a lot of normal people would be incorrectly diagnosed as diabetics.

2 At *y* units some diabetics would be 'missed', and some normal people would be included as diabetics.

3 At *z* units, a lot of diabetics would be 'missed', but *no* normal people would be incorrectly diagnosed.

What is clear from this is that there is no perfect solution, because people both with and without a disease share some features. On the whole, simple, quick and cheap tests are unable to make subtle distinctions. Given that no screening test can be completely valid, it is necessary to be able to assess its *level* of validity to decide whether it is worthwhile using. This is done by considering two questions.

□ Can you suggest what they are?

■ 1 To what extent does the test detect *all* those people who have the disease?

2 To what extent does the test *only* detect people with the disease, and thus avoid incorrectly including normal people?

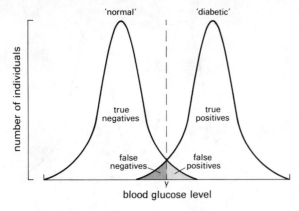

Figure 8.4 Outcome of screening for diabetes using a blood glucose level of *y* units as the cut-off level.

These are known, respectively, as the *sensitivity* and *specificity* of a test. Suppose that a screening test for blood glucose uses *y* units as the cut-off level to distinguish diabetics from normal people. The people will be included in one of four possible categories (Figure 8.4) based on whether their test result is normal (referred to as negative) or abnormal (positive). Diabetics with blood glucose levels above *y* units will be detected as diabetics (referred to as true positives). However, some diabetics who have levels below *y* units will be declared incorrectly as normal (known as false negatives). Normal people with levels below *y* units will be correctly identified as normal (true negatives) while some with high levels will be incorrectly diagnosed as being diabetic (false positives). The calculation of the sensitivity and specificity of the test is then quite simple:

$$\text{sensitivity} = \frac{\text{true positives}}{\substack{\text{all those with the disease} \\ \text{(i.e. true positives + false negatives)}}}$$

$$\text{specificity} = \frac{\text{true negatives}}{\substack{\text{all those without the disease} \\ \text{(i.e. true negatives + false positives)}}}$$

As you may have realised, the sensitivity and specificity of a test will depend on where the cut-off level is placed. This can be seen in Table 8.1 which shows the sensitivity and specificity at different levels of blood glucose obtained in an American study.

☐ What is the effect of raising the cut-off level?
■ The sensitivity falls and the specificity rises.
☐ How would you decide what cut-off level to use for a screening programme?

■ The decision would depend on which was more important — missing people with the disease or including people without the disease.

For example, if the disease being screened for was rapidly fatal and could only be successfully treated if detected early, then it would be more important to detect everyone with the disease even if that meant incorrectly diagnosing some normal people (i.e. sensitivity would be more important than specificity). If, on the other hand, the treatment for those found to be positive by the test involved a dangerous procedure in which 5 per cent of people died, it would be more important to avoid subjecting normal people to it (i.e. specificity would take priority over sensitivity).

So far this discussion has been concerned with the validity of a test from the point of view of the population as a whole. While this is of some interest to individuals, of greater concern is the *predictive value* of a test — the extent to which a positive result really does mean that an individual has the disease and conversely, that a negative result can be taken as reassuring. The predictive value of a test depends not only on the relative proportions of true and false results but also *on the prevalence of the disease in the population.* Even when the sensitivity and specificity are high, the predictive value of a test can be relatively low. Consider the example of screening for breast cancer shown in Table 8.2.

Table 8.1 Sensitivity and specificity of a blood glucose test (two hours after a meal) for 70 true diabetics and 510 non-diabetics at different levels of blood glucose.

Blood glucose level (mg/100ml)	Sensitivity (percentage diabetics so identified)	Specificity (percentage non-diabetics so identified)
80	100.0	1.2
90	98.6	7.5
100	97.1	25.3
110	92.9	48.4
120	88.6	68.2
130	81.4	82.4
140	74.3	91.2
150	64.3	96.1
160	55.7	98.6
170	52.9	99.6
180	50.0	99.8
190	44.3	99.8
200	37.1	100.0

(Source: United States Public Health Service, 1960, p.21)

Table 8.2 The results of a screening test and biopsies for breast cancer in 1 000 women.
(Note that only those women with a positive screening test result had a biopsy. However, in addition, three women with a negative screening test subsequently developed a breast lump that was found to be positive (cancer) on biopsy.)

| | | Results of biopsy | | |
		positive (cancer)	negative (no cancer)	total
Results of screening test	positive	13 (true positives)	37 (false positives)	50
	negative	3 (false negatives)	947 (true negatives)	950
	total	16	984	1 000

(Source: based on Shapiro, 1977)

□ What is the sensitivity and the specificity of the screening test?

■ Sensitivity is the proportion of people with the disease (16) who are detected by the test (13): $13/16 \times 100 = 81\%$. Specificity is the proportion of people without the disease (984) who are correctly identified by the test (947): $947/984 \times 100 = 96\%$.

□ One of the fifty women who has a positive screening test result has a biopsy (a small amount removed for detailed examination) of a suspicious lump which has been detected. What are the chances of the lump turning out to be cancer?

■ About one in four, as only thirteen of the fifty women found positive on screening have a positive biopsy.

In other words, the predictive value of a positive screening test result is only 26 per cent. Why is it so low? The reason is that despite the high specificity of the test (96 per cent) leading to the correct identification of 947 women *not* having breast cancer, the other 4 per cent of women who were incorrectly identified by the test (false positives) amounts to thirty-seven individuals, nearly three times larger than 81 per cent of sixteen (thirteen). If the prevalence of the disease were higher than sixteen per 1 000, then the predictive value of a positive test result would be higher also. Similarly, if the prevalence were lower, so would be the predictive value. For example, a screening test for coeliac disease (a disorder of the small intestine resulting in its failure to absorb food into the body) was shown to have a sensitivity of 79 per cent and specificity of 95 per cent. However, even in the areas of highest prevalence (two per 1 000), the test would identify thirty false positives for every true positive — a predictive value of about 3 per cent (cited in Barker and Rose, 1984).

We have considered validity in some detail because it lies at the heart of deciding whether or not to use a screening test. However, as you will see in a moment, even tests which have been shown to be valid may be rejected on other, equally important criteria.

The effect of early treatment

It is not enough for a screening test to be safe, repeatable and valid if it does not lead to an improvement in outcome for people with the disease. The introduction of a screening programme is only justifiable if it reduces mortality, morbidity or disability. In other words, there has to be a demonstrable benefit from early detection. It is important to ensure that any such benefit does not simply arise from advancing the point in time at which diagnosis occurs, known as increasing the *lead time*. For example, if a cancer has a certain duration from inception until it results in death, the earlier it is diagnosed, the longer will be the measured survival of patients *diagnosed* as having the disease (even if treatment has no effect). Screening may simply lead to increased periods of time that individuals have to live with the knowledge of an untreatable cancer.[*]

It is therefore important to know about the natural history of the disease. The lack of such knowledge has been a major problem, for example, in assessing the value of screening for cervical cancer. The screening test involves scraping some cells off the cervix and examining them under a microscope. Broadly speaking there are three possible findings: a normal appearance; obvious invasive cancer, in which the cells show clear signs of malignancy; and pre-invasive cancer, also known as carcinoma-in-situ, in which the cells are abnormal in appearance but are confined to the surface layers of the cervix. While it is clear what action needs to be taken with either of the first two findings, the significance of pre-invasive cancer is uncertain. This is because the natural history of the condition was never established before the widespread introduction of the screening test. While most experts in the subject would agree that most pre-invasive cancers become invasive, it is believed that as many as 25–30 per cent revert spontaneously to normal. It is now unlikely that it will ever be acceptable

---

[*]The detection, diagnosis and treatment of cancer is discussed further in *Experiencing and Explaining Disease, ibid.*

to either doctors or the public, to stop treating pre-invasive cancer so as to study the natural history to find out which women benefit from treatment and which do not. This experience has led people to be more cautious about the premature introduction of other screening programmes, such as mammography, for breast cancer.

Not only must early treatment be effective, it must also be *available* and *acceptable*. There is no point in detecting pre-symptomatic disease if the effective treatment is so expensive as to be unavailable. Similarly, it is important to ensure that the service is well organised so that all positive test results are adequately followed up. This has not always been the case, as the following newspaper report illustrates.

> ## Cancer victims not told results of early warning tests
>
> The cases of three women who developed cervical cancer because they were not told the results of early warning smear tests are to be investigated by Dr Donald Acheson, the Government's chief medical officer. One woman died and the other two are seriously ill.
>
> (Alan Copps, *Daily Telegraph*, March 18, 1985)

Screening tests must also be acceptable. This has been a major issue in pre-natal tests in which severe fetal abnormalities, such as neural tube defects (NTDs), are screened for in early pregnancy. The 'treatment' for such conditions is abortion, and while most people find such an action ethically acceptable, others do not.

Prenatal screening and abortion raises other questions. Is there any point in people who reject abortion in any circumstances being included in such a screening programme? Or if you did systematically ask this question in advance of screening, might it perhaps deter some women from undergoing the test who would in fact have chosen an abortion when faced with the knowledge that their child was severely deformed?

The economic efficiency of screening

You have already seen in Chapter 7, the difficulties of economic appraisal of health care activities. This is equally true when attempting to evaluate the economics of screening. The costs and benefits both to the individual who is screened and to the health care system, and therefore society as a whole, must be assessed.

The efficiency of any screening programme will be largely dependent on two aspects of the disease, its prevalence and its severity. The impact of *prevalence* on the costs to the health care system can be seen by comparing screening the newborn for phenylketonuria (PKU) with screening for Wilson's disease. In both diseases, an inherited lack of an essential enzyme leads to the accumulation of harmful chemicals in the body resulting in mental deterioration. While the prevalence of PKU is about one in 10 000 live births, that of Wilson's disease is about one in 100 000. The low *yield* that would result from screening for Wilson's disease means that the benefits are not felt sufficient to justify the costs. In contrast, screening for PKU is now well established in the UK.

Sometimes it is possible to increase the yield of a screening test by restricting the programme to those known to be at increased risk. For example, in most parts of the UK, pre-natal screening for Down's Syndrome is restricted to pregnant women over the age of 35–40 years for whom the incidence is much higher than for younger mothers. This may seem unfair, but the costs to the health service (and, indirectly, to all of us) have to be balanced against the benefits. Such a comparison has been done for prenatal screening for neural tube defects by comparing the costs of the programme with estimates of the additional use of health care and other services made by affected individuals. The benefits of screening were estimated to exceed the costs by at least 40 per cent, and depending on which costs and benefits are included in the calculation, may be by as much as 300 per cent (Henderson, 1982). In this sense, screening for NTDs has proved a success. By contrast, the failure to direct a screening test towards those people most at risk has been one of the reasons for the relative failure of the cervical cancer screening programme in the UK.

> ## Cervical cancer check system aims to halve death rate
>
> A properly organised cervical cancer screening programme could save 1000 women's lives a year, scientists said yesterday ... Women were willing to have smears taken — 3 million tests were performed annually — but no system existed to ensure that the right women were screened.
>
> (Andrew Veitch, *The Guardian*, June 14, 1983)

While the programme has been successful in screening young women, it has failed to attract older women, who are at much greater risk of the disease. As a result, it has been estimated that the cost of preventing one death from cervical cancer may have been as high as £300 000 (at 1980 prices).

Compared with assessing the costs and benefits of screening to the health service, their assessment from an individual or broader social point of view is much more difficult. On the whole, for individuals who are *correctly* identified by a screening test (true positives and true negatives), the benefits will outweigh the costs incurred in being screened. However, this might not be so for those incorrectly identified (false positives and false negatives).

☐ What costs might someone incur who is wrongly diagnosed as having a disease?

■ Considerable unnecessary anxiety, loss of time and discomfort in having to undergo further investigation and possibly treatment. In addition to the person directly involved, anxiety and other costs may be incurred by friends and relatives.

In contrast, there is a sense in which people who are defined as false negatives are no worse off than if they had not been screened. However, it is possible that the reassurance of the negative test result will engender a false sense of security in them, leading them to ignore taking any other preventive action from which they might have benefited. Again, these effects may be spread well beyond the person directly involved. When the economics of a screening programme are being considered, all such costs should be taken into account. In practice, often only the costs and benefits to the NHS are considered. It may well be that having done that, the costs outweigh the benefits. It then becomes necessary to decide whether other unquantifiable benefits, such as the prevention of discomfort and distress can justify the use of resources that could be put to other uses. Such decisions are extremely difficult to make in practice.

The acceptability of a screening test

How acceptable are screening tests to the public? Assessing the acceptability of a screening test differs from that of other aspects of care provided by health services in one important way: screening results from health services approaching people rather than being initiated by patients. The importance of this difference has been explained by Thomas McKeown:

When the patient seeks medical advice, the doctor's ethical position is relatively simple: he attempts to do his best with the knowledge and resources available to him ...

The position is quite different in screening ... there is a presumptive undertaking not merely that the abnormality will be identified if it is present, but that those affected will derive benefit from subsequent treatment or care. (McKeown, 1976, p.145)

Consider, for instance, a woman who detects a lump in her breast and fears she has cancer. If she approaches her doctor, she will probably accept the need for an anaesthetic and biopsy. If, however, the breast lump is detected on screening, it is the health services which have initiated her fear, anxiety, anaesthetic and biopsy. If it transpires she has cancer, screening can be regarded as justifiable in her case. However, suppose it turns out not to be cancer. Would the fear, anxiety and medical treatment she has suffered have been justified? Would the benefit gained by other women, who on screening were found to have cancer, more than compensate for her 'unnecessary' suffering?

Screening poses several other ethical issues. One arises during prenatal screening. It is generally considered acceptable to use amniocentesis to screen pregnant women who are over the age of thirty-five to forty years for Down's Syndrome. But this procedure also allows doctors to determine the sex of the fetus. Suppose the parents desperately want a daughter and discover from the amniocentesis that their child is a boy. Are they justified in requesting a termination? At present most people would find such a suggestion unacceptable, but attitudes to this and other reasons for selective abortion may, and probably will, alter in the future.

The screening of adults to detect carriers of abnormal genes is another controversial area.* Tay-Sachs disease was the first disorder for which carrier screening was done in the USA. By screening the Ashkenazim Jewish population, in whom there is a relatively high prevalence of the disease, the frequency of the disease has been significantly reduced and couples who are known to be at risk have through genetic counselling (advice about the chances of their children being affected by a genetic condition) been able to ensure having healthy children by means of prenatal amniocentesis and selective abortion. However, some genetic screening and counselling programmes, have met with fierce criticism from the population for whom they were established. This was true of a programme for sickle cell disease in the black population in the USA. People identified as carriers of the gene complained of having suffered a blow to their self-esteem; some reported that they were discriminated against for purposes of marriage, employment and insurance; and the programme had the unfortunate effect of exposing instances of non-paternity, the fathering of a child by someone other than the presumed father. In some states, laws were passed requiring sickle testing at birth, school entry or prior to marriage, which even led to charges, by some blacks, of attempted genocide.† Elsewhere, programmes to eliminate genetic

---

*The genetics of disease is discussed in *The Biology of Health and Disease*, Chapters 4 and 12, *ibid*.

†The management of sickle cell disease and carriers is discussed in TV11, 'Asian rickets, the English disease'.

disorders have led to people questioning definitions of 'abnormality' and rejecting the idea that people born with severe disabilities have any less right to live than more able bodied people.

As you have seen in the case of sickle cell disease, there is a danger that screening tests may lead to the stigmatisation of people. For example, the current interest in screening people to assess their risk of coronary heart disease involves identifying 'high risk' individuals. These people have subsequently to live for the rest of their lives with the threat of a serious disease which they might never actually suffer. And if health services cannot offer them any effective action to reduce significantly the risk of the disease occurring, is there sufficient justification to screen them in the first place? In addition, there is the danger that people's employment prospects may be jeopardised by the results of screening tests: a person's level of risk of heart disease could be used by employers as a criterion of employment. This already happens to people with established diseases such as diabetes. These sorts of issues reinforce the need for screening tests to be carefully assessed from a wide range of viewpoints before their introduction. The temptation in the past has been to introduce a programme if it appeared to provide some help to at least a few people. Nowadays a more cautious approach is advocated, as in the case of screening for breast cancer: the 1980s are seeing the results of some major research studies which were set up in the 1960s and 1970s. These are demonstrating that the early detection and treatment of breast cancer, is beneficial. At the time of writing, a national policy for breast cancer screening is awaiting the assessment of economic and other criteria.

Although deciding whether or not to establish a screening programme can be difficult, and despite the failure of some programmes, there have been several highly successful examples. Table 8.3 lists the programmes currently available, or at least advocated, in many parts of the UK. In addition there are others, such as breast cancer screening which have been established in some places, though they have not yet fully met the criteria discussed above. Nevertheless, despite the success of some of the tests shown in Table 8.3 it is clear that screening is only appropriate in the case of a relatively small number of diseases. Moreover, this is likely to remain so, given the stringent criteria which a screening programme should meet before it is considered worth establishing. Thus, although screening may initially seem the answer to many contemporary health care problems — and as such is enthusiastically advocated by some — a careful consideration of all the many complex issues which screening involves suggests that it is far from being a panacea. Indeed, even where screening is appropriate, screening programmes which are carelessly introduced may in fact create as many problems as they solve.

Table 8.3 Conditions for which screening is widely available, or advocated, in the UK, 1985.

Prenatal		
(a) maternal conditions	syphilis	
	rubella immunity	
	diabetes	
	pre-eclampsia	
(b) fetal conditions	neural tube defects	
	haemolytic disease (eg. Rhesus disease)	
	genetic disease (e.g. Down's Syndrome; Tay-Sachs disease; sickle cell disease)	
Newborn babies	phenylketonuria (PKU)	
	hypothyroidism	
	haemoglobinopathies (in select groups)	
	congenital dislocation of the hip	
Infants	general development	
	hearing defects	
	vision defects	
Children	hearing defects	
	vision defects	
	abnormal growth rate	
	general development	
	scoliosis (curvature of the spine)	
Adults	cervical cancer	
	hypertension	
	genetic 'carriers' (eg. Tay-Sachs; sickle haemoglobin)	

Objectives for Chapter 8

When you have read this chapter you should be able to:

8.1 Explain what screening involves and describe the four aspects of a screening programme which should be considered when deciding on whether or not to set one up: the nature of the screening test; the effect of early treatment; the economic efficiency of screening; and, finally, its social acceptability.

8.2 Explain why some screening tests have been established while others have not, and the disadvantages of setting up screening tests prematurely.

Questions for Chapter 8

1 (*Objectives 8.1 and 8.2*)

Call for blood pressure tests for children

Annual blood pressure tests for schoolchildren starting at the age of four were urged by doctors at a conference in London yesterday. They said the tests would pick out children who might otherwise be at high risk of heart attacks in much later life.

(David Fletcher, *Daily Telegraph*, April 20, 1983)

What factors would you need to consider in order to decide whether or not to start screening schoolchildren's blood pressure?

Preventive health care

This chapter concentrates on contemporary aspects of preventive health care. An account of the historical development of public health and personal hygiene measures appears in Book VII, *Caring for Health: History and Diversity*, Chapters 2–4. During this chapter you will be asked to read two articles in the Course Reader: 'Cancer and work: guidelines for workers taking collective action over health hazards', prepared by the General, Municipal, Boilermakers and Allied Trades Union (Part 7, Section 7.7) and 'A new kind of doctor', by Julian Tudor Hart (Part 3, Section 3.4). There is also a television programme (TV 11) 'Asian rickets: the English disease' and an accompanying audiotape sequence (Band 4, AC 808) that relate to material in this chapter.

The Fence or the Ambulance
'Twas a dangerous cliff, as they freely confessed,
Though to walk near its crest was so pleasant:
But over its terrible edge there had slipped
A duke and many a peasant;
So the people said something would have to be done,
But their projects did not all tally:
Some said, 'Put a fence round the edge of the cliff';
Some, 'An ambulance down in the valley'.

Then an old man remarked, 'It's a marvel to me
That people give far more attention
To repairing results than to stopping the cause
When they'd much better aim at prevention;
Let us stop at its source all this mischief,' cried he.
'Come, neighbours and friends, let us rally;
If the cliff we will fence, we might almost dispense
With the ambulance down in the valley.'
(Joseph Malines, 1953, p.24)

Prevention is the modern fashion. Faced with the mounting dilemma of providing ambulances which are both effective and sufficient in number, many professional and lay people have rallied to the building of fences. But is all this enthusiasm and optimism actually justified? Can prevention really solve many of the dilemmas that confront health care?

Before attempting to answer these questions, we need to consider briefly what we mean by 'prevention'; what its relationship is to cure; the different approaches that have been adopted; and the range of people, both professional and lay, who are involved in attempting to prevent disease and promote health. Against that background we will then consider a series of case studies, the subjects of which have been some of the major targets for prevention in the UK over the last ten to twenty years. However, the subjects were not only chosen because of the large amount of attention they have received, but also because each one vividly illustrates one or two key aspects of the different guises that prevention can adopt, such as legislation or fiscal measures. As a result, none of the case studies attempts to provide a *comprehensive* account of its subject. The final part of the chapter examines what is not only one of the major strategies for prevention, but also one that generates considerable controversy and debate: health education — is it effective? Is it education or propaganda? Is it simply a cosmetic exercise concealing government's lack of action in tackling the underlying issues?

To start, let us consider what we mean by 'cure' and by 'prevention'. They are commonly viewed as distinct alternatives. Cure is portrayed as unattractive — it happens only when prevention has failed or not been attempted; it is also highly expensive, needing ever more new, high technology equipment. Prevention on the other hand is thought to be cheaper, to rely on fairly simple forms of technology and also to be ethically superior: it is better to prevent than to cure disease. However, such a clear distinction ignores several key aspects. First, much so-called curative work has the objective of *preventing* disability rather than providing a full cure, and conversely, as you have seen in the previous chapter, some prevention is concerned with the detection and early treatment of disease rather than stopping its initial appearance. Furthermore, some prevention isn't cheap or simple, for example, screening newborn infants for PKU requires the use of elaborate equipment combined with technical and scientific expertise in carrying out the tests. Finally, assessing whether prevention is cheaper than cure depends entirely on the definitions we use. Should we include expenditure on road safety, on better housing and on education? Once we start to do this, prevention can look as expensive as cure.

Such difficulties have led to several ways of classifying health care. One such system views *all* health care as being concerned with prevention. On this scheme, different activities are defined as either primary, secondary, or tertiary prevention. *Primary prevention* means avoiding the onset of disease and covers the everyday meaning of 'prevention' — activities such as discouraging smoking and legislation to control pollution (Figure 9.1). *Secondary prevention* refers to the early detection and treatment of disease which thereby, prevents established diseases from advancing any further. As you have seen in the previous chapter, these measures can take two forms.

☐ What are they?

■ 1 Mass screening, in which the whole or part of the population is tested for the presence either of a disease or of a risk factor (such as high blood pressure).
2 Individual screening, or case-finding, which may occur in routine consultation with health professionals.

Finally, there is *tertiary prevention*, which aims to prevent the worst effects of those diseases which are already

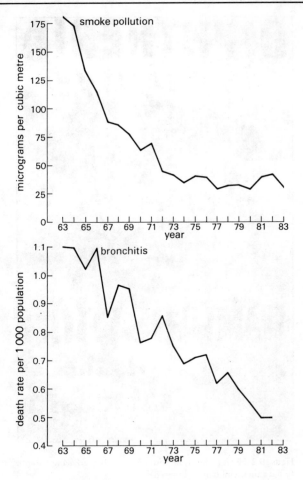

Figure 9.1 Reduction in deaths from bronchitis that accompanied the decline in levels of air pollution following the Clean Air Act in Sheffield.
(Source: Sheffield Health Committee, 1984, p.8)

established. For example, immobility resulting from osteoarthrosis of the hip joint can be prevented by replacing the joint with an artificial one; death from appendicitis can be prevented by removing the appendix; and in a few cases, death from a severely damaged heart can be prevented by a transplant operation.

Our concern in this chapter is with primary prevention — with preventing the onset of disease. This includes activities ranging from immunisation programmes (Figure 9.2) to the impact that subsidies for public transport have on road accidents, from sex education to national economic policy (which may have a considerable effect on inequalities in health). This is an extraordinarily diverse range of activities. Is it possible to classify them any further?

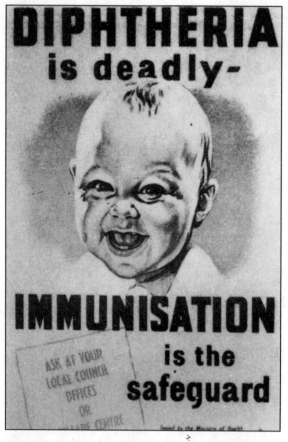

DIPHTHERIA is deadly—

IMMUNISATION is the safeguard

ASK AT YOUR LOCAL COUNCIL OFFICES OR

Issued by the Ministry of Health

Figure 9.2 Health education poster in the 1940s advising parents to have their children immunised.

The first distinction that can be made is between those measures where disease prevention is the *principal* goal, such as immunisation and stopping smoking, and those in which it is *incidental* — merely one of a number of effects, such as the reduction in deaths on the road when public transport is subsidised (a product of the smaller number of private vehicles). Although the distinction between these categories is often unclear we shall, in this chapter, concentrate on those measures which have prevention as their principal objective.

Another distinction that can be drawn is that between measures aimed primarily at *environmental* change and those aimed at *individual* behaviour. The distinction is classically embodied in the two nineteenth-century phrases '*public health*' and '*personal hygiene*'; the former focusing on measures such as improved sanitation, water and housing, the latter on things such as personal cleanliness and making sure that food is stored and cooked properly. But although the distinction is easy to make in theory, in practice, the two are often interwoven.

Finally, a distinction can be drawn between measures that rely on individuals changing their own behaviour — as with health education that encourages people to give up smoking — and measures such as legislation on car seat belts that force people to change their behaviour. The first relies on *individual choice*, responsibility and motivation, the second on *external compulsion*.

The point to note is that no single form of classification is entirely satisfactory. On the one hand, drivers can refuse to belt up when driving, factory owners can ignore safety legislation and, on the other, health education can have an important element of compulsion — some campaigns aim to shock and frighten people into compliance.

Having reviewed some of the ways of classifying approaches in primary prevention, we must briefly consider the main people involved in such activities. Within the NHS all health professionals have a role. Every consultation that takes place either in primary care or in hospital provides an opportunity for health professionals to advise their patients on preventive measures. And, in the case of health visitors, prevention is their primary role, particularly in the area of child care. However, prevention is also handled in other ways. Within health districts, the planning and overseeing of preventive programmes is one of the responsibilities of the community physicians. Centrally involved in such programmes is the district's health education unit staffed, on average, by two or three *health education officers*. Being so few in number, most units try to work through other people — school teachers, health visitors, health and safety officers in industry, and community workers — rather than directly with the public.

Another important occupational group is the *environmental health officers* — the descendants of the nineteenth-century public health inspectors. Employed by the District Councils, they are responsible for maintaining the purity of food and of water supplies, for housing standards, and the surveillance of air pollution (including noise levels). Over the years their work has become increasingly scientific and technical.

But prevention is not left entirely to the discretion of health and local authorities. Apart from the enactment of new legislation, central government is involved, issuing priority documents, such as the *Prevention and Health* series which started in 1976, and influencing the pattern and style of health education through the Health Education Council (HEC) in England and Wales, and the Scottish Health Education Group. These partly autonomous organisations (commonly known as '*quangos*' — short for 'quasi-non-governmental organisation') are funded by the government. Up until the early 1980s they concentrated on producing materials such as leaflets, posters and TV advertisements which essentially tell people what to do. Since then, however, they have begun to change their role

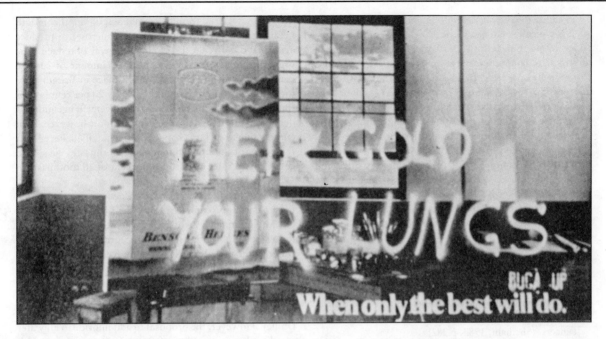

Figure 9.3 Aerosol protest by BUGA UP, an Australian anti-smoking group.   (Source: Taylor, P. 1984, opp. p.171)

— funding more research and trying to alter the climate of public opinion through debate. In practical terms they also provide some support for local NHS and other staff.

Finally, there is one other type of organisation involved in active prevention: pressure groups such as ASH (Action on Smoking and Health). Such groups come in a wide variety of forms — ASH is run under the auspices of the Royal College of Physicians; trade unions campaign for health and safety at work; while some other groups take direct action. One of these is BUGA UP (Billboard Utilising Graffitists Against Unhealthy Promotions), an Australian group who 'improve' billboards by transforming Dunhill into 'Lung Ill' and Rothmans into 'Rot Mans' (Figure 9.3).

There are, then, a great range of people and organisations with an interest in prevention. Prevention is a powerful lobby with many forces behind it — health professions, trade unions, government organisations and groups of activists. And these are joined by some important commercial interests such as those who promote and sell health foods. But, as you will see in the case studies, set against all this are some equally or even more powerful groups and organisations whose activities obstruct those of the prevention lobby. These include the tobacco and drinks industries, government departments who may put a higher priority on such issues as employment rather than prevention, members of the public who may oppose restrictions on their personal freedom to behave in whatever way they wish, and people who oppose measures on religious or ethical grounds (Figure 9.4).

League of National Life.

53, VICTORIA STREET, LONDON, S.W.1.

Telephone No: VICTORIA 3920

Official Organ of the League: "National Life"
(quarterly) price 3d., or 1s. 4d. a year, post free.

OBJECTS.

1. To uphold the honour and blessing of Parenthood.

2. To Combat the theory and practice of Contraception.

3. To oppose any form of State or Municipal assistance for the promotion of Contraception.

The League stands for :

THE PHYSICAL AND MORAL HEALTH OF THE INDIVIDUAL.

THE WELFARE AND SAFETY OF THE HOME, THE NATION, AND THE EMPIRE.

THE NATIONAL TRADITION OF REVERENCE FOR MARRIAGE AND PARENTHOOD.

THE TRUTH AS TAUGHT BY SCIENCE AND RELIGION.

Figure 9.4 Publicity leaflet produced by the pressure group, League for National Life, which campaigned against contraception in the 1920s and 1930s.

In short, the pressure from one kind of group, such as ASH is typically matched by pressures from other groups. As a result, policies on prevention are shaped by a multitude of contradictory pressures. As such, campaigns to alter behaviour have to utilise a huge variety of different approaches. For example, attempts to reduce the prevalence of cigarette smoking have involved the prescribing of nicotine-containing chewing gum, lobbying Parliament for an increase in the level of excise duty, campaigning for no-smoking areas in public places, setting up smoking-cessation clinics to help smokers quit, and challenging tobacco companies during meetings of shareholders. Likewise the pro-smoking lobby has done battle wherever it can. The case studies that follow examine the various aspects of such complex struggles in more detail.

Fluoridation and seat-belts

> Each year over 30 million teeth are filled and five million extracted by 20 000 dentists at a cost of over £400 million. Caries costs more to treat than all cancers. (Sheiham, 1983, p.282)

Dental caries appears to be a modern disease associated with changes in diet which have taken place during the last hundred or so years (Figure 9.5). Its increased prevalence is related to the increased consumption of sugar: in England from 19 lbs per person per year in 1850 to over 100 lbs by

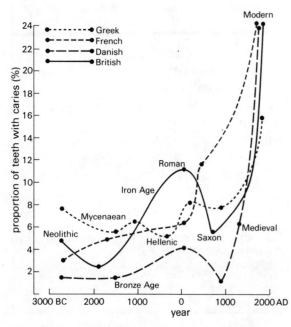

Figure 9.5 Rates of dental caries from neolithic to modern times in Britain, Denmark, France and Greece.
(Source: Wells, 1964, Fig. 19)

the 1960s.* Caries results from bacteria in the mouth breaking down sugars (in particular, sucrose) to produce acids that dissolve the teeth. Thus, one way of reducing the prevalence of caries is to reduce the amount of sucrose consumed. This has certainly taken place in Britain since the 1960s — consumption has fallen by 20 per cent — and this has been accompanied by an improvement in children's dental health. This improvement has not, however, been entirely due to dietary changes. It is generally believed that the use of fluoride-containing toothpaste has also contributed. Sales rose from 4 per cent of all toothpaste in 1970 to 95 per cent in 1977.

While most children have benefited from fluoride toothpaste, approximately 15 per cent have also benefited from living in places which have high levels of fluoride in the water supply (either naturally occurring or added by the water authority). In such areas an even more impressive reduction in caries has taken place. For example, children in Birmingham (fluoridated) experienced a 54 per cent reduction in the incidence of caries between 1964 and 1977 compared to a 32 per cent reduction in non-fluoridated Dudley. However, the proposal to add fluoride to all water supplies has met very effective resistance from such pressure groups as the Pure Water Society.

The debate about fluoridation reached a climax in 1978 when legal action was taken by a Glaswegian woman to prevent Strathclyde Regional Council adding fluoride to the local water supply. The case lasted 201 days (over 1980–1982) and cost about £1 million, making it the longest and costliest case in Scottish legal history. Fluoridation was opposed on the grounds that it was an infringement of *individual freedom* — the freedom to drink 'pure' water. After spending a year considering a massive amount of evidence the judge, Lord Jauncey, decided in 1983 that under the then existing laws, an individual did indeed have the right to choose how to care for his or her own body and that fluoridation would contravene that right. However, he also concluded that fluoridation was both effective and safe and that the laws governing water supplies needed to be changed so that advantage could be taken of this public health measure. As a result in 1985 new legislation giving water authorities throughout the UK the right to add fluoride to their supplies is being considered by Parliament.

The enforcement of such legislation will be relatively easy as it does not require the active cooperation of individuals — if you live in a fluoridated area you are forced to use fluoridated water, unless you choose to buy a bottled variety. In contrast, legislation that requires the *cooperation* of individuals can present the enforcing authorities (such as the police) with considerable difficulties.

*Historical changes in nutrition are discussed in greater detail in *The Health of Nations*, Chapter 12, *ibid*.

□ Can you suggest why some laws may be difficult or even impossible to enforce?

■ Most laws depend on the majority of citizens abiding by them. The police can only cope if law-breakers are few in number.

Difficulty in law-enforcement in the prevention of disease has a long history. Carlo Cipolla, an economic historian, has described how the Church repeatedly defied the public health magistrates during an outbreak of plague in Tuscany in 1630. When the magistrates tried to isolate a small town to reduce contagion (which they believed was the means of transmission of the disease), clerical leaders in the town organised a mass procession during which the town gates were broken down.

Two centuries later, in 1864, laws to control the movement of smallpox victims, a disease that claimed over 9 000 lives in the UK that year, were being hotly debated. Sir James Simpson, the professor of obstetrics in Glasgow and an advocate of legislation, argued as follows:

The legislature has no scruples in some other diseases to as great or indeed to a greater extent. It enforces, for instance, the isolation of any individual affected with insanity, be he rich or poor, who is a homicidal lunatic endangering the lives of others. If, by a law which no one thinks harsh or severe, lunatics are prevented from destroying the lives of their fellow-men, why should it be thought harsh or severe that people affected with smallpox should be prevented from dealing out destruction and death ...? (cited in Haggard, p.227)

And similar arguments were used by the National Association of Health Authorities (NAHA) a century later, in 1979, on the question of seat-belt legislation:

The community will have to pay a heavy price if the Bill to make the wearing of seat-belts compulsory does not become law ... If legislation goes through in this country, we can hope to avoid some 9 000 cases every year of fatal or serious injury ... We hope that Parliament will recognise the extent to which the driver's freedom in this respect creates a volume of avoidable injury which effectively denies or delays the giving of badly needed health care to other members of the public. (NAHA, press release, March 3, 1979)

□ How was the issue of individual freedom handled by those such as NAHA, who were in favour of legislation?

■ By arguing that the resources used in treating injuries caused through the failure to wear seat-belts were thereby not available for others who also needed health care.

However, not only were the opponents of legislation fighting to protect freedom to drive without wearing a belt, but also they were expressing their anger at the loss of another type of liberty, defined by the political philosopher, Isaiah Berlin, as *positive liberty*. Positive liberty is the liberty to decide how much freedom one has. In other words, they also resented the fact, so they claimed, that their opinions were not even considered and that their destinies were being decided by people over whom they had no control: bureaucrats and experts. Resistance to issues such as seat-belt legislation is to some extent both an expression and a symbol of this resentment at the loss of positive liberty.

The seat-belt saga also illustrates another obstacle — the need for *empirical evidence* for the measure being introduced. The supporters of seat-belts claimed that legislation would increase the use of belts from around 30 per cent (the most that had been achieved through health education campaigns) to about 85 per cent — the average wearing rate in the twenty-three countries in which it was already compulsory in 1979. This, they claimed, would lead to 9 000 fewer fatal and serious injuries with a potential saving in health care costs and damage to property of £60 million per year (in 1979). Such claims were largely instrumental in generating sufficient support in Parliament for legislation to reach the statute book. In February 1983 the law came into operation. Have these claims been borne out in practice?

Judged on the first eight months following legislation (February to September 1983), the claims appear to have been well-founded. During that period approximately 95 per cent of people wore seat-belts and there were 350 fewer deaths and 4 500 fewer serious injuries among front-seat occupants of cars and vans than in the previous year. The impact on hospital services was dramatic, as one surgeon reported:

Whereas before the legislation we expected to see four or five patients a week with a range of serious injuries such as very severe facial lacerations, severe bruising, and head and neck injuries, we now see only one such case every few months, and these in the main have been front-seat occupants not wearing seat-belts. (Baderman, cited in Burningham, 1984, p.533)

□ Is it reasonable to conclude that the introduction of seat-belt legislation caused the decline in deaths and serious injuries? If not, why not?

■ Not without first checking for other possible factors. For example, there might have been fewer vehicles on the road in 1983 than 1982; the weather conditions might have been better in 1983; and there may have been less drinking-and-driving in 1983.

Study of these other possible factors suggests that the decline in deaths and injuries was almost certainly due to the wearing of seat-belts. However, this success story was marred by one potentially worrying finding — an increase in the number of casualties amongst other road users, such as cyclists, during the same period. It is not clear whether this was associated with the seat-belt legislation, although it has been suggested that one effect of wearing a seat-belt is to increase the driver's sense of personal safety with the unfortunate consequence that drivers tend to then drive faster and take more risks. How far this hypothesis is true is at the time of writing not known.

Controlling alcohol

Doctors launch drive against alcohol abuse

One in five male patients in hospital medical wards are there because of excessive drinking, senior doctors said yesterday. They blamed the growth of heavy drinking for a range of deaths and accidents, including 40% of road accidents involving pedestrians.

(David Fletcher, *Daily Telegraph*, September 16, 1983)

The excessive consumption of alcohol can kill and injure in a variety of different ways — directly through conditions such as cirrhosis of the liver and indirectly through road traffic accidents, domestic violence and, when heavy drinkers lose their jobs, through a deterioration in living standards. As some of these examples indicate, heavy drinking can have serious effects for others besides those doing the drinking. The issue of alcohol is further complicated by two other aspects: the vast majority of the population drink alcohol without any serious ill-effects (indeed, low levels of consumption are thought to be beneficial); and any reduction in alcohol consumption might lead to increases in the use of other, possibly more harmful, drugs.

Given the complex range of effects that alcohol has, any calculation of its overall effect on mortality is bound to be difficult. On standard estimates, it is thought to cause somewhere between 5 000 and 10 000 premature deaths in the UK every year. Two economists, Rebecca McDonnell and Alan Maynard, have put the minimum social cost of alcohol abuse in 1983, from absenteeism from work and demands on health services, police and judiciary, in excess of £1 500 million.

The current increase in alcohol consumption in the UK

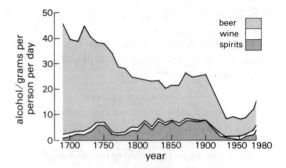

Figure 9.6 Alcohol consumption in the UK, 1690–1980. (Source: Spring and Buss, 1977, p.571)

started in about 1960. But it may help to take a longer-term view (Figure 9.6). There have been significant changes in the consumption of different types of alcoholic drink over the past three centuries. Beer consumption reached a maximum of 832 pints per person per year in 1869, since when consumption has dropped fairly steadily to the present day. Increases in the consumption of spirits (mostly gin) in the middle of the eighteenth century, and again for most of the nineteenth century, make the present rise in consumption seem minor in comparison. It has very tentatively been suggested that there may be a cycle whereby one or two generations learn to drink heavily, the next then react to the increased damage with controlling measures, but then as the subsequent generations forget the damage caused by alcohol they begin to drink more and so start the cycle again.

While there is little agreement about why some people drink to excess, and whether alcoholism is a 'disease' or simply a response to personal or social difficulties,* there is agreement on some other aspects. The more alcohol that a population consumes, the higher the prevalence of alcohol-related diseases. And three factors are known to influence the amount a population consumes — price, legal availability and advertising. The influence of *price* can be seen in Figure 9.7.

   □ How does the price of a litre of alcohol in 1979 compare with the price in 1949?

   ■ A litre of alcohol costs in real terms less than half what it cost in 1949.

In other words, alcohol has become progressively cheaper over the last few decades, mainly because the excise duties levied by the government have been increased by less than the rate of inflation. The treasury is well aware of this as it has published figures on what are termed its *price* and

---

*Drinking problems are discussed further in *Experiencing and Explaining Disease*, Chapter 12, *ibid*.

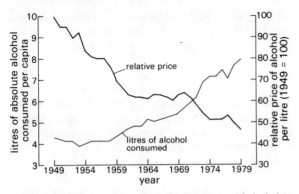

Figure 9.7 Alcohol consumption and relative price of alcohol in Britain, 1949–1979.
(Source: Office of Health Economics, 1981, Figure 10, p.40)

income elasticity. Price elasticity is the percentage change in demand that occurs in response to a percentage change in price. Income elasticity is the percentage change in demand that occurs in response to a percentage change in income. The price elasticity figures in Table 9.1 show the percentage by which average consumption would change in response to a 1 per cent increase in price, and the income elasticity figures show the percentage by which average consumption would change in response to a 1 per cent rise in disposable income.

□ What would be the effect on consumption of a 10 per cent increase in the price of (1) beer, and (2) spirits?
■ 1 Consumption of beer would fall by 2 per cent (i.e. −0.2 × 10).
2 Consumption of spirits would fall by 16 per cent (i.e. −16 × 10).

Thus, at current levels of consumption, changing the price is more effective at controlling the consumption of spirits than beer. Given that the government has such a powerful tool at their disposal, why have they failed even to maintain the real cost of alcohol? First, the government's principal concern is raising revenue — negative price elasticities mean that an increase in price would lead to a reduction in consumption, and as a result, maybe a reduction in revenue. The government seeks to find the *optimal* price level — the price at which they gain the greatest amount of revenue. In addition, it has to consider the wider economic consequences of a fall in consumption. In 1984 the drink

Table 9.1 Price and income elasticity for sales of alcoholic drinks in the UK, 1980

	Beer	Spirits	Wine
Price elasticity	−0.2	−1.6	−1.1
Income elasticity	0.7	2.2	2.5

(Source: HM Treasury, 1980)

trade provided about 700 000 jobs, the government raised £4000 million in taxes and excise duty (about 6 per cent of total revenue raised) and there was a balance of trade surplus of £500 million due to the export of products such as gin and whisky.

Another reason why the government has not maintained the real cost of alcohol is that although people would favour tougher sentences for drunken driving, they would oppose large increases in price (Table 9.2). Since two-thirds of the population drink regularly, substantial increases in price would damage the electoral prospects of a government. In addition, alcohol expenditure is included in the Retail Price Index, the main indicator of the inflation rate and a key influence on wage-bargaining. A substantial increase in alcohol prices would increase the inflation rate, something that all governments would be reluctant to do. And if alcohol were removed from the Retail Price Index, as some medical bodies have argued, there would be criticism that the government was falsifying the true extent of price increases — akin to removing rain from weather reports. Finally, some governments are reluctant to increase indirect taxes (such as VAT and excise duty) because they are seen as *regressive*; that is, the increase is the same for everyone regardless of their income.

If control of consumption through price regulation is attractive neither to consumers nor governments, then other means of governmental control need to be considered. One possibility is to change the *legal availability* of alcohol. The experience of prohibition in the USA illustrates how dangerous such changes can be, if taken too far.

On January 17, 1920, the Volstead Act officially prohibited the manufacture and sale of all 'intoxicating liquors', although it did not make consumption illegal. The effects were dramatic. Because there was still a huge public demand for alcohol, its supply was taken over by criminal

Table 9.2 Public opinion about action to curb drinking (1 058 people polled by MORI, December 1980)

	Percentage in favour
Tougher sentences for drinking and driving	87
Random breath tests	66
More health education on dangers	63
Health warning on all cans and bottles	55
Tougher licensing laws	50
Ban on advertising drink on TV	46
Ban on alcohol sales in supermarkets	37
Total ban on drink advertising	29
Large increase in price of alcohol	26

(Source: Lipsey, 1980, p.1)

organisations. Indeed, the basis for the enormous power of organised crime in modern American life was created by this extraordinary business opportunity. Not only was crime set on an entirely new footing (during the fourteen years of prohibition 703 gang murders in Chicago were officially attributed to the alcohol trade) but the government itself and its agents became criminalised. By 1923, on another official estimate, no less than 60 per cent of the Chicago police force were themselves involved in the liquor business.

There are problems even with minor alterations to the law, as it is not clear what changes would be necessary to achieve a decrease in morbidity and mortality. Advocates of more restrictive laws point to France where bars are open at all hours, and the death rate from cirrhosis is over ten times that of the UK. However, this view has its opponents. In 1976, the licensing laws in Scotland were relaxed in an attempt to change the pattern of 'binge' drinking that was felt to be partly responsible for some of the harm resulting from alcohol. In addition, the official commission of inquiry into drinking habits in Scotland (the Clayson inquiry) suggested that an attempt should be made to change the image and atmosphere of bars from that of male drinking dens to places which would attract wider custom. Although the effect of such changes on health are not yet clear, there is evidence that a reduction in alcohol-related crime has resulted.

A third approach is that of greater control of *advertising*. The drinks industry spent around £100 million in 1984, compared with the £1–2 million spent by health educators (Figure 9.8). Would restrictions on advertising be effective in reducing the harm caused by alcohol? The drinks industry, like the tobacco industry, argue that advertising is only aimed at getting consumers to switch brands. While this is clearly a major objective of advertising, many health educators and some advertising experts believe that the effect is to increase consumption, whether or not it is an objective.

Besides controlling consumption through price, legal availability and advertising, there is one other approach to consider: limiting the damage alcohol can cause. Tougher legislation on drinking and driving and the use of 'breathalysers' had a dramatic effect when they were first introduced, but this has faded as time has passed, and the actual danger of getting caught has turned out to be low. There is still, however, widespread support for the

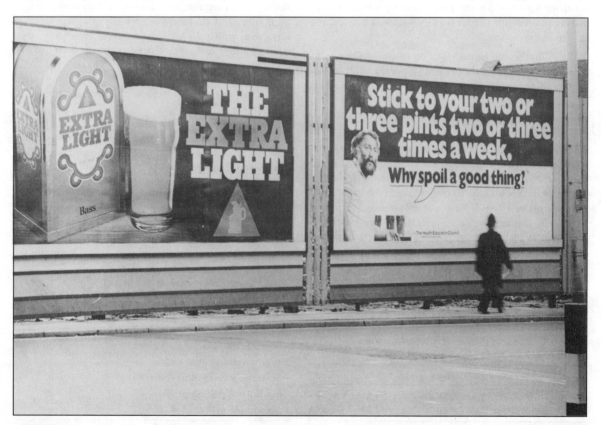

Figure 9.8 Contrasting messages on alcohol.

introduction of random breath tests (see Table 9.2), though the police remain worried about alienating law-abiding citizens whose cooperation they depend on in much of their work, and many people would feel that the introduction of such a measure was an unacceptable infringement of their personal liberty.

It appears, therefore, that there is no simple, acceptable solution to counteract most of the harm of alcohol abuse. Although different countries have taken very different routes to limit alcohol consumption — in Finland, drinkers can only buy one drink at a time in bars and there is therefore no buying of rounds — no country can claim any great success for the measures it has introduced. Alcohol may be a problem for some, but attempts to limit its damaging effects run up against the pleasure and liberties of the rest of the population.

Controlling tobacco

Although alcohol has been brewed and distilled for thousands of years, tobacco was only imported into Europe at the end of the sixteenth century and it was only towards the end of the last century that machines were invented to mass-produce a cheap, readily available form: the cigarette. With respect to men, cigarette smoking spread rapidly in North America and Europe during the first decades of this century (Figure 9.9). For women, the habit became widespread only after the First World War. By 1945, two out of three adult males in the UK were cigarette smokers.

□ When did the upward trend in cigarette consumption among men level off, and why?

■ In the early 1960s (it was still rising in the 1950s following the dramatic slump during the immediate

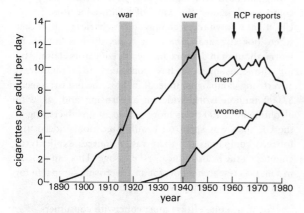

Figure 9.9 Cigarette consumption in the UK, 1890–1981, given as the average number per adult per day irrespective of whether they smoke or not. The arrows indicate the date of the first three reports of the Royal College of Physicians warning of the dangers of smoking.
(Source: Royal College of Physicians, 1983, Figure 1.1, p.1)

post-war period of austerity). This is generally attributed to the early reports of the harmful effects of smoking.

In 1962, the Royal College of Physicians (RCP) published their first report, *Smoking and Health*, which concentrated almost entirely on men (the worst effects in women had been delayed by their later adoption of the habit). The most important piece of evidence came from a study of British doctors conducted by an epidemiologist, Richard Doll, and a statistician, Austin Bradford Hill. They demonstrated that, compared with non-smokers, men who smoked twenty-five or more cigarettes a day had about thirty times the chance of dying of chronic bronchitis and twenty-three times the chance of dying of lung cancer, and this has subsequently been confirmed by other studies. Moreover, since the first study in 1962, it has been shown that smoking not only increases the risk of chronic bronchitis and lung cancer, but also coronary heart disease (CHD), stroke, and cancers of the larynx, oesophagus, mouth, pancreas, bladder and cervix. Smoking during pregnancy is associated with lighter babies, and in women who smoke the menopause occurs an average two to three years earlier than in non-smokers. Finally, there is evidence that the health of non-smokers is damaged by *passive smoking* — the involuntary inhalation of others' smoke. Children of parents who smoke are particularly liable to suffer in this way.

In England and Wales, it is reckoned that about 95 000 people die prematurely each year as a result of smoking. It has been estimated that out of 1 000 young men who smoke in the UK, one will be murdered, six will die in road accidents and 250 will die as a result of smoking. Of all the known avoidable risks to health, smoking is in a league of its own.

Stopping smoking reduces the risk both of lung cancer and coronary heart disease. Although the risk of lung cancer declines quite rapidly in the first few years after stopping smoking, it takes about twenty years for the risk in ex-smokers to reach the low levels found in non-smokers. In contrast, the risk of coronary heart disease falls rather more rapidly after giving up — by about 50 per cent in the first two years, then declining rather more gradually, so that after ten years it is similar to that in non-smokers.

The Royal College of Physicians' report in 1962 appears to have stemmed the growing consumption of cigarettes. This suggests that part of the answer lies in health education. However, an additional factor that has been shown to effect the level of consumption in the UK is that of increases in excise duty (Figure 9.10) — larger increases tend to be associated with larger reductions in consumption. By 1984, total sales of cigarettes had fallen to around 100 000 million from their peak of 137 000 million in 1973.

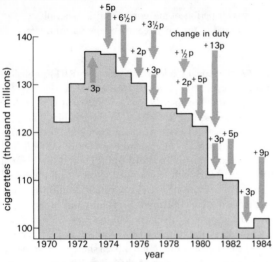

Figure 9.10 Sales of cigarettes in the UK, 1970–1984. Changes in the level of excise duty on a standard pack of 20 cigarettes is shown. Changes in VAT are excluded.
(Source: Simpson, 1984, Figure 4, p.25)

Over the same period the proportion of smokers declined both in men (from 52 per cent to 36 per cent) and women (from 41 per cent to 32 per cent).

☐ What are the principal differences noted so far between the consumption of alcohol and the smoking of tobacco?

■ First, smoking is far more dangerous. Second, even a small amount of smoking may be harmful, whereas small quantities of alcohol may actually be beneficial. Third, whereas the consumption of alcohol has risen since the 1950s, that of tobacco has fallen quite sharply, though there is still a vast number of smokers.

☐ What are the similarities in the problems facing those who wish to curb these activities?

■ There are several: further legislation is opposed on the grounds of the infringement of individual freedom; both legislation and the use of fiscal measures would be electorally unpopular for a government; any major reduction in consumption would have serious consequences for the national economy; both the tobacco and drinks industries have extremely powerful and effective lobbies in Parliament; and both alcohol and tobacco are addictive.*

Successive governments have been reluctant to take more action to combat smoking. Here, for example, is how the government of the day reacted to the news, in 1955, that there was a link between cigarette smoking and cancer. As

*Addiction is discussed in greater detail in *Experiencing and Explaining Disease*, Chapter 10, *ibid*.

you will see there is a shift of emphasis between the private and public statements:

> ### Cabinet ignored cancer link with smoking
>
> The Cabinet was first told of the link between smoking and lung cancer in a report from the Government Actuary thirty years ago. But no action was taken because of the tax revenues from cigarettes and a £250,000 grant to the Medical Research Council from the tobacco industry. The decision to ignore the evidence is disclosed among the official documents released under the 30-year rule at the Public Record Office. (In a cabinet meeting) Mr Ian MacLeod, the Minister of Health said that: 'There was no doubt in his own mind that a relationship between smoking and lung cancer had been established'. But Mr MacLeod said, in the Commons: 'I would draw attention to the fact there is so far no firm evidence of the way in which smoking may cause lung cancer or of the extent to which it does so'.
>
> (Pearce Wright, *The Times*, January 7, 1985)

The tobacco industry has many other powers besides granting money for medical research. Ever since the link between smoking and cancer was established, it has fought a long and hard campaign against government attempts at control and against the work of health educators. In the UK, it has its own research bureau which tries to show that when looked at from the right angle, there is far less to worry about than doctors and health educators claim. And for the consumer, it has continued to mount vast advertising campaigns; indeed, in 1982 the industry spent $2 000 million world-wide on advertising and, as with alcohol, about 100 times more was spent on advertising in the UK than was spent on health education. Indeed, the tobacco companies use their vast resources explicitly to counteract the health educators' message. This can be seen in a market research report for an advertising campaign for an American brand known as 'Viceroy':

> The marketing efforts must cope with consumers' attitudes about smoking and health, either providing them a *rationale* for smoking a full flavour VICEROY or providing a means of *repressing* their concerns, about smoking a full flavour VICEROY. (Viceroy Strategy, 1976; cited in Taylor, 1984, p.180)

The tobacco companies have been highly versatile in their attempts to evade restriction. Although cigarette advertising was banned from television in the UK in 1965, the tobacco companies have been able to circumvent the legislation, and in 1981 commanded 247 hours of television time through their sponsorship of a range of sporting events. This should be judged alongside the total time of *all* TV advertisements in a year of 510 hours. This form of advertising is also incredibly cheap. As the advertising magazine, *Campaign*, has noted, the snooker championship sponsored by the Imperial Tobacco Company ('Embassy' brand) 'must rank as the best media buy of the century': in 1980 £50 a minute compared with £140 000 a minute for peak time commercials. Moreover, the commercial health of the tobacco companies is not dependent solely on their advertising; direct pressure for the right to smoke can come from smokers themselves.

Smoke fear

A smoking ban on single-decker buses in Newport, Gwent, is to be dropped after five years because staff say they are frightened of being assaulted when they try to enforce it.

(*The Guardian*,
October 5, 1984)

☐ Given the increasing evidence of the dangers of passive smoking, should the authorities in Newport have dropped the smoking ban?

■ It is unreasonable to expect staff to have to put up with threats of assault. Until the vast majority of the public are prepared to abide by the ban and maybe openly support the staff, the authorities have little option but to drop it.

In short, there is a powerful combination of demands for personal liberty, of vast and determined commercial power, of addiction, of party-political fears about losing votes in elections and of governmental concerns about treasury revenue (equal to one third of the cost of the NHS), all of which has been dubbed 'the smoke ring' by Peter Taylor, an investigative journalist. Despite this there has been a decline in the prevalence of smoking in the UK since the early 1970s, largely as a result of health education, supported occasionally by substantial increases in excise duty. In addition, there has been a steady increase in the elimination of smoking from public places, and an acceptance that people have a right to work in a smoke-free environment if they so wish. Is there anything more that could be done to accelerate the decline in smoking?

Some critics of government policy have argued that more use should be made of fiscal measures. They argue that despite concerns about obtaining money from cigarettes sales, there is no evidence that increasing the duty would lead to a fall in government revenue, at least in the short term. Unlike alcohol, the price elasticity of tobacco is such that a 20 per cent increase in price would lead to a 10 per cent decrease in consumption, and no reduction or even an increase in overall revenue raised (Cohen and Henderson, 1983). As for the argument that excise duty is a regressive tax, they argue that some of the extra revenue generated from increasing the duty could be redistributed, through changes in direct taxation (such as income tax) and social security, to the poorer members of society to counteract the increased inequities which the change in duty may initially cause. While this may be attractive in theory, there is always the danger with such schemes that the redistributive component may never be carried out — it is much easier to impose a regressive tax than to institute redistribution.

Occupational and environmental protection

On an average working day in this country four workers will die, and over 3 000 will be injured seriously enough to lose three or more days from work. The total number of injured runs into millions every year. (TUC, 1975, p.5)

Ever since the Health and Morals of Apprentices Act in 1802, legislation protecting people's health in their place of work has steadily increased.* The multiplication of Acts has been matched by attempts to review and rationalise existing legislation. The best example of this process is the 1974 Health and Safety at Work Act (HSW) which brought together, and extended, legislation covering such diverse settings as factories and nuclear installations, mines and quarries, shops and offices. Moreover, for the first time, the jobs of over eight million people including postmen, photographers, teachers, doctors, nurses, clergymen and many more, gained some protection.

One of the key questions regarding health and the workplace is who should be responsible for ensuring a high degree of safety — employers or employees, or both?

☐ Suppose that someone working in a very noisy environment suffers damage to their hearing. Who would you consider was at fault?

■ Most people would consider it was the employer's responsibility to protect his or her employees.

---

*The working environment and health is discussed in *The Health of Nations*, Chapter 10 and *Birth to Old Age*, Chapter 12, *ibid.*; and the history of occupational legislation is covered in *Caring for Health: History and Diversity, ibid.*

☐ But suppose the employer had supplied protective ear muffs, which the employee had not used. Now who do you think was responsible?

■ You may feel it was the employee because he or she failed to use the muffs.

☐ You then discover that not only are the muffs uncomfortable to wear, but the employees claim that when they wear them they can no longer hear other sounds that spell danger, such as the machinery jamming or somebody shouting a warning. Now who do you think was responsible for the damage to the employee's hearing?

■ This is a difficult question — the employers may be under tight financial constraints and claim to be unable to afford alternative measures (though noise is often one of the cheaper hazards to control). Equally, the employee's decision not to use the muffs was understandable in the circumstances.

While the question of responsibility may not always be clear cut at the level of the shop floor, the HSW Act is quite clear that in principle it is the employer who is responsible. However, unless employees take action, little may be done. While some trade unions have made relatively little effort in this area, others have established sophisticated methods of monitoring the health both of their current and retired members. The General, Municipal, Boilermakers and Allied Trades Union (GMBATU) have, for example, mounted a campaign to prevent occupational cancers. An edited version of material produced by the union to guide its safety representatives in the investigation of possible carcinogens appears in the Course Reader. You should read this article now.

☐ In what way does the union's view of a *possible* carcinogen in the workplace differ from that of employers or government?

■ The union assumes that chemicals and other agents are dangerous until proved otherwise, whereas employers and government tend to assume there is no problem until clear proof of harm is demonstrated.

☐ Why does the union claim that only a low level of proof of carcinogenicity is required before action can be taken?

■ If workers wait for a high level of proof to become available, several of them are likely to have become victims of the carcinogen before any action is taken.

☐ Can you suggest any disadvantage there might be for the workforce if this approach were pushed hard by the union?

■ Since the carcinogenicity of many industrial materials is not known, it could lead to large numbers of suspect chemicals and other agents being abandoned. If alternatives were either more expensive or maybe not

even available, then the future of the plant and everybody's jobs could be put at risk.

In practice, trade union involvement in monitoring safety has, in some industries, led to much needed improvements in working conditions. There are, however, some notable exceptions, such as the continued existence in the clothing trade of small backstreet sweatshops in which conditions are often unhealthy or even dangerous. Although the HSW Act gives workers the right to appoint their own safety representatives, this is only feasible if the workforce is unionised, something that is seldom the case in those places of work that are most in need of reform.

Traditional levels of health and safety in factory and workplace have undoubtedly been too low. But even if those levels are dramatically improved, certain problems will remain. Suppose, for example, it is decided to raise tenfold the safety margin for exposure to a carcinogen: from one in 100 000 to one in 1 000 000. Even with this major improvement there is still an element of risk. Precisely where should we stop and just how much are we prepared to pay to avoid such risks? In the early 1980s, around £5 million had to be spent on modifications to the main hospital in Liverpool to meet new fire regulations. Would that £5 million have been better spent on providing health care or combating smoking? What level of risk are we prepared to accept, given that a risk such as fire damage can never be completely eliminated? Just as tragic choices have to be made regarding curative services, so the same is true for prevention.

Health education

During the case studies, we have discussed the role of the different preventive approaches available, with the exception of one: health education. While British governments have varied in their views about the use of such approaches as legislation and fiscal measures, there has been unanimity about health education. In 1976, the government (at that time Labour) restated its commitment in a key consultative document:

> There is much potential for prevention in health education aimed at altering people's attitudes towards such things as tobacco, alcohol and exercise — persuading them in effect to invest in their own health. (DHSS, 1976b, p.87)

The underlying belief was that 'the onus of making decisions in order to safeguard health must necessarily rest on the individual'. When the Conservative Party came to power in 1979, they too emphasised the same themes, as the following statement from Geoffrey Finsberg, Under

Secretary of State for Health and Social Services, makes clear:

> This government is committed to the goal of better health for everyone. We believe that in a free society this can only be achieved by the informed exercise of personal responsibility. (Finsberg, 1982, p.8)

This policy has, however, met two serious criticisms. The first has concerned the content and style of health education: critics have argued that the message is often badly put across and may even sometimes do more harm than good. The second is political: health education can be a device by which governments and health professionals distract attention from the real causes of health problems. Let us consider each in turn.

Muir Gray, a community physician, has suggested several possible ways in which poor technique may let health education down. The first is that of the *linguistic* aspects of educational material. Clearly any type of teaching depends on the target audience sharing the same meanings of words as the teacher. For example, health educators often attach the word 'risk' to activities that they want people to avoid, such as smoking. But to many young people 'risk' has connotations of adulthood.* Rather than avoidance, they might actually be encouraged to seek out such activities. Similarly, threats about the consequences of taking risks may prove ineffective in young people. To someone of fifteen, the argument that people who smoke sometimes die suddenly at the age of fifty-five may have little impact if the prospect of being fifty-six is not only difficult to imagine but has little appeal.

Communicating the size of any risk can also prove difficult. By its nature, health education has to consider and communicate the likelihood of ill health and death associated with different activities. The difficulty of the task is compounded in mass campaigns which attempt to address people of different ages, sexes, social classes and ethnic groups, each of whom may attach a different shade of meaning to the same word.

In addition to linguistic difficulties, there are *psychological* barriers to be overcome. One aspect of health education is to raise people's level of anxiety about the subject to stimulate them to take some action. But there are dangers in raising it too high. The smoker who cannot stop may be converted from a happy smoker to an unhappy, anxious, guilt-ridden smoker. For example, what happens to pregnant women who find they cannot give up smoking and yet continue to be confronted by health education literature (Figure 9.11) about the dangers to their baby?

*This is discussed in *Birth to Old Age: Health in Transition*, Chapter 10, *ibid*.

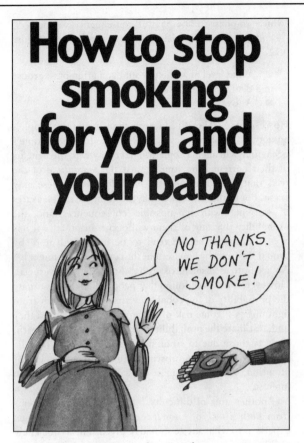

Figure 9.11 Anti-smoking education for pregnant women produced by the Health Education Council.

This was true for about 40 per cent of women in a study by Hilary Graham, a sociologist. This was the response of one woman:

> I've cut down and I'm down to ten a day. If I cut down any more I take it out on my son which isn't fair on him so it's one bairn or the other. (Cited in Graham, 1983, p.345)

Graham concluded that the traditional health education message exhorting mothers to be more responsible was unlikely to be effective and might even engender feelings of failure and guilt. How might one avoid this? A partial solution was suggested in much earlier research by two American psychologists, Irving Janis and Seymour Feshbach, in 1953. They gave different sorts of illustrated talks on dental hygiene to various groups and measured the proportion of people who subsequently adhered to the recommended practices. They used three levels of anxiety arousal — minimal (which rarely alluded to the consequences of tooth neglect), moderate (which included a mild description of the dangers of neglect), and strong (which emphasised the painful consequences of neglect) — and compared the effects with a control group (Figure 9.12).

☐ What level of anxiety would you attempt to arouse in a dental hygiene education programme?

■ A low level.

However, even if health educators manage to raise people's anxiety to this optimal level, it does not follow that people's behaviour will alter. People still have to weigh the benefits of their current behaviour against the *magnitude* of the risks that it involves and the *probability* that these may occur. For example, smokers have to compare the pleasures of smoking with its possible consequences and the probability that any of them will occur. In practice it has been found that people tend to be influenced more by probability than by how serious the consequences might be. An accurate assessment of probability is therefore crucial. However, it has been found that people often overestimate the probability of improbable events, such as death from lightning (a lifetime risk of about one in 40 000), and they underestimate the probability of common causes of death, such as those due to smoking (Table 9.3). This may be because deaths from obscure causes attract a lot of attention, whereas common causes generate little or no interest.

Another area of difficulty for health education stems from both a *lack of knowledge* and *agreement* amongst experts as to what advice should be given. This is not a new problem:

So much has been written and taught of late years on the principles of a healthy diet that the ordinary person might be excused if he were to find the wealth of information bewildering and fall back in despair upon the easiest and most haphazard method of satisfying his appetite. (Lane, 1934, p.269)

Although written over fifty years ago, this view could equally well have been expressed today. The difficulties in

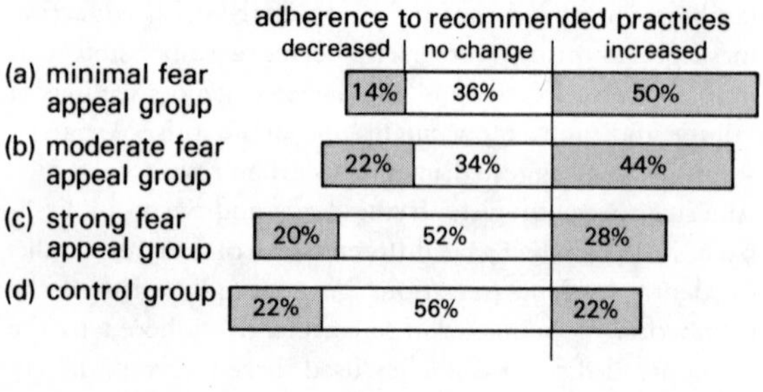

Table 9.3 True rate of causes of death in the USA compared with judged rate

Cause of death	True rate per million	Judged rate per million
flood	1.0	4.3
pregnancy	2.2	9.6
appendicitis	4.5	4.4
poisoning	12.8	6.5
fire	36.9	19.0
leukaemia	72.7	14.0
suicide	123.0	333.7
breast cancer	155.8	18.0
car accident	276.7	169.4
lung cancer	379.2	48.6
stroke	1 045.5	53.3
cancer	1 640.0	2 376.1
heart disease	3 690.0	1 295.0

(Source: Lichtenstein, cited in Hallett, 1980, p.503)

giving dietary advice will be considered further in the discussion of coronary heart disease in Chapter 11.

Criticism of the techniques of health education are not restricted to its content and style: some critics have argued that an even more serious problem is the lack of interest shown by health professionals.

The first physicians by debauch were made;
Excess began and sloth sustains the trade.
(John Dryden (1631–1700))

As Dryden's couplet suggests, doctors (and most other health staff) have a financial interest in disease. But even where there is no such incentive, which is broadly true for practitioners within the NHS, it remains the case that what most staff are trained in is the management of disease. Health and health promotion come very far down the list of priorities.

Here, then, is a further major opportunity — so it is argued — for prevention. Health education should be more than a matter of pamphlets and posters, it should be something that *all* health professionals are trained in, and not just health visitors, community physicians and health education officers. That such ideas may have some practical benefit is demonstrated by work such as that of Mike Russell and his colleagues at the Institute of Psychiatry in London. They compared the effectiveness of four different strategies for giving up smoking in a group of smokers attending their general practitioners. The strategies and the percentage of smokers who gave up smoking, and were still non-smokers one year later, in each of the four groups is shown in Figure 9.13. The authors of the study calculated that if all GPs in the UK adopted the

adherence to recommended practices

	decreased	no change	increased
(a) minimal fear appeal group	14%	36%	50%
(b) moderate fear appeal group	22%	34%	44%
(c) strong fear appeal group	20%	52%	28%
(d) control group	22%	56%	22%

Figure 9.12 Effect of fear appeals in an illustrated talk on dental hygiene practice.
(Source: Janis and Feshbach, 1953, Table 6, p.84)

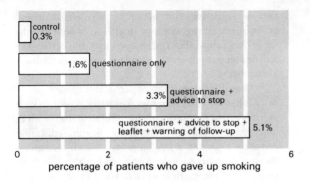

Figure 9.13 Proportion of patients who gave up smoking for at least one year in response to various health education strategies from their GP.
(Source: Russell, *et al.*, 1979, p.231)

most successful strategy, the result could be an additional half million ex-smokers a year.

Research such as this has suggested to some of those working in primary care, that its whole orientation ought to be shifted much more radically in a preventive direction; that far from sitting in the surgery and just seeing what turns up, general practitioners should be actively monitoring the health of their entire practice and intervening before disease gets a grip on their patients. One prominent advocate of this position is a general practitioner, Julian Tudor Hart. Extracts from his article 'A New Kind of Doctor' are contained in the Course Reader (Part 3, Section 3.4) which you should now read.

☐ What does Hart see as the advantage of the 'new kind of doctor'?

■ They would be more likely to encounter disease in its early stages or even prevent it from occurring.

☐ What are the possible disadvantages?

■ It may be argued that this new vision of doctoring is an infringement of personal liberty. Should doctors have the right to monitor their patients' lives so intensively and then tell them what to do?

In short, more active attempts at prevention have been viewed by some people as yet another form of *medicalisation* — the extension of the influence of medicine over people's lives. This remains a largely academic dispute, as few GPs have adopted Hart's suggestions yet. What is clear is that for this and other reasons, health education faces considerable difficulties if it is to be successful. And even if, or when, it has overcome the technical difficulties it would still find itself subjected to political criticism. Why should this be so? Consider once more the phrase used in the 1976 consultative document, *Prevention and Health*:

☐ If 'the onus ... rest[s] on the individual', what is implied about the cause of illness when it arises?

■ The cause must be the failure of the individual to safeguard her or his health.

☐ Is this a plausible analysis of disease arising from alcohol or tobacco consumption?

■ There is clearly an element of truth in it; after all some people do manage to reduce consumption or give up. But such remarks obscure the government's own revenue interest in alcohol and tobacco sales, not to mention the enormous pressure applied by the industries.

As a result, critics of government policy have argued that such statements amount to mere *victim-blaming*: pinning the responsibility on the individual who actually suffers the disease and ignoring the crucial role played by others. Indeed, they argue that victim-blaming is a standard part of many health professionals' view of patients. This includes health education that attempts to get patients to use health services 'properly'. Consider, for example, a woman who fails to attend an antenatal clinic. This may be seen by staff as evidence that she is unreliable, irrational, unconcerned about her future child and even, perhaps, culpably negligent. Thus, she might be viewed as in need of serious re-education.

☐ What alternative interpretation could staff make about women who fail to attend antenatal clinics?

■ That there is something wrong with the way the clinics operate, so that women do not use them.

Thus, although it is possible that some pregnant women are selfish and irresponsible, this ignores the difficulties many women face in travelling by public transport to the clinic, having to wait two hours to be seen, only then to be seen for five minutes by a doctor whose interests may be more in her pregnancy than in her as a person. In these circumstances it might be argued that what is surprising is that so many women *do* attend.

In other words, critics argue that the emphasis in health education on personal responsibility serves the interests of governments and health staff by deflecting attention from their own failings. Indeed, a body such as the Health Education Council has been viewed simply as a device to get governments off the hook:

government ministers from both sides of the House, along with their civil servant advisers, have consistently used the HEC as an instant, highly visible, relatively cheap and superficially plausible means of responding to pressure to 'do something' about a particular health problem ... the quango image and the illusion of independence of the HEC allow programmes initiated for political reasons to be carried out behind a smokescreen of professional and scientific justification. (St George, 1981, p.51)

☐ What points might be cited in response to these allegations?

■ You might argue that smoking and drinking do carry at least some measure of personal responsibility; that there are huge public pressures on governments to act and yet their opportunities for action are often severely circumscribed; and that getting people to change their lifestyle is much cheaper than improving their living conditions.

Both sides in the debate can therefore point to powerful arguments in their support. However, the critics of conventional health education have yet another argument: that the current notion of health education is far too narrowly conceived. 'Yes,' they say, 'people do need information about the causes of disease and what they can do about them; and, yes, health education — as in the seat-belt campaign — can play an important role in changing public opinion; and, yes, indeed, people do need information about how to use health services; but the information they are currently given and the mannner in which they are given it is wholly inadequate.'

What, then, is an appropriate form for health education? In 1980 a group of health researchers at the Unit for the Study of Health Policy in London suggested three related roles (Draper, *et al.*, 1980). The first concentrates on the individual, the family and on personal responsibility for health. The researchers suggested that rather than advising and instructing people on how to behave, health education at this level should be concerned with providing biological and physiological information about the human body. Second, they proposed a role for education about health services, but one oriented to informing people about what is available and how to gain access to it. In addition, they suggested, this type of health education should be extended to explanations of why services are the way they are and the difficult, sometimes tragic, choices about resource alloca-tions that, as you have seen in Chapter 3, have to be made by health authorities. This would not only help people to understand the underlying issues confronting those responsible for making decisions about the provision of services, but would also lead to wider participation in that process. And finally, health education should attempt to inform people about those aspects of the environment that damage their health in the hope that a wider awareness of such factors might lead to pressure for environmental changes. This might include pressure for increased safety at work and in the home, fluoridation of water supplies, and even reductions in the level of unemployment.

☐ What benefits can you see in this alternative model of health education?

■ The more that people know about the biological and social determinants of health and disease, the more they may strive for action (both personal and environmental) to improve matters. Moreover, the more they know about health services, the better they will be able to both use them and take part in the debates about them.

☐ What difficulties can you see in this model?

■ First, though a greater level of participation in such debates might be produced, not everyone may wish to participate. Second, if current health education provokes criticism, a new approach which focuses on the social and economic aspects of health is likely to prove even more controversial because of the overt political nature of such criticism.

Conclusion

Primary prevention has some big advantages — in particular, it offers the only real hope of combating the major killer of our times, smoking. But, for all this hope, preventing disease is not always as easy as it might first appear. There are many barriers. Legislation can be hard to enforce. Fiscal measures, while effective in some cases, are rarely electorally popular. Commercial, governmental, and popular interests may act as serious barriers to reform. And, as you have seen, health education has its critics — on the one hand, it is not always effective, on the other hand, it too, just like legislation, can sometimes prove both an intrusion on personal liberty and an unwarranted accusation of individual culpability.

There are, then, many dilemmas to be resolved. But might it be that the biggest difficulty of all is simply that we do not spend enough on health education; that the NHS is, as has often been said, merely a 'National Illness Service'? Have we got the entire balance of spending wrong? To answer this we first need to know the answer to another question: just how much do we spend on prevention?

☐ Why might this be a difficult question?

■ It all depends on how you define 'prevention'.

Taking 'prevention' as those activities discussed in this and the preceding chapter, two health economists, David Cohen and John Henderson, calculated that in 1980/81 almost £1 000 million was spent in the UK (Table 9.4). As you can see, they allocated a proportion of various NHS budgets to prevention (such as 40 per cent of community services) and identified areas of expenditure in other central and local government departments. The total of around £1 billion compares with about £13 billion spent on NHS curative and caring services in 1980/81. However, these figures do not include a whole host of other measures that have the prevention of ill-health and injuries as one of their goals: improvements in road design, enforcement of speed limits, construction of new houses, maintenance of sewers and water supplies, and many others.

Table 9.4 UK expenditure on prevention (£'000) 1980/81.

NHS		
Community services	(40%)	312 652
General medical services	(10%)	75 978
General dental services	(20%)	101 533
Hospital services	(0.8%)	59 385
Non-NHS (public sector)		
Ministry of Agriculture, Fisheries and Food		34
Health and Safety Executive		72 167
Department of the Environment		268
DHS (including health education, public health laboratories)		19 882
Home Office		45
Northern Ireland Office		109
Scottish Office		1
Department of Trade		30
Central Office of Information		100
Environmental health (local government)		309 000
Private and voluntary bodies		15 500
	Total	966 648

(Source: Cohen and Henderson, 1983, Tables 1, 4 and 5)

Indeed, prevention can go wider still. Throughout this chapter one key aspect of health has largely been ignored: the inequalities in health that exist between the sexes, age groups, social classes, ethnic groups and geographical locations. Some of these inequalities arise from differences in recognised risks — the prevalence of smoking is greater in men than women, and in lower than higher social classes. However, such differences in recognised health hazards only *partly* explain the inequalities in mortality and morbidity rates between social groups. Thus, however effective the sorts of preventive measure discussed in this chapter might be, there will still be little impact on the major social inequalities in health. To affect those it will be necessary to tackle the underlying factors: the relative positions in society of men and women, black people and white people, and higher and lower social classes. Suggestions about dealing with social class differences is the subject of the next chapter.

Objectives for Chapter 9

When you have read this chapter you should be able to:

9.1 Explain why the enactment of legislation often requires a long political struggle, for it may be challenged on the grounds of restricting individual freedom, diminishing positive liberty, being based on insufficient evidence, being difficult to enforce, and risking alienating large numbers of law-abiding people.

9.2 Describe the different ways in which commercial interests that are deemed to be health-damaging may be restricted: by fiscal measures, legal restrictions on the availability of the product and control of advertising.

9.3 Explain how legislation to control environmental hazards raises issues both of apportioning responsibility and of deciding on what is an acceptable risk in the light of the costs of protection.

9.4 Describe the contribution that health education has made in preventive health care; the difficulties it faces as regards content, style and lack of professional interest; and the ways in which it might be reformed to avoid a victim-blaming approach.

Questions for Chapter 9

1 (*Objective 9.1*) 'The only purpose for which power can rightfully be exercised over any member of a civilised society is to prevent harm to others. His own good, either physical or moral, is not a sufficient warrant' (J.S. Mill, 1859; cited in Gray, 1979, p.157). Would the banning of smoking in public places be justifiable according to John Stuart Mill's philosophy?

2 (*Objective 9.2*)

> ### End 'cant' about alcohol and raise drink prices doctors urge government
>
> Alcohol abuse is costing Britain at least £1,600 million a year, and ministers are talking 'cant' in telling doctors to do more when the answers lie in government policy, a conference on alcohol was told yesterday.
>
> (Nicholas Timmins, *The Times*, November 29, 1984)

What are the 'answers' that lie in government policy? How might such 'answers' affect the personal lives of doctors?

3 (*Objective 9.3*) Table 7.2 shows the value of a human life implicit in four decisions to control environmental hazards, made by the British government. What factors may account for such dramatic differences?

4 (*Objective 9.4*) 'Today the most serious health problems arise from personal lifestyles — smoking, misuse of alcohol, bad diet, lack of exercise. They can be overcome only by individuals accepting greater personal responsibility for their own well-being' (Finsberg, 1982, p.2). What obstacles may health education face when trying to persuade individuals to accept a greater personal responsibility for their own well-being by reducing their alcohol consumption?

10

'To make the poor less poor'

During this chapter you will be asked to read an article in the Course Reader entitled 'Inequalities in health: the Black Report and reactions to it' (Part 7, Section 7.4).

Reflecting in 1890 on progress towards 'that great system of Preventive Medicine which is hoped for by the Sanitary Reformers', Sir John Simon, one of the leading health reformers of nineteenth-century Britain, turned his attentions to the question 'how far the poor can be made less poor?':

> In the whole range of questions concerning the Public Health, there is not, in my opinion, any one to be deemed more important ... whenever I reflect what chief factors have to be desired for progressive improvement in our conditions of public health, I doubt if any can be considered more essential, or ought to be hoped for with more ardent hope, than that the poverty of our poorer classes may be lessened. (Simon, 1890, p.444)

Since Simon made these observations, much has changed. Medical science has held out an ever-increasing range of treatments; a national health service has been created with the intention of providing comprehensive health care to poor and rich alike; a welfare state has been developed to remove the worst features of social insecurity; and economic growth has greatly increased the material standard of living. The health of poorer sections of the population in the UK has dramatically improved since the nineteenth century, and poverty and disadvantage no longer exist on the scale familiar to Simon.

In the light of these changes, it is perhaps not surprising to note that many contemporary policies towards public health and prevention pay little attention to the issues that concerned many nineteenth-century reformers. Indeed, as the previous chapter showed, many of these contemporary policies define the health problems they seek to tackle in such a way as to exclude social inequalities in health: personal behaviour, rather than age or class or gender or ethnicity, is frequently identified as the relevant dimension of analysis.

Not everyone, however, agrees with this trend — Jerry Morris, a community physician has argued that John

A Worker's Speech to a Doctor
(an extract)

Are you able to heal?
When we come to you
Our rags are torn off us
And you listen all over our naked body
As to the cause of our illness.
One glance at our rags would
Tell you more. It is the same cause that wears out
Our bodies and our clothes.

The pain in our shoulder comes
You say, from the damp; and this is also the reason
For the stain on the wall of our flat.
So tell us;
Where does the damp come from?

Too much work and too little food
Makes us feeble and thin.
Your prescription says:
Put on more weight.
You might as well tell a bullrush
Not to get wet.

Bertolt Brecht

Simon's question is no less relevant to health policy today than it was a century ago:

> late in the twentieth century — we are still beset by nineteenth-century type problems of deprivation. If we are to be rid of social inequalities in health these will have to be resolved at the same time as more focussed education and health service measures are instituted and the initiatives provided for changes in lifestyle, diet and exercise and smoking and drinking behaviour. (Morris, 1980, p.1003)

The term '*social inequalities in health*' refers to the variations in the experience of health and disease which are apparent between different social groups in the population. While biological factors help to explain part of these variations, such as some of those related to age and sex, the different social and economic circumstances in which people live account for most of the differences between social classes, the married and the unmarried, men and women, geographical areas and ethnic groups.* Such inequalities extract a considerable toll. If for example the mortality rate for social class I had applied to social classes IV and V during 1970–1972, there would have been 74 000

*These differences are discussed in detail in *The Health of Nations*, Chapters 9 and 10, *ibid*.

fewer deaths amongst people under the age of seventy-five, including 10 000 fewer among children.

However, while the evidence of continuing inequalities in the social distribution of ill-health is incontrovertible, there is very little agreement about the reasons why they exist, and even less about what can or should be done. And these disagreements raise many issues other than the prevention of ill-health. If social inequalities in health have persisted despite the existence of a welfare state, has the welfare state been a failure? If so, how has it failed, and why? Should it be improved or abandoned? How much should health policy have to do with the whole question of social, political and economic reform? These are some of the questions addressed in this chapter.

The chapter begins by tracing the intentions, achievements and failures of post-war welfare policies in the UK. It then examines the main strands of opinion, both from the left and the right of the political spectrum, on the lessons that can be drawn from the experience of these policies. Finally, the chapter looks at prospects for social and economic policies that may in the future reduce social inequalities in health.

The dawn of a new era: the social legislation of the 1940s

> Over the greater part of Western Europe, the common values for which we stand are known and prized. We must indeed beware of defining these values in purely nineteenth-century terms. If we speak of democracy we do not mean a democracy which maintains the right to vote but forgets the right to work and the right to live. If we speak of freedom we do not mean a rugged individualism which excludes social organisation and economic planning. If we speak of equality we do not mean a political equality nullified by social and economic privilege. If we speak of economic reconstruction we think less of maximum (though this job too will be required) than of equitable distribution ... The European house cannot be put in order unless we put our own house in order first. The new order cannot be based on the preservation of privilege, whether the privilege be that of a country, of a class or of an individual.
>
> (Editorial, *The Times*, July 1, 1940)

This editorial comment from *The Times* in 1940, with its calls for a new order, economic reconstruction and equitable distribution, provides telling evidence of the influence of war on attitudes to social reform. Evacuation, the Blitz, rationing and conscription produced an unprecedented degree of social intermingling, and made obvious to all the extent of the poverty and disadvantage that had, for many people, blighted the inter-war years. At the same time the extensive government control and planning involved in organising the war effort illustrated what was possible. Indeed, the war created amongst many Britons, from all ranks and conditions, an extraordinary sense of social cohesion, of national and social unity.

Hopes for a better future were given concrete form in the now famous report of William Beveridge (Figure 10.1), an ex-civil servant turned academic and government adviser, who had been involved in the formulation of social policy since the early years of the twentieth century. The *Report on Social Insurance and Allied Services*, published in 1942, set out a plan for a system of *social security* which was intended to abolish poverty. But Beveridge's vision was broader than this. In an appendix to the report he argued that:

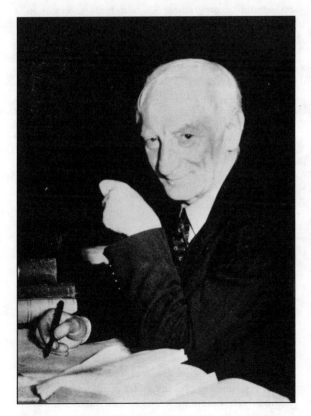

Figure 10.1 William Beveridge (1879–1963). Social reformer, economist and civil servant.

The plan for Social Security is put forward as part of a general programme of social policy. It is only part of an attack upon five giant evils: upon the physical Want with which it is directly concerned, upon Disease which often causes that want, and brings many other troubles in its train, upon Ignorance, which no democracy can afford among its citizens, upon the Squalor which arises mainly through haphazard distribution of industry and population, and upon Idleness which destroys wealth and corrupts men... (Beveridge, 1942, Appendix A, paragraph 83)

An attack upon each of these evils was not just desirable but also necessary, for success on one front was seen to be dependent on success on others. With regard to his plan for social security, for example, Beveridge proposed three related developments. The central feature was a scheme of *Social Insurance* whereby people in employment would pay a *flat-rate* weekly contribution in return for which they and their dependants would receive a basic cash benefit, as of right, when earnings were interrupted or lost. The scheme was to be as comprehensive as possible, both in relation to its coverage of the population and in relation to the causes of the poverty it sought to relieve: chief amongst these being sickness, unemployment, old age, disability and maternity. The second element was a scheme of *National Assistance*, which would provide cash benefits for those who had no other source of income and who were not covered by the insurance system. Finally, individuals were to be encouraged to take out *voluntary insurance* to provide additions to the basic minimum.

Two separate principles for paying out social security benefits were contained within these proposals: *universalism*, in which everyone receives benefits regardless of their wealth or income, and *means-testing*, in which benefit is only paid after detailed examination of a person's 'means'. This distinction has a long history and is central to all debates about social security: means-testing had been an important part of services provided in the nineteenth century under Poor Law legislation. Some of the arguments for and against each principle were as follows: that means-testing in practice often involved humiliation, loss of self-respect and official snooping into private affairs, whereas universal entitlement avoided these problems and involved few administrative costs; that means-testing might direct benefits to those most in need whereas universal entitlement would allow people to obtain services and benefits they did not really need.

Although the proposals of Beveridge included some means-tested benefits, such as the 'safety net' of the National Assistance scheme which was only paid if claimants could prove they had no other source of income, the general tenor of the proposals was universalist. The respective merits and drawbacks of these principles have continued to be debated fiercely and form an important part of arguments in the 1980s both over the past and future of social policy.

Beveridge's plan was not, however, restricted to a system of social security. Indeed, he was adamant that the success of such a system depended upon three further developments: the introduction of a *child allowance* to be paid to all families to help with the cost of child rearing; the provision of a comprehensive health and rehabilitation service;* and the avoidance of mass unemployment. The need for a child allowance was based on the findings of social researchers, such as Seebohm Rowntree, who some years earlier had argued that the risk of poverty was not just related to the level of savings, but also to the number and age of children in a family. Each of Beveridge's proposals were interrelated — the absence of one would jeopardise the success of the others.

☐ In what ways do you think the social insurance scheme depended on the other proposals?

■ The social insurance scheme required people to pay regular contributions while in employment. Both the provision of a health and rehabilitation scheme and avoiding mass unemployment would help ensure that people were able to make these contributions. They would also reduce the number of claims for benefit, and the size of the claims.

While the establishment of social security schemes and health services depended largely on the provision of sufficient funds, how was the other major plank of Beveridge's plan to be achieved — the maintenance of full employment? It had long been evident that a business cycle of 'boom and slump' recurring approximately every four to seven years was a characteristic and inherent feature of the British economy (in common with other capitalist economies). The instability this cycle created in the livelihoods of large parts of the population had been an important reason for the growth of friendly societies and insurance systems in the nineteenth century, for such schemes reduced uncertainty. But the slump that had occurred in the inter-war period had been quite unprecedented both in severity and international impact: in the USA, for example, industrial production fell by 45 per cent from its peak in 1929 to its trough in 1933 (the previous largest fall had been less than 15 per cent in the 1870s). Between the wars, unemployment had become not only widespread but stubbornly persistent, and the lesson seemed clear to some that the only way to break out of semi-permanent recession was through *conscious economic management by governments*.

*The establishment of the NHS is discussed further in *Caring for Health: History and Diversity*, Chapter 5, *ibid*.

The economists who did most to work out the implications of the anguished inter-war lesson were a Swede, Gunnar Myrdal, a Pole, Michael Kalecki, and above all an English economist, John Maynard Keynes. The nub of Keynes's contribution was to persuade western economic policy-makers that a 1930s-style slump *could* be avoided after the war if governments used their powers of taxation and expenditure to regulate the level of demand in the economy and if they could agree to a strong framework of international cooperation in economic policy. Such *Keynesian* policies were widely adopted in the aftermath of the war, and the 1944 White Paper on employment policy in the UK held out the promise of ensuring one of the preconditions for the success of Beveridge's welfare policies — full employment.

Armed with these new intellectual weapons and impressed by the success of the wartime state control of the economy, the post-war Labour government embarked on massive social and economic reconstruction. This included an extensive programme of nationalisation, eventually involving public ownership of the Bank of England, airways, coal, gas, electricity, railways, canals, ports and the iron and steel industries. They also promised a massive housebuilding programme — four million houses in a decade. The Education Act of 1944 had already provided for a comprehensive national education system up to the age of fifteen; and in 1946 universal child allowances of five shillings a week were introduced for every second and subsequent child.

Finally, on 5 July 1948, the central pillars of what was to become known as the '*Welfare State*' came into operation — a comprehensive national health service and a system of social security providing both a range of universal benefits, such as retirement pensions, unemployment benefit and disability benefit, and means-tested benefits under the National Assistance scheme. The role of the last was defined in the House of Commons by Aneurin Bevan:

The amount to be left to the [National] Assistance Board, after the whole of needs have been met by all the other measures — insurance allowances, old age provisions, sickness benefits — will be very small indeed. Only the residual categories will be left. (*Hansard*, 1948)

☐ How, therefore, were 'the poor to be made less poor' by all this?

■ By the public provision of *minimum standards* of income, housing, health and education, which they would receive as of right; and by state intervention in the economy along Keynesian lines in an attempt to prevent slumps and maintain full employment.

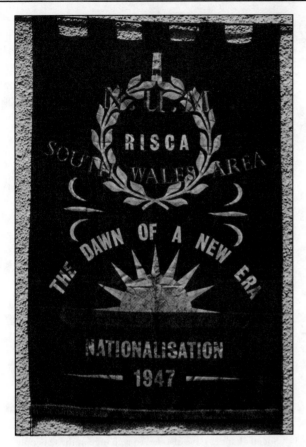

Figure 10.2 Banner of the Risca branch of the National Union of Mineworkers celebrating nationalisation of the coal mines in 1947.

For some, as the banner of the National Union of Mineworkers declared in 1947, it was to be the dawn of a new era (Figure 10.2).

The performance of public welfare

How did the social security system work in practice? We noted earlier that it was only one of a number of interdependent policies, and it follows that it is difficult to isolate any one component and look for failings. Many aspects of the performance of the social security system can only be understood in a wider context. Nevertheless, two particular problems can be described which dogged the system almost from the beginning: the first relating to its *cost*, the second concerning its inflexibility in the face of *changing social conditions*.

The impact of cost can be seen in Table 10.1 which compares estimated and actual expenditure from the 1940s to the 1960s.

☐ How would you describe the relationship between actual and expected expenditure on social security over the period covered by Table 10.1?

■ Initially, actual costs were substantially below the estimates, but by the 1960s actual costs were 50 per cent higher than had been estimated (although inflation accounted for half of this).

By the time the scheme started, the unemployment rate had fallen further and stayed lower than Beveridge, or indeed Keynes, had expected: the new policies of economic management seemed to be achieving more than anyone had predicted. But whereas Beveridge had proposed gradually phasing in retirement pensions over a twenty-year period, they were introduced more rapidly. In addition, the number of pensioners in the population also grew (from 4.2 million claimants in 1950 to 7.4 million by 1970). By 1965 over 80 per cent of the difference between actual and estimated expenditure was due to retirement pensions. Rather than increase taxation to meet these increasing demands on the system, successive governments chose to increase the flat-rate insurance contributions deducted from wage-earners' pay. Under this scheme all wage-earners paid the same

Table 10.1 Social security expenditure: estimated and actual

| | Beveridge's estimates (£m) | | | Actual expenditure (£m) | | |
	1945	1955	1965	1948/9	1955/6	1965/6
Social insurance						
retirement pensions	142	214	339	176.6	312.2	658.8
unemployment	124	123	121	15.2	11.3	26.2
other benefits	148	161	166	89.1	137.8	270.2
all insurance benefits	414	498	626	280.9	461.3	955.2
National assistance	53	46	36	34	76.6	133.9
Children's allowance	127	125	115	65	83.1	80.7
Total expenditure	594	669	777	379.9	621	1 169.8

(Source: adapted from Dilnot, Kay and Morris, 1984, Table 1.2, p.16).

amount, regardless of level of pay. This meant that people on lower income were increasingly paying proportionately more. It was therefore decided to revise the scheme and link the level of contributions to level of pay, making the whole system more like a tax and essentially abandoning the insurance principle. Repeated increases in national insurance contributions have resulted in a significant rise in the proportion of the total wage and salary bill of the country going to the insurance scheme: from 5.5 per cent in 1949 to 16.3 per cent in 1982.

The problems of cost did not only relate to the overall amount. Other problems arose, related to entitlement. For example, while insurance benefits, other than pensions, were not increased in line with inflation, means-tested national assistance benefits were, and more and more people became entitled to claim them. Rather than being, as Bevan had suggested, a 'residual category', national assistance became a crucial part of the whole system, and by 1981 one third of people claiming social insurance benefits were also claiming *supplementary benefits* (the new term for national assistance). Simultaneously, the social insurance scheme turned out to be far less universal in its coverage than intended: by 1981, 47 per cent of people receiving supplementary benefits — some 1.8 million people — had no entitlement to social insurance at all.

So much for the problems of rising costs and lack of entitlement. What of the impact that changing social conditions made? With the benefit of hindsight it is clear that a number of the assumptions underlying the plan introduced in 1948 was unwarranted. Four of these would appear to be particularly important. First, the scheme assumed a model of a two-parent family, with a male breadwinner and a dependent wife. The husband and wife were assumed to work as a team with the wife dependent on the husband for entitlement to insurance benefits. As Beveridge noted:

> On marriage a woman gains a legal right by her husband as a first line of defence against risks which fall directly on the solitary woman. (Beveridge, 1942, p.49, para.108)

The three other assumptions were that the labour force was primarily made up of full-time male workers who would be employed largely uninterrupted all their working lives; that they would earn enough in employment to keep themselves, a dependent wife and one child (child allowances would subsidise other children); and that full employment would be maintained. These assumptions had a number of important consequences: a large number of people who were unable to get regular employment, such as those disabled from birth, were excluded from the insurance scheme altogether as were part-time workers earning below an officially defined weekly minimum wage; no insurance

provision was made for women who were divorced or separated and in need of support but who had no independent entitlement to benefit; and no social security provision at all was provided for the working poor with one child.

Despite these obvious shortcomings, the *family model* underlying the system has continued to influence the design of new benefits. For instance, in the middle of the 1980s married women were unable to receive an Invalid Care Allowance because it was assumed that they would be at home anyway and therefore providing such care could not interrupt their employment and earnings. These assumptions weakened the system from the outset, but the weaknesses have become more pronounced with the passage of time: the increasing number of families headed by a divorced or separated woman, and until recently the increasing number of married women in paid employment, have undermined the assumed family model. Similarly, the return of an extraordinarily high level of unemployment has excluded many young people from the labour force altogether and severely disrupted the employment patterns of many other people. In 1978, an EEC directive instructed the British government to introduce, by 1984, equal treatment within the social insurance system for men and women regardless of marital status (at the time of writing this has yet to be done). However, the assumption of women's dependence on men is still very much a feature of means-tested benefits, and past discrimination has left an important legacy.

Social changes have also led to a change in those people who are at greatest risk of poverty. In 1948, the group most at risk were the elderly, but by 1981 most people living on low incomes were below pensionable age. Those groups most at risk in the 1980s are single parents, the low paid and the unemployed.

☐ Can you suggest why single parenthood might involve a disproportionate risk of poverty?
■ Sole responsibility for child rearing imposes considerable restrictions on a person's availability for work. Additionally, the majority of single parents are women and they are particularly disadvantaged in the labour market being over-represented in low-paid jobs.

Low pay has always been an important cause of poverty, but during periods of high employment, wages tend to be pushed up because of labour shortages and therefore the problem becomes less acute. In recent years, however, with rising unemployment the number of low-paid jobs has increased. In addition, since 1948 the problems of low-paid people, particularly those with dependent children, have been exacerbated by two other developments.

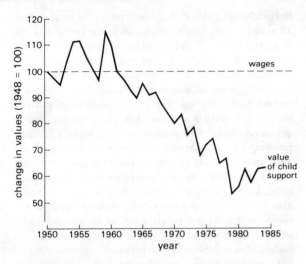

Figure 10.3 The value of child support compared to wages for a two-child family, 1948–1982.
(Source: Dilnot, Kay and Morris, 1984, Figure 1.4)

Table 10.2 Changes in tax rates and thresholds for a two-child family of male manual worker in manufacturing industry (1955–1982)

Year	Tax threshold as a percentage of average earnings*	First tax rate payable (%)
1955	99.5	9
1974	57.1	33
1982	41.4	30

* Includes family allowance/child benefit.

(Source: Walker, Winyard and Pond, 1983, Table 3.2, p.19)

☐ Considering Figure 10.3 and Table 10.2, what have these two developments been?

■ 1 Child support has failed to be increased in line with wages (Figure 10.3).

2 The level of income at which income tax becomes payable has fallen over time. In 1955, for example, a man with a two-child family on average earnings in manufacturing industries received 99.6 per cent of those earnings tax free but by 1982 the figure had fallen to 41.4 per cent (Table 10.2). And while the proportion of income exempt from income tax has fallen, the rate of tax first encountered on the way up the income scale has increased.

The collapse of the final 1948 assumption — that full employment would be maintained — has, however, been the most significant factor affecting the nature and extent of poverty in the UK in recent years. Between 1948 and 1966 registered unemployment averaged 1.7 per cent of the labour force. But by 1974, the numbers of registered unemployed had risen to almost 3 per cent, and by 1985 it had topped 3.1 million — almost 14 per cent of the labour force. Moreover, because so many who are unemployed have been out of work for more than a year (between 25 per cent and 50 per cent depending on the age group), and because universal entitlement to insurance benefits ceases after twelve months' unemployment, increasing numbers of the unemployed have had to rely on supplementary benefits — again, the social security system has proved unable to cope with changed social and economic circumstances.

So a combination of increasing cost and changing social and economic circumstances have placed the social security system under enormous strain. And what of the original aim of abolishing poverty? Beveridge's definition of 'poverty' was that of complete and utter destitution. His concern was therefore to provide benefits simply for *subsistence*, that is, a minimum income necessary for physical survival. However, as the welfare state grew, so it also grew more ambitious. It has increasingly been argued that poverty is not an *absolute* concept, rather it should be defined *relative* to those standards which are common and customary to society. By this definition, the level of income at which people are defined as living in poverty and in need of state benefit will change as the average standard of living in a society changes.* And yet, although the level of supplementary benefits has increased relative to average earnings — from around 54 per cent in 1961 to 62 per cent in 1983 — it is far from clear that the standard of living provided by such benefits has in fact been adequate to protect health or mitigate hardship. A considerable body of research has demonstrated that the levels of income involved are insufficient to ensure a 'healthy' lifestyle. A recent review of this research concluded that:

The evidence from many studies is that living at . . . the supplementary benefit levels of income does mean *real* hardship; going without necessary food, clothing, household goods, etc, living under constant strain and being vulnerable to debt. (Brown and Madge, 1982, p.299)

The plan for social security implemented in 1948 has therefore failed to eliminate poverty. Social insurance does not provide comprehensive protection for the loss or interruption of earnings and an increasing number of people are having to depend in whole or part on means-tested benefits. Though the system has undoubtedly protected the poor from the deprivations experienced in previous decades, poverty, in the sense of a lack of

*These issues are discussed in more detail in *The Health of Nations*, Chapter 10, *ibid*.

necessary financial resources, continues to be a problem for people living on benefit.

What has been the response of governments to this situation? Up until 1985, it has been one of piecemeal changes rather than fundamental reform. The intention of many of these changes has been to try to reduce the demand for the major means-tested benefit, supplementary benefit. In practice, most changes have involved the increasing use of means testing to obtain access to other benefits. By 1977, the National Consumer Council could identify no fewer than forty-four separate means-tested benefits, including such recently introduced benefits as family income supplement for low-paid people who have dependent children. This retreat from the principles of universalism

Table 10.3 The experience of social security

Married couple, one child

'All I'm allowed is £37 for myself, wife and child. The rent is £13 a week. I also have to pay out quite a lot of money for clubs. After all that we do not have much money to live on. We are all right at the weekend but when it comes to during the week, there's no money at all for food. We have to keep borrowing. Also out of that money we have to keep at least £6 or £7 for electricity and gas ... I go out regularly looking for a job and there is nothing about.'

Married couple with two children. Unemployed for three months

'After paying rent, rates, electric and gas bills and a few HPs I have about £25 a week to live on which I can assure you is no joke ... I have to borrow large amounts of money just to keep going which is getting me further and further into debt, and it is getting me even more depressed with each passing week without a job to ease the problems.'

Couple with children

'During the winter, my husband and I never built the fire up for the evening once the boys were in bed ... I never felt the house was really warm enough for the children ... I was fortunate as my parents provided winter coats and boots and wellingtons for the children. Had they not done so, I just would not have managed to keep them warm. I cannot rely on this for future years as my parents are both now near retirement age ... I ensure that the children have good meals and that is all I can do with my money. There is nothing left over for other necessities such as clothing, adequate heating and "treats" are unheard of. My husband and I eat poor meals ... to ensure more money in the "kitty" for the children.'

Married couple with four children. Unemployed for just under a year

'Our worst heartbreak is when the kids come home from school and say there is a daytrip somewhere with the school. We have to say "no" as we just have not got the funds ... Our kids have never had a holiday, it is heartbreaking ... When we last had a joint of meat I just can't remember. Unless I bake there is no way we could afford a cake ... I try to make a lot of their clothes but it breaks your heart when you see other kids really well dressed and ours have to get hand me downs.'

(Cited in Burghes, 1981, p.93–4)

has produced two problems in particular. The first has been an increase in the failure to take up benefits — that is, the proportion of those entitled to benefits who do not claim them. In 1983, for example, around 28 per cent of people entitled to claim supplementary benefits were not doing so; the total amount of money not claimed was estimated at around £2 000 million. There are a number of possible reasons for this. It is clear than many people find it demeaning to have to prove poverty in order to receive benefits. The procedures for determining entitlement are also often extremely complicated and the combination of stigma and complexity deters some people from making a claim. Lack of knowledge about what one is entitled to is also likely to be a factor. In 1983, about £3 million was spent on advertising entitlements to health and social security benefits — a trivial amount compared to the total budget of over £35 000 million for social security that year, but at least it represents an indication of some concern with the problem of incomplete take-up.

The second problem has arisen as a consequence of lowering income tax thresholds (illustrated in Table 10.2). These changes have combined to create what is termed a '*poverty trap*'. Many families are now considered poor enough to receive a state benefit, but rich enough to pay taxes. In 1981, for example, over 90 per cent of the 147 000 families receiving family income supplement were paying all or part of it back in taxes. These inconsistencies in the provision of benefits make the administration of the system inefficient — high administrative costs are a feature of means-tested benefits. Thus over ten pence in every pound paid out as supplementary benefit in 1981 went on administration, compared to 1.5p in every pound paid out for retirement pensions.

Benefit office closure sparks clashes

Eight people were arrested yesterday after clashes between social security claimants and police outside a closed London benefits office. Staff at the office in Regency Street, Victoria, had walked out claiming they feared for their safety ... following a stabbing in the waiting room on Thursday.

(David Rose, *The Guardian*, April 27, 1985)

In the mid 1980s, therefore, there is a crisis of confidence in the public welfare system. As the quotations in Table 10.3 show, many recipients of public welfare are themselves disillusioned with the experience, finding it frustrating, demeaning or inadequate (Figure 10.4). Some aspects of this system were flawed from its inception, others have been overtaken by events. But taken together, these failings have become a major part of the evidence in evaluating the welfare state. Indeed, many commentators look no further, treating the public welfare system we have been examining as identical with the welfare state, or at least as its central component. It is now time, therefore, to look more closely at the meaning of the much-used phrase 'welfare state'.

The welfare state and the social division of welfare

The first recorded use of the phrase 'the welfare state' appears to have been in 1941 by the Archbishop of Canterbury, Dr Temple. It is likely that it was coined as a deliberate contrast to the phrase used to characterise Nazi Germany — the 'warfare state' — and these origins give us the first clue about its meaning: it began life, less as a description of anything very specific, more as a slogan of wartime propaganda — a statement of the hopes for a new society which would truly be a 'common wealth': a society in which everyone worked together.

One of the key theorists of the new welfare state, and someone who made a highly influential attempt to pin down just what it might involve, was a social policy analyst, Richard Titmuss. In 1955, he argued that one of the outstanding social characteristics of the twentieth century was the increasing specialisation and division of labour, whereby:

> ... more and more people consciously experience at one or more stages in their lives the process of selection and rejection; for education, for work, for educational training, for professional status, for promotion, for opportunities of access to pension schemes, for collective social benefits, for symbols of prestige and success, and in undergoing tests of mental and physical fitness, personality, skill and functional performance. (Titmuss, 1976, p.43)

This division of labour implies a high degree of social and economic *dependency* in modern industrial societies; that is, specialisation necessarily entails the exchange of the products of specialisation, and a highly interdependent social system. In addition, there is a range of other more universal forms of dependency; for example, the dependencies of childhood, old age, child bearing, ill-health and incapacity. These states of dependency change, both over the lifetime of an individual and over time in society as a whole, and give rise to various 'needs'. It is in response to those needs that various welfare services develop. As Titmuss points out in his article, 'The Social Division of

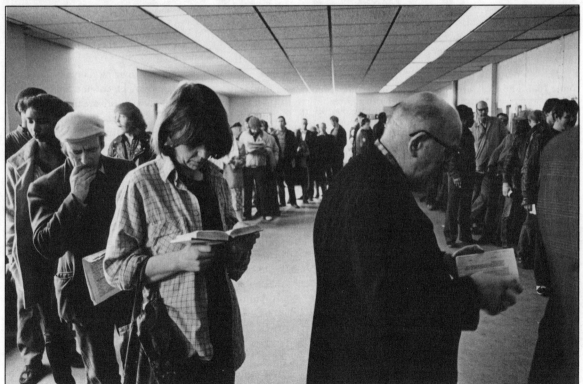

Figure 10.4 Waiting in the dole queue.

Welfare', social or *public welfare* is only one part of a wide range of services, which have similar objectives, but which are seldom thought of as being part of the welfare state; public welfare is 'only the most visible part of the real world of welfare' (*ibid*. p.53).

What else, then, does this 'real world of welfare' include? There are several different components, the most significant being the fiscal welfare and occupational welfare systems.

Fiscal welfare takes the form of income tax relief and allowances which recognise a variety of states of dependency and responsibilities. In other words, while public welfare consists largely of direct cash payments to people, fiscal welfare largely consists of a decision not to collect tax for certain specific reasons. Table 10.4 shows the main items subject to tax relief in the UK, and the amount of money involved. Total tax revenue foregone in 1985 was equivalent to almost one third of public expenditure on social security. A married man, for instance, is allowed to earn a greater income before he begins to pay tax than a single man, on the assumption that he has a non-working, dependent wife. Similarly, someone buying their own house can claim income tax relief on the interest paid on the loan. Their tax is reduced and so their net resources are increased, as if they had been given a grant.

Despite the fact that a system of *direct taxation* of income has the potential to reduce inequalities in income by taxing wealthier people more heavily than the poor (termed a *progressive tax*), the system, as it presently operates,

maintains, and in some instances actually enlarges, inequalities in living standards in the UK. Over time, as you saw earlier, the level of income at which tax has become payable — the tax threshold — has been falling, so that many people receiving means-tested state benefit are also paying income tax. At the same time, allowances and tax relief once restricted to the lowest paid are now available to all. In addition, recent trends have reduced the progressive nature of income tax by cutting taxes paid by higher earners — the number of people paying any income tax above the standard rate fell by half between 1978 and 1985. Not only that, but *indirect taxes* such as VAT and excise duties, which are *regressive* in that they affect everyone the same way regardless of their income or wealth, have increasingly been used by governments to raise revenue. In 1985, the British government raised a higher proportion of its revenue through indirect taxes than any other western country. So even if the public welfare system we examined earlier was redistributing resources towards the poor, the fiscal welfare system appears to be re-distributing resources towards the better-off.

Let us turn now to *occupational welfare*. This system is comprised in the main of *fringe benefits*, that is, benefits in cash or in kind that supplement earnings. They are provided both by employers for employees and trade unions for their members.

☐ What sorts of fringe benefits can you think of that could be included under the umbrella of occupational welfare?

■ There are, in fact, an amazing number of services and benefits, in cash or kind, which should be included: occupational pension schemes, private use of company cars, subsidised meals or vouchers, free or cheap goods, social or sports facilities, travel and removal expenses, private medical insurance, cheap loans, school fees, holiday and sick pay, and accommodation.

Table 10.5 shows the proportion of total remuneration which was made up of fringe benefits in a variety of different manufacturing industries in 1981. A number of things can be gleaned from this table: first, that in all the industries listed, fringe benefits represent a significant part of total remuneration; second, that they are much more significant in some industries than others; and third, that their importance seems to increase in line with the overall level of total remuneration: well-paid industries tend also to have higher fringe benefits, and vice versa.

Like fiscal welfare, the available evidence tends to suggest that occupational welfare maintains or accentuates rather than lessens the existing patterns of income distribution. Table 10.6, for example, shows the fringe benefits expected by employees in different income groups in the late 1960s.

Table 10.4 The fiscal welfare system: costs of tax relief

| | Tax revenue foregone in: | | |
	1978/9 (£m)	1984/85 (£m)	increase (%)
Married allowance	6 600	11 700	77.3
Single person's allowance	3 200	6 750	109.3
Mortgage interest relief	1 110	3 500	219.8
Occupational pension relief (max.)	450	3 400	655.6
Wife's earned income relief	1 800	3 100	72.2
Life assurance policies	260	725	178.8
Self employed: annuities	70	500	614.3
age allowance	265	420	58.3
Interest on National Savings Certificates	70	350	400.0
Non-residents' gilt-edged	100	300	200.0
Schedule E work expenses	–	275	–
Charity income	120	270	125.0
Separate husband/wife taxation	90	190	111.0
Statutory redundancy payments	25	175	600.0

(Source: *Sunday Times*, January 27, 1985, p.57)

Table 10.5 Fringe benefits by manufacturing industry, 1981

Industry	Average value of total remuneration (£ per hour)	Fringe benefits as a share of total remuneration (%)
Coal and petroleum products	5.47	26.8
Chemical and allied industries	4.30	24.2
Vehicles	4.01	21.8
Food, drink and tobacco	3.39	20.4
Instrument engineering	3.57	20.4
Metal manufacture	4.23	19.2
Mechanical engineering	3.54	19.0
Electrical engineering	3.47	18.9
Shipbuilding	3.61	18.2
Other manufacturing industries	3.11	18.1
Bricks, etc.	3.40	18.0
Paper, printing and publishing	3.99	18.0
Metal goods not elsewhere specified	3.25	17.6
Textiles	2.68	15.2
Timber and furniture	3.03	14.7
Clothing and footwear	2.25	13.7
Leather, etc.	2.52	13.5

(Source: Smail, *et al.*, 1984, Table 2, p.8)

Table 10.6 Membership of occupational pension schemes, based on secondary analysis of data from Townsend (1979).

Household income bracket	Proportion of employees expecting a pension from their employer (%)	Proportion of employees expecting a lump sum upon retirement (%)
Top 20%	45.8	16.1
Second 20%	44.1	15.0
Third 20%	40.0	10.8
Fourth 20%	31.5	9.2
Bottom 20%	13.5	3.7

(Source: Smail, *et al.*, 1984)

☐ How would you summarise the information in Table 10.6?

■ Employees in the highest income bracket have much higher expectations (around four times higher) of receiving an occupational pension and a lump sum on retirement than employees in the lowest income bracket.

As with fiscal welfare, occupational welfare serves to redistribute resources on a major scale. Indeed, the two systems overlap: Table 10.4 shows that the fringe benefit of occupational pension schemes attracted tax relief estimated at £3 400 million in 1985. The true scale of fringe benefits is unknown, for many go unrecorded. There is similar uncertainty about fiscal welfare, as British governments have been reluctant to publish detailed information on the precise extent of many tax concessions and reliefs. Nevertheless, it is clear that both fiscal and occupational welfare are not only very extensive, but also that they exhibit some of the same defects and failings that you saw earlier in the public welfare system. One of the most striking is the deep-seated *gender division* in the way in which benefits are distributed.

Fiscal welfare is based on the same assumptions about men's and women's roles in the family that were discussed earlier. This reinforces women's dependence on men. For example, what is known as the 'aggregation rule' defines a woman's income to be her husband's for tax purposes, while married men receive a 40 per cent higher tax allowance than single men, whether or not they have a dependent wife or children, on the assumption that income within the family is shared. Likewise, within the occupational welfare system similar inequalities on the basis of gender exist. In one survey of employers in 1979, 71 per cent of firms offered pension benefits greater than those in the state scheme but only 38 per cent allowed part-time workers to join. As over 90 per cent of part-time workers are women, these benefits inevitably discriminate against women.

It seems evident, therefore, that any examination of the contemporary structure of public welfare, and the relation this has to inequalities in health, must take a wide view of what is meant by 'welfare'. The public welfare system is only one part of this structure, and the other welfare systems we have examined, far from reducing inequalities and redistributing resources to the poor, seem to be organised at present in such a way as to reinforce and accentuate inequalities. Equipped with this broader definition of 'welfare', let us now look at some of the main currents of opinion on the lessons to be drawn from Britain's post-war welfare experience.

What went wrong? Welfare in post-war Britain

Although there was never complete agreement in the UK about the mechanisms or objectives of welfare policy, successive post-war governments shared a broad commitment to the maintenance both of the public welfare system and full employment, and the notion that government had an active role to play in economic management and the provision of services. The same could be said of other western industrialised countries, and by the 1960s many people were expressing the view that the problems of poverty, unemployment, slump and deep social inequality had been banished never to return. Some, such as American sociologist Daniel Bell, argued that the distinctions between left and right, socialism and capitalism, east and west, had become outmoded and redundant and that 'the end of ideology' had occurred; others suggested that convergence was taking place between east and west.

Similar ideas were expressed in Britain. In 1956, the Labour politician Anthony Crosland published an influential book entitled *The Future of Socialism*. In it, he pondered the changes that had occurred in British society, concluding:

> And so, to the question 'is this still Capitalism?' I would answer 'No' ... One cannot imagine today a deliberate offensive alliance between Government and employers against the Unions ... or, say, a serious attempt to enforce, as so often happened in the 1920s, a coal policy to which the miners bitterly objected ... We have now enjoyed more than ten years of consecutive peace-time full employment — not only in Britain, but in most other major countries also. This suggests that a world-wide change in the economic climate has occurred ... Electorates now believe that full employment can quite well be maintained, and are consequently in no mood to tolerate a failure to maintain it. Any government which permitted appreciable unemployment for more than a short period would court certain defeat at the polls. (Crosland, 1967, pp.42, 14–15, 289–90)

Such comments serve as a useful warning of the dangers of neglecting a historical perspective: it is apparent from the history of health care, that the past is full both of sharp discontinuities and of events unfolding over centuries, thus to extrapolate into the indefinite future from the experience of a mere ten years is wantonly hazardous. The context

within which writers such as Bell and Crosland propounded their ideas was a sustained period of expansion in the world economy that was historically unique. Table 10.7 shows some salient features of this expansion.

☐ What does Table 10.7 reveal about economic growth in the post-war period?

■ It falls distinctly into two phases: the period from 1950 to 1973, where growth rates were on average 2½ times higher than the interwar period (and in a country such as the UK substantially higher than those experienced even at the height of the Industrial Revolution), and the period after 1973, when the rate of growth was on average only one-half of that in the preceding phase.

☐ What does the table reveal about the economic performance of the UK relative to other industrial countries?

■ The UK's rate of growth has been below average since 1870, and in the post-war period has been just a little over one-half of the average.

Such aspects of post-war Britain have become inextricably bound up with the debate over welfare policies. Although the UK was slipping behind other countries in terms of economic growth, and although societies such as Sweden and West Germany were far outspending the UK in the provision of health and welfare services, nevertheless there was sufficient growth in the British economy up to 1973 to distract attention from issues of distribution. If the size of the cake was growing, then no matter how it was divided up everyone would gradually get a bit more. Economic growth was at the heart of Crosland's views on social policy, and as you saw earlier in this book, the growth mentality also permeated the fabric of the NHS, holding out the promise of painless changes in priorities.

Since 1973, as Britain's economic growth has slowed, unemployment has soared (Figure 10.5), and the country's

Table 10.7 The growth of gross domestic product per person in eight industrialised countries, 1700–1979

| | Average annual rate of growth of GDP per person in constant prices | | | | | | |
	1700–1820	1820–1870	1870–1913	1913–1950	1950–1973	1973–1979	1820–1979
France	0.6	1.4	1.7	1.0	5.1	3.0	2.0
Germany	–	2.0	2.8	1.3	6.0	2.4	2.6
Italy	–	–	1.5	1.4	5.5	2.6	–
Japan	–	0.4	2.5	1.8	9.7	4.1	2.7
Netherlands	0.1	2.4	2.1	2.4	4.8	2.4	2.7
Sweden	–	1.6	2.8	2.8	3.8	1.8	2.5
UK	1.1	2.4	1.9	1.3	3.0	1.3	2.0
USA	–	4.4	4.1	2.8	3.7	2.7	3.8
Arithmetic average	0.6	2.1	2.4	1.9	5.2	2.5	2.6

(Source: derived from Maddison, 1982, Table 3.1, p.44)

comparative position has deteriorated rapidly, so the post-war consensus on welfare has disintegrated. From the political right it has been argued that the pursuit of egalitarian welfare policies, the use of Keynesian economic policies, and the growth of public expenditure have been seriously damaging to economic prosperity and threatening to personal freedom. From the left it has been argued that Keynesian economic policies could not postpone indefinitely the inevitable working out of certain inherent contradictions in capitalism, and that welfare spending has contributed to a fiscal crisis in the capitalist state. Many others hold intermediate positions, or remain wedded to the ideas and policies of pre-1973 consensus, or are simply uncertain: the crisis in the world economy, and particularly in the British economy, has its counterpart in an intellectual crisis. Let us look at these strands of thought in more detail.

The radical right

In 1944, the same year that legislation was in full swing to create Britain's post-war welfare system, the Austrian philosopher and economist Friedrich von Hayek published a book entitled *The Road to Serfdom*. Heavily influenced by the appalling wartime experiences of Eastern Europe, Hayek's work focused on the efficiency of different types of economic system and the legal framework within which they operate. This led him towards the conclusion that rational economic planning by a central authority was both impossible — because the knowledge required to make rational decisions was too dispersed — and deeply injurious to personal liberties. The most rational form of economic system was one that was as *decentralised* as possible, and the best way of promoting political freedom was by guaranteeing *economic freedom*. Decentralisation and economic freedom, he argued, were the essential characteristics of markets, and consequently the more extensive the market — and the smaller the role of the state, organised labour unions, and other limits on the market — the better.

Hayek's stress, in common with others from this strand of the radical right, was essentially on rights, liberties and the independence of the *individual*. Whereas Titmuss emphasised the values shared in common by the members of a society, theorists from the radical right emphasise the very different likes and dislikes of different individuals. Society to them is simply a collection of differing individuals and the good society is that which enables them to satisfy their individual preferences most satisfactorily.

The ideas and writings of Hayek have exerted a strong influence on many leading right-wing theorists, and particularly on the American economist Milton Friedman. Friedman's economic analysis, and his political and social views, are based primarily upon his arguments concerning the merits of the market mechanism, and the damage that

he believes occurs by interfering with it. That massive programmes of government expenditure will do more harm than good is the charge Friedman has levelled at welfare spending:

> The [welfare] bureaucrats spend someone else's money on someone else. Only human kindness, not the much stronger and more dependable spur of self-interest, assures that they will spend the money in the way beneficial to the recipients. Hence the wastefulness and ineffectiveness of the spending ... The waste is distressing, but it is the least of the evils of the paternalistic programs that have grown to such massive size. Their major evil is their effect on the fabric of our society. They weaken the family; reduce the incentive to work, save and innovate; reduce the accumulation of capital; and limit our freedom.
> (Friedman and Friedman, 1980, pp.117 and 127)

Friedman believes that individuals must be free to make choices, though he also acknowledges that in such a system chance will also play a large part in determining the distribution of income:

> The amount each of us owns is partly the result of chance, partly of choice by ourselves or others. Chance determines our genes and through them affects our physical and mental capacities. Chance determines the kind of family and cultural environment into which we are born and as a result our opportunities to develop our physical and mental capacity. Chance determines also other resources we may inherit from our parents or other benefactors. Chance may destroy or enhance the resources we start with. But choice also plays an important role. Our decisions about how to use our resources, whether to work hard or take it easy, to enter one occupation or another, to engage in one venture or another, to save or spend — these may determine whether we dissipate our resources or improve and add to them. Similar decisions by our parents, by other benefactors, by millions of people who have no direct connection with us will affect our inheritance. (*Ibid.*, pp.21–2)

The essential diagnosis by the radical right of what went wrong with post-war welfare is that the free market was displaced by an ever-expanding government, creating lack of freedom, inefficiency and an artificial income distribution; and their prescription for action is a reduction in government expenditure and the removal of barriers to the operation of the market.

The Marxist left

On the left as well as the right, recent years have seen attempts to interpret the welfare state and its problems by drawing on somewhat older bodies of thought. Here we will concentrate on the work of Ian Gough, who has attempted to provide a Marxist analysis of the post-war welfare state. Before looking at his arguments it is worth stating as simply as possible some of the most distinctive features of Marxist analyses.

First, just as Hayek and Friedman see economic activity as being of fundamental importance in human affairs, so too do Marxists. Indeed, the latter go even further — economically productive activity is seen as being of central importance in determining the shape of all aspects of the social world, such as law, religion, culture, intellectual thought and language.

Second, whereas the radical right seek the most free market possible, Marxists view such markets as integral to capitalism, which is merely one *mode* or type of production which was preceded by others and will in turn be replaced.

Capitalism is seen as having the following features: widespread exchange relationships — including the buying and selling of labour as a commodity; the private ownership of the means of production; and the exploitation of labour by capitalists (that is, the private owners of capital). Exploitation, on this analysis, provides the mainspring of the system, for it is through exploitation that the owners of capital can accumulate more capital, and accumulation is what the system is directed towards.

Thus, whereas free-market theories emphasise competition between *individuals*, Marxist theories stress the importance of conflicts between powerful *groups*: in a capitalist society the interests of capital and labour, of ruling class and working class are fundamentally opposed. These contradictions will ultimately lead to the overthrow of the capitalist state and its replacement by a new socialist mode of production.

Finally, note that from a Marxist perspective, the differences between Keynes and Friedman are of relatively minor importance; both are products of contemporary capitalist society and their theories reflect and sustain the system of ideas, thought and values — in short the *ideology* — that supports capitalism. They make legitimate the existing social world rather than explaining it. Thus, for example, both Keynes and Friedman make the fundamental assumption that individual human beings are essentially competitive — by contrast, Marxist theory sees this not as a universal human trait but rather as a product of capitalism.

So how is state expenditure on welfare viewed by Marxists? According to Gough, capitalism requires labour, which in turn must be maintained and reproduced. This can be facilitated by state expenditure on housing, food, health and education. Non-working parts of the population must be included, not least because they may become part of the working population in the future (e.g. children), or

are part of a 'reserve army of labour' (e.g. the unemployed). But Gough also draws attention to what he sees as positive aspects of welfare expenditure. In Britain particularly, he argues, much of the welfare state was part of a post-war settlement, a set of concessions won by the working class in return for their support in the war-effort. Welfare expenditure does contain progressive features as well as coercive features, is liberating as well as repressive, and meets genuine needs of people using the services as well as the long-term requirements of capital accumulation. And:

> once the contradictory nature of the welfare state and its contradictory impact on capitalism is appreciated, then the political strategy of all who work in it, use it or are concerned with it can be refined. The positive aspects of welfare policies need defending and extending, their negative aspects need exposing and attacking. (Gough, 1979, p.153)

The future of welfare

For all that the arguments of the radical right and left are based on different premises and arrive at quite different conclusions about future strategies, it has been pointed out that many of the charges levelled by them against Keynesian welfare and economic policies are strikingly similar:

> Both emphasise how full employment has strengthened labour against capital. Both sets of literature describe the public sector as 'unproductive'. Although the meanings attached to this word are very different, the vocabulary clearly communicates a view of the public sector as a burden. There is a shared contention that the present strains engulfing western societies can only be resolved through radical action (respectively the rolling back of the state or socialist revolution). (Heald, 1983, p.276)

Although the period of Keynesian economic and welfare policy is regarded by one camp as a dangerous flirtation with socialism that threatened to destroy the viability of capitalism, and by the other as a diversion from genuine socialist change that rescued capitalism in its hour of need, both share a hostility to the concept of political accommodation or compromise.

In addition, feminist critics have pointed out that both the critiques of the right and the left share another feature — a failure to identify the *gender* inequalities that exist in the welfare state and the benefit system. Two social policy analysts, Hilary Land and Hilary Rose, have argued that the welfare state is posited on the 'compulsory altruism' of women and so benefits not only capitalists but men in general.

Faced with such a sustained barrage of criticism, what remains of the arguments that brought the welfare state of

Keynes and Beveridge into being in the first place? Many supporters of such policies have travelled a long way towards their critics in agreeing that, *in practice*, things did not work out as intended. The economist Julian Le Grand, for example, has studied in detail the impact of public expenditure on the distribution of a range of services — health, education, housing and transport.

☐ Le Grand's findings on the distribution of health care between socio-economic groups on the basis of their needs were discussed in Chapter 7. What was Le Grand's main conclusion?

■ That when differences in the level of need for health care between socio-economic groups were taken into account, people in higher groups received significantly more care than those in lower groups.

Overall, Le Grand has concluded that public expenditure has done little to reduce inequalities and in some instances has exacerbated them:

There is so much evidence from so many different areas that, almost regardless of the method of provision, the better off will always be able to make more effective use of even freely provided services than the less well off. In that sense, the strategy of attempting to create equality through the provision of services that are free, or at a subsidised price at all, seems fundamentally misconceived. (Le Grand, 1982, p.137)

Supporters of Keynes and Beveridge have also accepted that the existence of occupational and fiscal welfare systems running parallel to the public welfare system has tended to redistribute income in an upward direction and that orthodox Keynesian policies have seemed to be unable to contain creeping inflation. While Britain 'had never had it so good', other countries were clearly having it better and moving further ahead in the great wealth race.

It would seem therefore that not only the theoretical basis of Keynes's and Beveridge's approach has been seriously undermined, but also the practical application of their policies have shown the theory to be flawed. This is not, however, necessarily the case. There is other empirical evidence that challenges and refutes some of the claims of the radical critics. For example, for all the criticisms of high public expenditure, the UK is neither top of the public expenditure league nor top of the taxation league (Figure 10.5). Not only that, but many of the countries with higher levels of taxation and public expenditure have also had higher rates of economic growth. In other words, it is by no means clear that high taxation rates have large disincentive effects, or that public spending slows down economic growth and reduces prosperity, or that welfare benefits provide a disincentive to work.

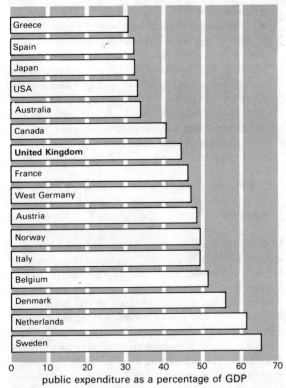

Figure 10.5 Public expenditure as a percentage of GDP in 15 member states of the Organisation of Economic Cooperation and Development (OECD) in 1980.
(Source: Heald, 1983)

Evidence such as this has contributed to the survival of Keynes's and Beveridge's view, albeit modified in the light of some of the criticisms already discussed. The best known and most influential example of this strategy in the field of health and social welfare is the report of a DHSS working group entitled *Inequalities in Health*, usually referred to as the *Black Report* after the group's chairman, Douglas Black.

The report was commissioned in 1977 to review information about differences in health status between the social classes, to consider possible causes of these differences and the implications for policy, and to suggest further research. Extracts from the report appear in an article in the Course Reader, 'Inequalities in Health: The Black Report and Reactions to it' (Part 7, Section 7.4). At this point you should read the part entitled 'The Black Report' (pages 326–30).

☐ The *Black Report* confirmed the existence of marked and persistent inequalities in health between social classes.* What explanations did the working

*Inequalities in health and possible explanations are discussed in more detail *The Health of Nations*, Chapters 9 and 10, *ibid*.

group offer for these inequalities?

■ The group felt there were several causes: 'specific features of the socio-economic environment' such as overcrowding and smoking; the availability and use of health services; and the more diffuse consequences of the class structure: poverty, working conditions and deprivation in various forms'.

□ These explanations were reflected in the group's recommendations for policy. What were the two main areas of policy recommendations?

■ 1 Measures relating to health and personal social services.

2 Wider aspects of social policy including both changes in welfare and alterations in wealth and income distributions.

Some of the ways in which health and personal social services could help alleviate inequalities are mentioned in the extract you have read in the Course Reader. Measures such as those to reduce smoking have already been considered in earlier chapters of this book. There was one innovative proposal, however: the suggestion of adopting an experimental approach in some geographical areas. Experimental programmes involving the provision of new services and costing around £30 million would, it was claimed, provide empirical evidence to substantiate or refute the claims of the working group. These programmes were primarily envisaged as opportunities to develop the role of existing statutory health and social services, as well as local involvement of trade unions, employers' organisations, and the local media. However, the opportunity to experiment, whether with different styles of management or varying patterns of health care organisation, is something that governments and the NHS have largely rejected to date. Instead, the policy of successive governments has tended to be broad, nationwide changes.

Having noted the suggestion for special experimental areas, let us turn to the second set of recommendations, those concerned with wider aspects of social policy. Broadly speaking, the report recommended a continuation of welfare measures in combination with some fundamental changes in the distribution of wealth and income between the social classes.

□ What recommendations could be seen as a continuation of the post-war welfare system?

■ A comprehensive disablement allowance; improvements in housing by local authorities; and the abolition of child poverty by increasing the value of child benefit, providing free school meals and milk, new education services for children under five and a new infant care allowance.

It was envisaged that these measures would not only give children a 'better start in life' but also provide women with more control over an independent source of income, while day care places and free school meals would provide a respite from unpaid domestic work and allow for the possibility of paid employment. In other words, while the report focused primarily on social class, the recommendations would not only be redistributing resources between classes. Inevitably, the strategy would also involve a redistribution of resources towards women as unpaid carers and as low-paid workers, towards people with children, towards members of minority ethnic groups to the extent that they too are disproportionately low paid, and towards disabled people. In the longer term, resources would also be redistributed towards the elderly in that people would be in a better position to accumulate reserves during their lifetime. There would therefore be considerable redistribution *within* different classes as well as *between* them.

As for more fundamental changes in wealth and income distribution, the group proposed several measures as part of an anti-poverty strategy:

While measures have to be taken to increase the living standards of poor people relative to those who are better-off, we believe that post-war history shows the inadequacy of the approach to this problem which has been followed by successive governments.

We believe that a new approach to the fairer distribution of resources needs to be developed on the following basis. The dispersion of resources is in fact very unequal, and the long-term objective of reducing by a moderate amount the proportionate share of, say, the top 30 per cent of income recipients, would substantially augment the sum redistributed at present to the poor. Though the political task will be difficult, greater restriction on the amount of wealth which may be inherited and accumulated, together with more effective measures to inhibit the growth of top incomes and reduce present differentials in incomes, preferably within the framework of nationally agreed and statutorily enforced maximum and minimum incomes, with appropriate adjustments for dependencies, will need to be developed.

The second part of a comprehensive anti-poverty strategy is to encourage self-dependence and a high level of individual skill and autonomy as a basis for creating a more integrated society. We believe that this is possible only by raising the standards and broadening the content of education so the need for advice or supervision from professionally trained personnel in medicine, nursing, law, housing, child care or administration is less marked or frequent and the capacity to undertake a range of skills greater; by improving individual access to information about, and control over, what goes on in the immediate community as well as society generally; and by conferring rights to employment and occupation and creating corresponding opportunities for such employment. (DHSS, 1980, paragraphs 9.6, 9.10 and 9.11)

☐ How does this anti-poverty strategy compare with the strategy proposed by Beveridge and implemented in 1948?

■ There are four main differences:

1 The *Black Report* is explicitly concerned with redistributing resources towards the poor, unlike the policy of 1948 which was more obviously a strategy to provide minimum standards.

2 Both strategies give high priority to the need to provide employment, but in very different ways.

3 The Beveridge strategy involved redistribution through public welfare and taxation whereas the *Black Report* suggests, in addition, state intervention to restrict the amount of wealth that can be inherited or accumulated and to reduce income equalities.

4 The *Black Report* places greater emphasis on the central role of education to encourage independence and autonomy, and to give people the necessary knowledge and skills to be able to gain more control over their own lives.

This last recommendation is sometimes referred to as *community development*. Though it has a long history, it gained contemporary popularity through experimental anti-poverty programmes in the USA in the 1960s and projects in the UK in the early 1970s. Table 10.8 lists the aims of one current community development project — the Waterloo Health Project which is part of a larger Community Resource Centre. The health project has been involved in a wide range of activities including a women's

Table 10.8 The aims of the Waterloo Health Project

1 To promote interest and understanding of positive health (WHO).

2 Develop a collective aproach to health.

3 Promote self confidence.

4 To enable greater access to health information and resources.

5 Promote positive changes in lay and professional relationships.

6 To encourage local people to identify and articulate their health needs.

7 To influence health policy at a local level.

8 To identify and influence factors affecting health.

9 To share the experience of the project with a wider audience.

health group which held regular discussions, made a video of local health services which generated a great deal of local discussion, and presented evidence to a planning inquiry which was considering a major redevelopment in the area. Poor housing, lack of play space and leisure facilities, and environmental pollution are other health issues that have been taken up by such local groups and pursued with the local authority.

Community health groups have been established in many parts of the country, some of them focusing on the problems of specific groups in the population, such as how racism affects minority groups, others concerned with specific diseases or conditions. They face many difficulties, in particular that of gaining the recognition and support of health professionals and of ensuring the continued participation of local people. Their importance lies in the fact that they represent an alternative to the top–down approach to health problems which is a feature of the large centrally-controlled services, such as the NHS. However, although, ideally, community development projects should arise from the community, once established they are often successful in gaining financial support from established sources such as health and local authorities and even central government.

Looked at overall, two strands of thought can be detected in the recommendations of the *Black Report*. On the one hand there is support for state welfare, a continuation of the views of Keynes and Beveridge which formed the basis of the post-war consensus in British politics. On the other hand, there is a recognition of the need for more radical measures if poverty is to be reduced successfully. Why was it that the working group adopted two somewhat contradictory solutions? As the report does not provide an answer we are left to decide for ourselves between two possible explanations. It may be that the members of the working group believed that it is possible to achieve radical change by means of *gradual* alterations, a view that the radical left would reject as fanciful. Alternatively, it may be that they recognised the impossibility of achieving a national consensus for radical change in the political climate of the 1980s and therefore accepted that a more pragmatic approach is the only practical solution. Whichever explanation is true, the report made no impact on the government of the day when it was published in 1980.

Closing the class health gap

The TUC has called for a variety of measures designed to close the gap in health between the social classes, including the reintroduction of free school meals, and the phasing out of sales of cigarettes over the next decade. In a report published yesterday it examines the findings and recommendations of the Black Report, published by the government just over a year ago, and notes that nothing has resulted from them.

(Penny Chorlton, *The Guardian*, September 9, 1981)

To understand why nothing resulted from the report during that first year, or indeed subsequently, it is necessary to consider its political background. By the time the report was published in August 1980, the Labour government that had commissioned it had been replaced in 1979 by the Conservatives; it was thus placed firmly in the centre of the changing attitudes to welfare policy and wider economic policy that this chapter has been considering.

The report was far from being a politically neutral document. Not only had it been commissioned by a Labour government, but two out of its four authors had very clear links to the Labour Party: Peter Townsend had conducted major academic studies of poverty, was also a founder of one of the most influential pressure groups, Child Poverty Action Group, and had been an advisor to an earlier Labour government, and Jerry Morris, had long been involved in left-wing health politics, an involvement that went back to the 1940s and the creation of the modern welfare state. The other two members of the working group had a much more neutral political stance. Cyril Smith, a sociologist, was secretary of the Social Science Research Council, while Douglas Black was Chief Scientist at the DHSS. None the less, although these last two members were not linked to the Labour Party, there were no members from other parties.

In most political commentators' eyes, 1979 marked the biggest shift in British politics since the Second World War. The continuing failure of the British economy relative to its competitors had led, so it was argued, to the end of the post-war consensus. Labour and Conservatives might have disagreed about many things in the thirty years after the war but there was general agreement about the welfare state. Now this could no longer be taken for granted. So the *Black Report* saw the light of day in a world that was radically changed. The Secretary of State at the DHSS in 1980 could not be guaranteed to be in favour of welfare. His response appeared as a foreword to the report, and is reproduced in the collection of articles and letters in the Course Reader. These extracts form only a small part of the public debate over the report and they focus primarily on the initial response of the new government and the counter-attack by some of those who had actually written the report or were committed to its recommendations. You should read these extracts now (pages 325–6 and 330–4).

☐ What were the three grounds on which the Secretary of State, Patrick Jenkin, challenged the report?
■ 1 That there was insufficient evidence to show that social inequalities *cause* differences in health between social classes.
2 That there was no evidence to prove that the report's recommendations would reduce inequalities in health.
3 That the cost of the recommendations was far too great to be afforded.
☐ To what extent were the wider political debates about the welfare state, which have been discussed in this chapter, present in the debate about the report?
■ There is hardly any evidence in these extracts of the wider aspects of the debate or the underlying theoretical differences between the adversaries.

The tone throughout is one of neutral scientific debate. Patrick Jenkin makes comments such as 'the difficulties they experienced are no surprise given current measurement techniques', while Jerry Morris urges that this is not a party political matter. In short, although the recommendations of the report touch on highly political matters, matters of belief and value as much as of fact, it is treated overtly as a non-political matter. Despite the fact that those involved differ markedly in their beliefs and values, it is very difficult to conduct public debate in these terms. As a result the debate focuses on matters of evidence, for here at least there is some real possibility of proof.

Despite this, it is the underlying differences of opinion, rather than scientific evidence, that often divide people in their views — disagreements that cannot be settled by recourse to empirical evidence. For example, what is the real nature of human beings? Are we inherently competitive or is this merely a product of the current mode of economic production? Statements that human nature will always be the same, or that it will all be different in the future, are merely statements of belief.

And just as our choices must be shaped by beliefs as well as facts, so they are also inevitably shaped by *values*. Which is more important, liberty or equality, the individual or the group? In the French Revolution, liberty, equality and fraternity were bracketed together, as if it were possible to have all three simultaneously. But since that date, the argument has grown more complex. Maximising individual freedom can seriously threaten equality and vice versa. Both are highly valued goals. But how far should one be pursued at the expense of the other? The decision admits of no easy solution, for different people place a different value on each.

The debate over the wider welfare state and its impact on health is not just a matter for academics, it is a political debate — it concerns everyone. But choices about health and social welfare have to be made in the context of choices about other aspects of our lives. Few people rank a concern with good health as the absolute priority in life. To argue that the consequences for health of economic and social policy have been unduly neglected in the past is one thing, to argue that economic and social policy is primarily about health is quite another.

Throughout this chapter we have primarily been addressing the question of *which* strategy should be pursued in view of the marked inequalities in health that exist. We end by considering a different though related question — *when* might a major change in strategy take place? As you have seen, the creation of the welfare state was helped greatly by the social cohesion and unity that in turn was a reaction to the massive external threat posed during the Second World War. The consensus that emerged in the immediate post-war years was maintained until the 1970s. However, in the early 1980s consensus has been lost. For the first time since the war a political atmosphere exists in which a radical shift in strategy on a whole number of issues, including the welfare state, can take place. Only time will tell in which direction and on what scale such a change will be.

Objectives for Chapter 10

When you have read this chapter you should be able to:

10.1 Describe in broad terms Beveridge's plan for a social security system based on social insurance, national assistance and voluntary insurance; the difference between universal and means-tested benefits; and the other key components of 1940s' welfare — Keynesian economics, nationalisation, comprehensive health care and full employment.

10.2 Explain how increasing costs and changing social conditions have placed the public welfare system under strain, and how aspects of fiscal and occupational welfare have contributed to a crisis in confidence in the system.

10.3 Compare and contrast the explanations and solutions for the crisis in the public welfare system put forward by the radical right and Marxist left.

10.4 Describe the key elements of the *Black Report* recommendations — changes in health and social services; alterations in welfare provisions; and an anti-poverty strategy; and the ways in which the public debate about the future of welfare reflects wider political beliefs and values.

Questions for Chapter 10

1 (*Objective 10.1*) What were the principal ways in 1948 in which social insurance differed from national assistance as regards the sources of revenue and methods of distribution and entitlement?

2 (*Objective 10.2*) What are the main changes in social conditions since 1948 that have contributed to a crisis in confidence in the social security system?

3 (*Objective 10.3*) On what grounds have the radical right and the Marxist left argued that the welfare system requires substantial revision?

4 (*Objective 10.4*) In what way may the recommendations of the *Black Report* be said to be contradictory? Suggest two possible explanations of this contradiction.

11

A cautionary tale

During Chapters 6–9 we considered the prospects for innovation, evaluation, screening and prevention. However, faced with limited resources, choices have to be made *between* these various options: money spent on surgery is not available for health education and so on. Sometimes such choices may be relatively easy to make. For example, while the treatment of lung cancer is largely ineffective, research studies have shown that around 90 per cent of cases are related to smoking tobacco. The principal approach should therefore be primary prevention: to reduce the amount of tobacco that is consumed.

However, for other diseases, the appropriate response is not so obvious. This is true of many of the conditions responsible for much of the mortality, morbidity and disability in industrialised countries. How do we make choices when treatments have not been adequately evaluated and the causes of the condition are not known? How do doctors, health service managers, the public, health educators and government proceed in such circumstances? To answer these questions, we shall take coronary heart disease as our example.

More than any other, coronary heart disease (CHD) is the disease of the moment. It accounts for about 30 per cent of deaths among men and 22 per cent among women. The estimated cost to the NHS of medical care for CHD was over £250 million in England and Wales in 1981 (OHE, 1982). Six thousand hospital beds were in constant use by sufferers of this condition, while the lives of tens of thousands were restricted by its disabling symptoms. So great are people's fears of CHD that many are prepared to change their lifestyle radically in the hope of avoiding a disease whose impact has been likened to plague.

Despite the considerable uncertainty that surrounds many aspects of CHD, there is no shortage of enthusiastic proposals for action:

The bypass road to recovery

Coronary artery bypass grafts are the sort of operation doctors would like to see more people with heart disease undergo. A meeting organised last week recommended that an extra 10,000 sufferers a year should be offered the operation.
(Olivia Timbs and Lorraine Fraser, *The Times*, November 27, 1984)

Scanner may end heart deaths

Coronary artery disease, which claims 180,000 lives a year, may be practically eliminated by new screening techniques and drug treatments, a leading heart specialist said yesterday. Mobile scanning trailers similar to those used by mass X-ray screening for tuberculosis could be introduced to provide early diagnosis, he suggested.
(Nicholas Timmins, *The Times*, September 21, 1984)

£60m programme urged to save 40,000 heart victims a year

Forty thousand heart disease deaths a year could be prevented, a group of health experts say. They urged the Government yesterday to spend £60m on a series of measures. They want changes in the nation's diet, better food in schools and workplaces, no cigarette advertising and improved food labelling.

(Thomson Prentice, *The Times*, April 18, 1984)

Innovations in surgery, screening for early diagnosis and preventive strategies all have their advocates, many of whom became highly committed to their own particular approach and dismissive of all others — the debate is quite acrimonious at times. However, before considering the arguments we need to review the basic biology* and epidemiology of the disease.

☐ What is coronary heart disease?

■ A condition in which the myocardium (heart muscle) receives insufficient oxygen because the coronary arteries fail to maintain a sufficient blood supply.

The main proximal cause of the insufficient blood supply is narrowing of the coronary arteries by fatty deposits, known as *atheromas* or *plaques*. These may start forming in childhood, but only give rise to symptoms when the inside of the arteries is considerably narrowed. The severity of the condition will depend on the location of the atheroma.

There are two main coronary arteries, the right and left, though the left main artery divides into two branches: the left anterior descending and the circumflex (Figure 11.1).

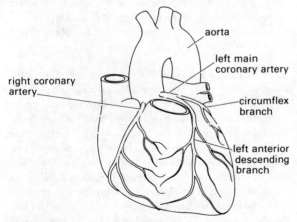

right coronary artery

aorta

left main coronary artery

circumflex branch

left anterior descending branch

Figure 11.1 Anatomy of the heart showing the two main coronary arteries (right and left) and the two branches of the left main coronary artery.

*The biology of CHD is discussed in *The Biology of Health and Disease*, Chapter 16, *ibid*.

The blood supply to the myocardium consists therefore of three arteries. It should be noted that the symptoms of CHD are also thought on occasion to result from *spasm* (sustained contraction) of the muscle in the arterial wall.

CHD affects people in three different ways. First, it may cause sudden death if the blood supply to the heart muscle suddenly stops, often as a result of *thrombosis* (a blood clot) on a plaque. Second, it may cause a *myocardial infarction* in which a portion of heart muscle is permanently damaged. This may lead to death, though in most cases the person recovers. These first two effects of CHD are often referred to as *heart attacks*. Third, it may cause *angina* (chest pain) which if severe and frequent can lead to considerable disability.

The current high mortality rates are a feature of the twentieth century. Deaths were rarely attributed to CHD before 1900, and there is a widely held view that many industrialised countries are currently experiencing an epidemic of the disease. To what extent this epidemic reflects changes in doctors' recognition of the disease rather than a real increase in its prevalence remains a matter for debate; a debate that may never be fully resolved, dependent as it is on inadequate historical material. This is obviously not true of the assessment of more recent changes in mortality rates. While CHD is the commonest cause of death in most industrialised countries, there are marked international differences in mortality rates (Figures 11.2

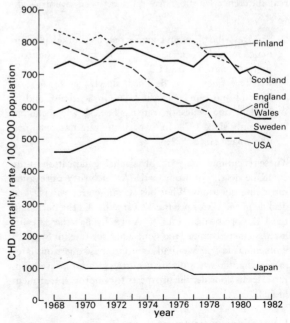

Figure 11.2 Coronary heart disease mortality rates for men aged 35–74 years, (age-standardised rates per 100 000 population), 1968–1982.
(Source: data supplied by Michael Marmot, UCH, London)

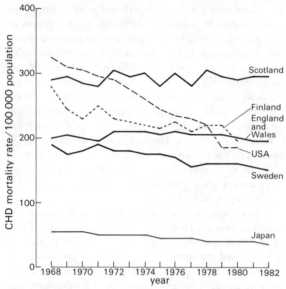

Figure 11.3 Coronary heart disease mortality rates for women aged 35–74 years (aged-standardised rates per 100 000 population), 1968–1982.
(Source: as Figure 11.2)

and 11.3). Some of the differences are undoubtedly due to differences in diagnostic practice. However, such factors do not explain all the differences and it is generally held that real differences in mortality rates between countries do exist.

☐ Describe the main changes that have taken place in male mortality rates since 1968 in the countries represented in Figure 11.2.
■ The rates have declined slowly in Japan and Finland and rapidly in the USA. In Scotland, and in England and Wales, the rate has been slowly declining, but only since 1978. In Sweden the rate has remained unchanged since 1971.

These recent data are probably a reliable indication of the changing death rate from CHD. As such they raise some intriguing questions. What has accounted for the marked decline in the USA since the 1960s? Why did the decline in the UK not start until 1978? And why has the rate for Swedish men remained the same while the rate for Swedish women has fallen? We shall return to these questions later in the chapter when discussing strategies for prevention. First, let us consider the prospects for improved treatment of CHD.

Innovations in treatment
The treatment of CHD has three main objectives. The first is prevention of death immediately after a myocardial infarction. This involves the use of drugs which strengthen

and regulate the heartbeat, and of life-support systems such as giving intravenous fluids and oxygen. However, such intensive treatment will help only a minority of patients to survive: it has been estimated that less than 5 per cent of people benefit from being admitted to a coronary care unit rather than simply being nursed in their own home. This is partly because most deaths occur in the first two hours after a myocardial infarction before it is usually possible to get someone into hospital, and partly because even the best medical care has little or no effect in many cases.

The second objective is to prevent people becoming disabled by severe angina. For most people this can be achieved with the use of drugs. However, for others who are seriously disabled, surgery is becoming increasingly popular.

The third objective is the prevention of further myocardial infarctions, thus prolonging the lives of people who are already suffering from the disease. Again, this can be attempted either with the use of drugs or of surgery.

It is not possible to discuss all aspects of treatment in greater detail, so we will consider just one procedure that exemplifies both the impact and the limitations that innovations in treatment might have — the surgical operation known as *coronary artery bypass grafting* (CABG: referred to by doctors as 'cabbage') introduced to relieve patients of severe angina.

☐ Is this a product or a process innovation?
■ A product innovation.
☐ From what has been said about the treatment of CHD, can you suggest an example of a process innovation in this field?
■ One such example would be the introduction of a means of getting people who have suffered a myocardial infarction into hospital faster so that treatment would be more effective.

The use of surgery to relieve angina is not new. Since 1916 attempts have been made to alleviate angina either by severing some of the nerve connections to the heart or by attempts to improve the blood supply to the myocardium. The latter have included pulling some of the tissue that supplies the intestines with blood up through the diaphragm and into the chest and attaching it to the heart, or by re-routing an artery from the muscles of the chest to the myocardium. These operations attempted to improve the blood supply to the whole myocardium rather than just the affected areas. This changed in the early 1960s when it became technically possible to produce accurate images of the coronary arteries and pinpoint the exact location of any obstructions in their supply. The method used was *coronary angiography* in which a dye that is relatively opaque to X-rays is injected into the coronary arteries so

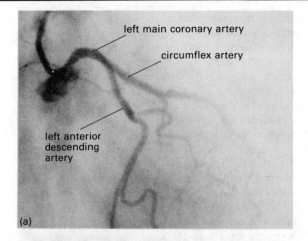

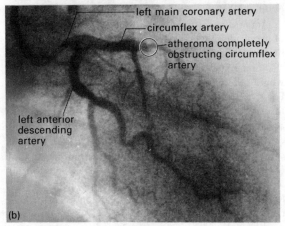

Figure 11.4 Coronary angiograms showing (a) a normal left coronary artery and (b) one in which the circumflex branch is completely obstructed by atheroma.

that the vessels show up on X-ray examination (Figure 11.4 (a) and (b)).

This newly-acquired ability led to an operation in which surgeons attempted to remove the obstructions within the arteries. This was partly successful, but was rapidly superseded by another operation, CABG, developed in Cleveland, USA in the late 1960s. Not only was the new operation highly effective in relieving angina sufferers of their disabling symptoms, it also *appeared* to increase the survival and life expectancy of patients. In this procedure serious obstructions in the coronary arteries are bypassed by grafting on a piece of blood vessel obtained from elsewhere in the patient's body, usually a vein from the leg (Figure 11.5).

One end of the graft is attached to the aorta (the main artery leaving the left side of the heart) and the other end to a coronary artery *beyond* the obstruction. To do this it is necessary temporarily to stop the heart contracting.

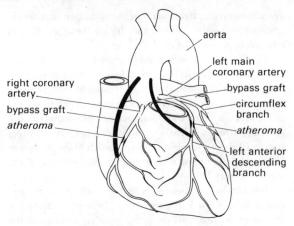

Figure 11.5 Heart and coronary arteries showing atheroma and two bypass grafts in position.

While the operation is being performed, blood has to be oxygenated and pumped round the body by a heart-lung machine. After the grafting is complete the heart is started again. After surgery, which lasts several hours, patients are placed in an intensive care unit where they can be carefully monitored. In most cases patients are able to leave hospital one to two weeks after the operation.

Given the high prevalence of CHD, it is perhaps not surprising that CABG has become the biggest growth industry in hospital medicine in the USA in the last ten years (Figure 11.6). (We shall discuss why the same has not been true of the UK in a moment.) But how effective is CABG? It is highly successful in relieving the victims of severe angina, of the disabling pain they suffer. About 90 per cent of angina sufferers gain immediate relief from the operation, though about 5 per cent relapse each year. Nevertheless, ten years after surgery 50 per cent of people will still be free of pain. However, while there is full

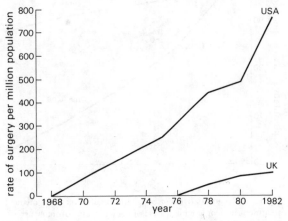

Figure 11.6 Rate of coronary artery bypass surgery in the UK and USA, 1968–1982.

agreement on the effectiveness of the operation in relieving angina, there is still considerable debate about its effect in improving people's survival.

This issue has been studied in three major randomised controlled trials (RCTs) in which CABG has been compared with medical (drug) treatment. These have shown that the effectiveness of surgery depends on the exact location, extent and number of obstructions in the coronary arteries. There is no doubt that surgery improves survival if there is an obstruction in the left main artery (see Figure 11.1) as can be seen in the results from one of the studies (Figure 11.7).

However, in only about 6 per cent of CABG patients is the obstruction in the left main artery. In most patients the obstructions are further on in the coronary arteries, in the two branches of the left main artery and in the right artery. In these patients the results of the RCTs have been less clear cut. The first American RCT reported in 1977 that CABG did not improve survival in these patients (Murphy, et al., 1977). However, it was argued that this was because the patients had undergone surgery in the early 1970s when up to 25 per cent of patients died as a result of the operation (as surgeons were still learning the new skills that were necessary). The results of the second trial carried out in Europe and published in 1980 seemed to confirm this view (ECSS, 1980). It found that surgery improved survival in those patients with all three branches of the coronary arteries affected (three-vessel disease) and in some patients with two-vessel disease (depending on the exact location of the obstructions). However, the third trial, which cost $24 million and was published in the USA in 1983, failed to show any improvement in survival in either two or three-vessel disease (CASS, 1983). The reason for the discrepancy

between the results of the second and third trials is a matter of considerable debate. There are two principal views. One is that drug treatment used in the third trial was so much better than in the second trial, that it wiped out any advantage of surgery. The other view is that the patients included in the third trial had less severe disease than those included in the second trial. On this basis people have argued that surgery would not be expected to make any difference to their prognosis.

As you can see, it is not easy to decide on the effectiveness of CABG. In 1985 the story of CABG is incomplete and still a matter for debate. However, there is sufficient evidence to show that many patients undergoing CABG in the USA (up to 20 per cent) gain no benefit from the operation. It has been estimated that this would have been true of about 25 000 of the 160 000 operations performed in the USA in 1982 (Kolata, 1983).

At the same time, there is no doubt that many thousands of people disabled by severe angina are restored to health by the operation. In addition, it has been estimated that in 1979 some 5 000 of 100 000 people operated on in the USA would otherwise have died (Aaron and Schwartz, 1984). For those 5 000, CABG has meant the difference between life and death. However, when viewed in the context of about 1.25 million deaths a year from CHD in the USA, the contribution of CABG is slight. In the UK, where the surgical rate in 1982 was one seventh of that in the USA (Table 11.1), the contribution of CABG in reducing mortality has been even less significant.

Why is the rate of CABG so much higher in the USA than the UK? According to Aaron and Schwartz, whose work was discussed in Chapter 2, there are two possible reasons. The first concerns the difference in the method of payment for health care between the two countries. As one American cardiologist put it:

> The entrepreneurial aspect of surgery in this country makes it imperative for surgeons to pursue the recruitment of patients aggressively. (Cited in Aaron and Schwartz, 1984, p.67)

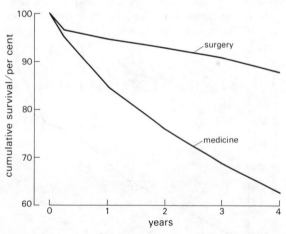

Figure 11.7 Cumulative survival with CABG and with medical treatment in people with disease of the left main coronary artery. Based on 1492 patients. P < 0.0001.
(Source: Chaitman, 1981, p.767)

Table 11.1 CABG — international comparisons

Country	Rate per million population
USA (1982)	770
Australia (1982)	410
Netherlands (1982)	377
West Germany (1983)	135
France (1983)	114
UK (1982)	110
Sweden (1982)	95

(Source: Wheatley, 1984)

In contrast, in the UK most surgeons are salaried employees of the NHS, whose resources are more limited and have to be competed for. However, while this restricts the number of NHS operations, it does not prevent many cardiac surgeons earning six-figure incomes by performing additional private operations — though even this is still only a fraction of the income of their American colleagues.

The second reason, which is related to the first, is the difference in attitudes of doctors: as one British physician noted:

> What impresses me is that in comparison with the UK it seems very seldom that the US physician ever states that there is no surgery that would help, no drug that is advantageous, and no further investigation that is required. There seems to be an irresistible urge to *do something*, even though in many cases the doctor concerned must realize that there is no possibility of benefit. (Cited in Aaron and Schwartz, 1984, p.66)

It seems unlikely that the rate of CABG will increase dramatically in the UK to match the American rate of surgery which in 1984 was a $375 million business. While innovations in treatment may make increasingly successful contributions to reducing the morbidity and disability resulting from CHD in the future, they are unlikely to produce more than a marginal reduction in mortality from CHD. It has partly been this realisation that has promoted so much interest in prevention.

Prospects for prevention

Ideally, prevention should be based on knowledge of the underlying cause or causes of a disease. Unfortunately, knowledge of the cause of CHD is incomplete. There is, however, considerable knowledge about *risk factors* — factors that are known to be associated with an increased risk of developing the disease. Some factors are unalterable: age (the risk increases with age), sex (more men than women are certified as dying from CHD), and a family history of the disease. However, others are amenable to change. For example, studies since the 1950s have suggested that *physical activity* reduces the risk of CHD. Comparisons of bus drivers with bus conductors, and postal delivery men with sorting clerks found people in the more active jobs suffered fewer myocardial infarctions. Taking vigorous exercise in leisure time has also been shown to protect against CHD. (Morris, *et al.*, 1980). Similar studies of women are still awaited.

Of the potentially reversible risk factors three are conventionally regarded as being of major importance: *smoking cigarettes* (Figure 11.8), having an *elevated blood pressure* (BP) (Figure 11.9), and having a *raised level of cholesterol* (a type of fat, or lipid) in the blood (Figure 11.10). From the point of view of prevention, we want to

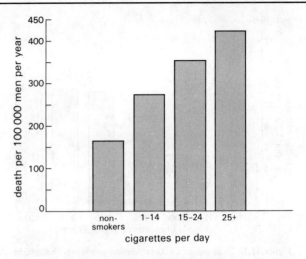

Figure 11.8 Mortality from CHD in non-smokers and cigarette smokers by level of consumption (men under 65 years of age). (Source: based on data from Doll and Peto, 1976, Table III, p.1527)

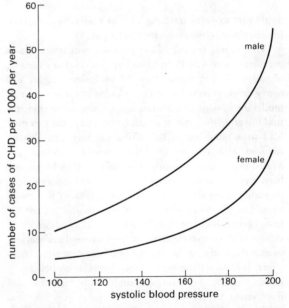

Figure 11.9 Incidence of CHD in relation to systolic blood pressure, for men and women aged 55–64 years. Annual incidence based on average over a 16-year period following blood pressure measurement being made.
(Source: Ball, 1979, Figure 9, p.7)

know the answers to two questions: are the associations causal, and what effect would control of these factors have on the CHD mortality rate?

As you have already seen in Chapter 9, it is possible to reduce the prevalence of smoking by measures directed either at the individual or the environment. There is little

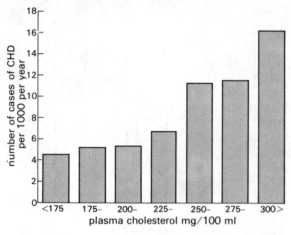

Figure 11.10 Incidence of CHD in relation to plasma cholesterol level in men aged 30–59 years at entry to study. Incidence based on first major events (myocrdial infarctions, sudden deaths) over a 10-year period. Plasma cholesterol refers to initial level.
(Source: based on data from Stamler and Epstein, 1972, p.27)

doubt that stopping smoking leads to a reduction in CHD. In other words, the association is causal.

This is not true of blood pressure reduction. Blood pressure can be reduced in a number of ways. For example, obese people can reduce their BP by losing weight, and heavy drinkers by reducing their alcohol consumption to a moderate amount. In addition, there is also some evidence that lowering the amount of salt consumed in the diet may lead to a reduction in BP. Blood pressure can also be reduced with the use of drugs. However, despite the availability of such measures, lowering people's BP has not been found to reduce CHD mortality (though it does reduce mortality from strokes — an interruption in the blood supply to the brain). There are three possible interpretations of these findings: that the risk of CHD associated with elevated BP is irreversible; that it is not a causal association; or that the studies were inadequate to demonstrate a small effect. Whichever is correct, there is little or no benefit, *as regards CHD*, in detecting people with high BP and intervening to reduce it. However, it is possible that preventing people from developing high BP in the first place may in time lead to a reduction in the CHD mortality rate for the population. It is with this in mind, that a reduction in the salt content of everybody's diet has been advocated by some experts in this field.

Even more controversy surrounds the third major risk factor — blood cholesterol. Although the mechanisms that determine the blood cholesterol level are not fully understood, two things are clear: that the amount of saturated fat (largely from meat and dairy produce) in the diet is *one* of the determinants of the blood cholesterol level, and that there is an association between the level of

blood cholesterol and the development of CHD (Figure 11.10). However, what is not clear is the effect on mortality of altering dietary fat intake. International comparisons reveal confusing and conflicting patterns. In Sweden, the consumption of saturated fat has decreased, while the CHD mortality rate in men has not changed. In Finland there has been no change in saturated fat consumption, but there have been falls in CHD mortality. And in the USA there has been a slight reduction in saturated fat consumption, and a marked reduction in CHD mortality. Overall there is little consistency between changes in saturated fat consumption and changes in CHD in international data.

Even more confusing have been the results of several RCTs of methods of lowering the level of blood cholesterol. These studies have taken two different approaches: the first has been based on *screening*, that is, targeted at the 5–10 per cent of the population at greatest risk. In all such studies, whether by dietary change or the use of drugs, blood cholesterol levels have successfully been lowered. However, in only one study was this accompanied by a reduction in CHD morbidity and mortality, and that partly resulted from a reduction in smoking as well (Hjermann, *et al.*, 1981). (In one other study the CHD mortality rate fell, but unfortunately this was balanced by an increase in deaths from other causes (LRCP, 1984).) Although the evidence from these studies is far from convincing, it does suggest that it might be possible to reduce mortality rates in people with very high blood cholesterol levels. However, even a major reduction in mortality in such a high risk group is only going to have a minor impact on the whole population's mortality rate, as *the majority of CHD deaths occur in people in whom the level of blood cholesterol is normal or only moderately elevated.*

Partly for this reason, some researchers have studied the effect of a second strategy: *mass intervention* — attempting to reduce the cholesterol levels of all members of the population. The results have tended to add to the existing confusion and uncertainty. In a major study in the Finnish county of North Karelia, a community-based programme was started in 1972. A neighbouring county, Kuopio, has been used as a comparison population to assess the effects of the programme. By 1979, although the annual decline in the rate of CHD mortality was higher in North Karelia (2 per cent in men, 2.3 per cent in women) than in Kuopio (1.4 per cent in men, 1.5 per cent in women), the difference was not statistically significant (Salonen, 1983). Despite this, these findings have been taken as evidence of the effectiveness of mass intervention by supporters of that approach.

Although the advocates of screening for high risk individuals and those who support mass intervention may disagree on the approach to be adopted, their strategies are not mutually exclusive. The former aims to reduce the high risk faced by a small proportion of people here and now, while the latter is a more ambitious long-term policy whose main beneficiaries (assuming there are some) are likely to be the young and the unborn.

Having discussed the nature of the associations, let us turn to the question of what effect we might expect on the CHD mortality rate if the three risk factors considered so far could be controlled. So far, when the *size* of risk associated with a factor has been mentioned, it has been referred to in terms of how much greater a person's chances are of developing CHD *relative* to a person who does not live with that risk.

☐ Looking at Figure 11.8, approximately how much greater is the risk of death from CHD for a person who smokes twenty-five or more cigarettes a day than for a non-smoker?

■ Approximately 2.5 times greater.

This figure is known as the *relative risk*. While it may be of use to an individual deciding on whether or not to smoke, by itself it is of no help to us if we want to determine what would be the effect on CHD mortality if everyone stopped smoking. To do this it is not the relative risk that is of interest, but the *attributable risk* — the contribution that a factor such as smoking makes to the total amount of CHD in a population. The only available estimates of attributable risk come from studies in the USA, in particular from a study carried out in Evans County, Georgia between 1962 and 1970 (Deubner, *et al.*, 1980). Making adjustments for differences in ethnic composition between the UK and Evans County (where approximately a third of the population were black) it is possible to demonstrate that even if everyone stopped smoking *and* their blood cholesterol level were reduced to less than about 210mg per 100ml, then the mortality rate for CHD would fall by about 8 per cent. It may be that if raised BP could be avoided in future generations, then the improvement could be as high as 20 per cent. However, that is pure speculation, for it is unclear whether or not such a change would accompany measures to control BP. In other words, just as you saw with the contribution of CABG, it appears that neither screening nor mass prevention based on the three major risk factors are going to solve the problem of CHD.

Evangelism, controversy and policy

While there is no doubt that innovation, screening and prevention all have a contribution to make, considerable uncertainty remains as to the impact each approach is likely to have.

☐ What similarity is there between the claims made in the newspaper stories at the beginning of this chapter?

■ The high level of optimism about the likely impact of each measure being advocated.

These stories all report the views of experts who are committed to a particular approach — *evangelists* who would not, at least in public, admit to having any doubts about the measures they are advocating. Evangelism is neither peculiar to experts in the field of CHD nor specific to health care in the 1980s. It is simply a characteristic of people with a belief in, and commitment to, a particular measure. As such, evangelists play an important part both in establishing and in maintaining debates about how health is currently cared for and in proposing alterations and developments which they believe would be of benefit. Although the experts cited in each of the newspaper stories hold different views from one another — some advocate more resources for surgery while others seek increased funding for prevention — they have several features in common. The first is their attitude to scientific validation of their views. Consider the following two quotations. The first comes from a leading British cardiologist, Celia Oakley, who believes that more coronary artery surgery should be provided:

It is unlikely that another massive trial will be mounted and in any case it would take another decade before it reported. In the meantime physicians will continue to apply their art where the science is lacking. The patients without severe symptoms are in the main quite happy with this and do not complain once they are dead. (Oakley, 1984a, pp.7–8)

The second quotation, from Frederick Epstein, an epidemiologist, concerns the decline in mortality rates that have occurred in the USA:

The only question is whether changes in nutrition in the direction of improving serum lipid patterns, better control of hypertension and less smoking can be held largely responsible for the change in mortality. This is indeed highly probable, unless one is willing to take recourse to mysterious forces which have hitherto escaped recognition. (Epstein, 1984, p.17)

☐ What similarities can you see in these two statements?

■ Both recognise the limitations of the scientific support for their views but believe the evidence is in their favour. They therefore demand that people should suspend their disbelief and have faith in either surgery or prevention. There is even a suggestion that everyone who does not agree with this must either be answerable to the victims of the disease or take refuge in supernaturalism.

Both specialities do of course face serious practical problems in obtaining scientific support for their views. As Oakley points out, any study of surgery will take at least ten years to produce meaningful results. In addition, there are the obstacles of cost — the third trial of CABG cost $24 million — and of size. It has been estimated that around 100 000 people would need to be included in an epidemiological study of the effect of changes in diet if reliable results are to be obtained. And even when a large scale study is funded and carried out, there is always the possibility that it will turn out to have been misconceived. For example, the failure of the major studies of dietary change to demonstrate any significant reduction in mortality from CHD are thought by some people to be because the 'wrong' studies were done. The consequences of this have been commented on by another leading British cardiologist, Michael Oliver:

> Whether the failure of these studies was due to the fact that too little was done too late will never be known and unfortunately no trials are ongoing to test the effects of doing more in younger adults. (Oliver, 1984, p.5)

Despite these methodological problems, and ignoring the exaggerated claims made for each approach, it is necessary that *some* strategy to combat CHD is adopted. What then are we to do? Do we have sufficient evidence to make policy recommendations? How certain do we need to be before prescribing action? Those who advocate prevention have been keen to point out that a similar dilemma was faced in the nineteenth century over the question of cholera:

> It is not unreasonable to adopt preventive policies that lack unequivocal scientific proof, provided they are very unlikely to do harm. There are precedents, dating back to the introduction of elementary sanitary engineering to control what subsequently became clear were water borne disease. (Bush, 1984, p.634)

Meanwhile advocates of a major increase in the provision of CABG are much more adamant:

> If we are going to save lives we have to diagnose coronary disease ... and obtain relief of ischaemia [inadequate blood supply to the myocardium] by surgical means when this is indicated. We must have the facilities to do this but will get them only if the profession wakes up to the realities and the message is not corrupted by those who work to obscure it. (Oakley, 1984b, p.1691)

> ☐ What similarity is there between the views expressed in these two quotes?
> ■ Both argue that we have sufficient knowledge to decide on what action should be taken.

The quote from Oakley reveals another aspect of the debate about a strategy for combating CHD — the attitude of evangelists to those who are not swayed by their proselytising.

> ☐ What is Oakley's view of those who do not agree with her?
> ■ Opponents are apparently not only unaware of 'the realities' of the effectiveness of CABG but are deliberately 'working to obscure' that reality.

Similar attitudes to non-believers are held by evangelists of prevention:

> The current wave of attacks against the risk factor theory is due in part to the fact that people dislike being overwhelmed, in this case by a compelling weight of scientific findings. (Epstein, 1984, p.18)

Those who fail to be 'compelled by the weight of scientific findings' find themselves accused of nihilism:

> No matter how many doctors recommend a diet low in saturated fat, some academic expert will disagree ... How can the damage be repaired? First the abominable no-men might be given less publicity. While the relative importance of diet, smoking, exercise, and treating hypertension may be debatable, the benefits of the total package can no longer be disputed. (*Times Health Supplement*, 1982, p.10)

Moreover, while calling for less publicity for the opposition, the envangelists of prevention are themselves busy urging members of the media 'to accept their important responsibility for promoting and protecting the nation's health' (HEC, 1984, p.xv). However, as one journalist has replied:

> Journalists are being enlisted to prescribe massive changes in lifestyle for millions of people on the basis of evidence about a relation between diet and CHD which is open to interpretation, to say the least. Am I thinking of a fabled golden age or was there a time once when a cautious view could be put forward without its instigator being accused of insanity or corruption? (Adams, 1984, p.1448)

So far we have only discussed the beliefs of the evangelists and the views of their opponents. There are, however, others in this debate who hold alternative views to those expressed so far. For example, some health professionals suggest that the call for more CABG ignores alternative treatments that centre on managing the psychological influences on the disease. They point out that the severity of angina may bear almost no relationship to the extent of atheroma in the coronary arteries, but may be heavily influenced by psycho-social aspects of a person's life. Others have pointed to the lack of adequate rehabilitation services for people who have suffered a myocardial infarction.

Similarly, in the field of prevention many of those who question the evangelists' belief in the 'holy trinity' of smoking, blood pressure, and cholesterol, argue that various psycho-social factors should also be taken into account. They point to the evidence that people with behaviour patterns characterised by intense ambition, competitive drive, constant preoccupation with deadlines and a sense of urgency (designated a *coronary prone personality*) experience more CHD than individuals with an opposite pattern of behaviour (Review Panel, 1981). The magnitude of this risk is roughly equivalent to that of smoking or having raised BP. Further support for the influence of behaviour patterns comes from a trial of a cholesterol-lowering drug. This study found that people who complied with medical instructions, regardless of whether they received the drug or a placebo, had a significantly lower mortality rate during the following five years than those who did not comply (15 per cent compared with 24–8 per cent) (Coronary Drug Project Research Group, 1980).

In addition to personality type, deaths from CHD also appear to be associated with periods of intense *stress*, such as being bereaved. 'Dying of a broken heart' may be more than just a romantic metaphor. It has also been suggested that stress could be the reason for the increased death rate from CHD in some migrant groups. Apart from psychological factors, one of the most powerful associations with CHD mortality is *occupational class*. In one of the largest studies of CHD mounted in the UK, over 17 000 civil servants working in Whitehall have been monitored since 1968. The CHD mortality rates for people in the four different occupational grades is shown in Figure 11.11

☐ How much greater is the risk of dying from CHD for unskilled workers compared with administrative staff?

■ Four times greater (relative risk of 4.0 compared with 1.0).

While some of this difference can be explained in terms of other risk factors (for example, the prevalence of smoking is higher in unskilled workers than in administrative staff), *most of it cannot*. The contribution that other recognised risk factors were found to make to occupational class differences is shown in Figure 11.11. Further evidence of the possible importance of social factors is the association between short stature and CHD, which might be explained by poor nutrition associated with poverty in childhood; the increased risk of CHD in the unemployed; and an association between the CHD mortality rate and fluctuations in the business cycle.* Given the extensive body of research on the influence of psycho-social factors, why is so

*This subject is discussed in *The Health of Nations, ibid.*

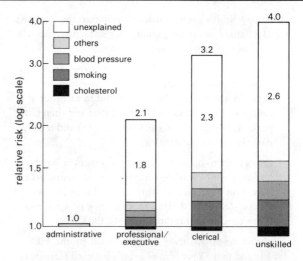

Figure 11.11 Relative risks of death from CHD according to occupational grade in the civil service. Note that a logarithmic scale has been used. Proportions of the differences between grades that can be explained by differences in known risk factors are shown. 'Others' include age, height, over-weight, leisure-time activity, and glucose tolerance (a test for diabetes). (Source: Rose and Marmot, 1981, p.17)

little attention paid to them? Two sociologists, Wendy Farrant and Jill Russell, have suggested a possible reason:

> this alternative model of CHD aetiology ultimately challenges orthodox medical practice by locating the appropriate point for intervention within the social and economic environment. (Farrant and Russell, 1985, p.14)

Not only that but as Peter Nixon, a cardiologist who is committed to the psycho-social model has indicated, part of the reason for a lack of support from researchers for this alternative approach is because of the considerable methodological problems it presents:

> The quality of sleep; the ability to modulate emotional arousal and sometimes to be still; the maintenance of a normal breathing pattern under stress; the choice of a salutary balance of rest and effort; and the security of confidence and self-respect may prove to be just as important as the conventional risk factors when we have developed the means of measuring them as readily as we can count cigarettes, units of blood pressure, and cholesterol today. (Nixon, 1984)

The alternative model would take the prevention of CHD outside of medicine and place it in the area of social and economic policy discussed in Chapter 10. Interestingly most health professionals would find such a shift more difficult to accept than would many lay people. Despite efforts by health professionals to promote the idea that CHD is caused by the 'holy trinity' of risk factors, many lay people hold different beliefs:

> It's always smoking ... they're always the same these things in books — they always go into smoking in detail, nothing else. There are bound to be other causes — but they say a bit about that and then have pages and pages about smoking. (16-year-old female, part-time shop assistant)

> ... its a lot to do with worry — if a woman has a husband out of work — unemployment means people have a lot of stress and worry ... and it creates lots of illness. (68-year old male, retired, railway worker) (Both cited in Farrant and Russell, 1983, p.31)

A market research survey commissioned by the HEC in 1981 found that 53 per cent of people believed stress was a major cause of heart attacks, a finding that the then HEC Director General Designate described as evidence 'that most of the public do not know what the important risk factors for developing a heart attack are'. Nevertheless, in the campaign that the HEC subsequently launched, entitled 'Beating heart disease', stress was mentioned, though somewhat grudgingly:

> ... it seems obvious that worry and anxiety, or frequent crises and rows, can make your blood pressure go up and lead to a heart attack. But *this is still difficult to prove*, partly because stress is almost impossible to measure and define. (HEC, 1982, p.11, our emphasis)

Similar concern about a lack of proof did not trouble the authors of the HEC booklet when discussing diet and blood pressure. While stress was at least acknowledged, the booklet's recommendations for action were, as Farrant and Russell have commented, firmly located in the sphere of individual change:

> Here, as elsewhere in the booklet, the role of the social environment is played down, whilst the individual, as a target for behaviour change or adaptation is emphasised. The available evidence was selectively presented to support a strategy of health education for individual change. (Farrant and Russell, 1985, p.28)

Apart from the debates between the evangelists and nihilists, and between a biomedical and psycho-social model, there is one further aspect to consider. Regardless of whether or not innovations in treatment are preferred to screening or to mass prevention, a more fundamental issue has to be faced — the relative merits of using resources in combating CHD rather than meeting other health needs. An indication of how limited resources might best be used can be obtained by cost-benefit analysis.

As you saw in Chapter 7, one way of doing this is by comparing the cost of different activities in producing the same amount of benefit, as measured in QALYs. As you may recall, the economists responsible for this approach found that in 1984 a QALY obtained by implanting a pacemaker cost £700, by replacing a hip joint £750, by a kidney transplant £3 000, and by a heart transplant £5 000. In comparison, they calculated that a QALY obtained from CABG cost between £800 and £3 000 depending on the severity and location of the atheroma. In other words, although no instances of CABG appear to be as good value as pacemakers and hip replacements, there are some indications for CABG being a better buy than kidney or heart transplants. While this study was very much a first look at the question of whether or not we should be investing in CABG rather than in other forms of health care, it illustrates the need to extend such debates to encompass a wide range of alternative strategies.

Just how practical will such an approach prove to be in the future? It seems likely that most decisions will have to continue to be made on the basis of incomplete information and a degree of uncertainty. Decisions about treatment, screening, prevention and wider aspects of public policy will continue to have to be made. The necessity of having to act today regardless of the greater wisdom we may possess tomorrow has long been recognised. The implication of this for the clinical management of patients was succinctly expressed by George Pickering, one of the most eminent of post-war British physicians:

> Intellectual nihilism is the very stuff of which scientists are made but it is scarcely convenient for a practising physician. (George Pickering, 1964; cited in Ferris, 1967, p.84)

Similarly in the field of prevention decisions still need to be taken in areas of uncertainty and doubt. As Alwyn Smith, a leading community physician has noted:

> Policy decisions have almost always to be taken against a background of scientific controversy since it is in the nature of science to be controversial while there must always be a policy, even if it is one of inactivity.(Smith, 1984, p.634)

The scientific controversy surrounding CHD illustrates just how polarised views can become. Researchers divide into opposing camps: surgery and medicine; treatment and prevention; screening and mass prevention; psycho-social and biomedical; individual and population. Given the complexity and contradictory nature of the subject, it seems unlikely that any single camp will solve the enigma of CHD. Indeed, the solution may be found by explaining the inconsistences in the story — a strategy that requires a multi-disciplinary approach that integrates biological, medical, sociological, economic and historical expertise.

Objectives for Chapter 11

When you have read this chapter you should be able to:

11.1 Explain the underlying pathology of CHD; the techniques involved in CABG; the difficulties in evaluating CABG; and why the rates of CABG are higher in the USA than in the UK.

11.2 Outline the risk factors associated with CHD and distinguish between relative risk and attributable risk.

11.3 Describe the similarities between the advocates of treatment innovations and of prevention; the domination of a biomedical over a psycho-social model of disease; the difficulties of scientifically evaluating their claims; a tendency to make exaggerated claims; and a rejection of opponents as nihilists.

Questions for Chapter 11

1 (*Objective 11.1*) Why has it proved so difficult to evaluate coronary artery bypass grafting?

2 (*Objective 11.2*) The relative risk of death from CHD for someone with a blood cholesterol level of over 300 mg/100 ml is much greater than that of someone with a level of around 210 mg/100 ml. But a policy that ensured that everyone had a level around 210 mg/100 ml would not have a marked impact on the population's mortality rate from CHD. Why is that?

3 (*Objective 11.3*)

> It's an illness I've got, sclerosis of the heart. It's the common illness of our time. I think its causes are chiefly moral. The great majority of us are forced to live a life of constant systematic duplicity. (Dr Zhivago in Pasternak, 1958)

Despite the limited success of the search for a biomedical explanation of the cause of CHD, there has been relatively little explanation of possible psychological and social factors. Why has this been so?

12
Futures

Thinking about the future is a universal human activity. The disciplinary term may change — astrology is out, futurology is in — but the practice remains. We all want to know what will or may happen next. We want to know what we should strive for and what we should avoid, what we should take into account and what we may safely ignore. And we want to know this not just for our own sake, but for those who come after us. So considering the future is a vital — though tricky — business. As such, it is central to both the study and the practice of health care. We may not know quite what will happen in health and health care, but we can reasonably assume that, whatever, does happen, some of it will be radically different from what has gone before. Equally, it is important to recognise that much will remain the same: hospitals have their origins in the Roman period; state involvement in social welfare is an ancient tradition; some aspects of health care, such as the sick role, are pretty much universal; and many very different societies have myths about some natural, uncorrupted ancient state in which people were healthy, happy and free of doctors. (Illich holds a contemporary version of this doctrine.)

Here, then, is the subject of this last chapter — some views of the future of health care: some cautious, others wild; some just a few years, decades or generations away, others cast in an utterly remote yet still (just) imaginable future. Before considering these views it is worth reflecting a little on the problems and more generally on the ways in which we think about the future.

Although we may now think far harder about the future than ever before, there is still no guarantee that we will get things right. Some things are confidently expected but never materialise; in their place comes something wholly undreamt of. Consider this definitive statement by a surgeon, J. E. Erichsen, made in 1873 at a surgical meeting at University College Hospital, London:

> That there must be a final limit to development in this department of our profession there can be no doubt ... An act may be modified, it may be varied, but it cannot be perfected beyond certain attainable limits. And so it is, and indeed must be, with surgery ... That we have nearly, if not quite, reached these final limits, there can be little question. (Cited in Graham, 1956, p.363)

During this chapter you will be asked to read an article in the Course Reader by Ruth West entitled 'Alternative medicine: prospects and speculations' (Part 7, Section 7.6). In addition, four other articles in the Course Reader are referred to: 'The flesh' by J. Desmond Bernal (Part 7, Section 7.1), 'Brave New World' by Aldous Huxley (Part 7, Section 7.8), 'High technology medicine' by Bruce Durie (Part 7, Section 7.2) and 'Biomedical research: changes and opportunities' by Sir MacFarlane Burnet (Part 2, Section 2.6). Although it is not essential that you read these in the study time available, each one of them extends the material in this chapter in interesting ways.

More recently, the spread of computers was wholly absent from visions of the future in the immediate post-war world. And there are countless other examples of mistaken prophesies. Although the human species has always considered the future (indeed this is one characteristic that distinguishes humans from other species), the ways in which this has been done have varied. Broadly speaking, two distinct methods can be identified — forecasts and projections. *Forecasts* involve studying the present and then, on the basis of the findings, extrapolating into the future. An obvious example, is that of forecasting the number of elderly people there will be in fifty years time — a straightforward task given our knowledge of the number of young people today. In contrast, *projections* are based on certain stated conditions or assumptions — if such and such happens, then the future will be so and so. As a result a projection such as the number of children there will be twenty years from now may be wildly inaccurate, based as it is on assumptions about changes in the birth rate. These examples of demographic changes will be discussed further in a moment.

The rise of science has not only transformed quantitative methods of viewing the future, but qualitative methods as well. Indeed, it has given rise to a specific genre, that of science-fiction. Qualitative methods have, however, considerably less academic respectability than quantitative methods — which is a pity, since from *Gulliver's Travels* (1726) onwards, it has regularly proved itself a profound vehicle for meditation upon human society and the human future. Indeed, some of the most interesting visions of health and health care are to be found here.

But just what is science-fiction? One central strand is *allegory* — much science-fiction contains a parable, a hidden meaning through which the events in some remote world have a vital relevance for today. That meaning can be either a beacon to draw us on or a terrible warning. In its first guise it is commonly termed a *utopia*, after the sixteenth-century book by Thomas More. For Oscar Wilde, writing in 1891, the production of utopias was itself a key way to shape a better future:

> A map of the world that does not include Utopia is not even worth glancing at, for it leaves out the one country at which Humanity is always landing. And when Humanity lands there, it looks out, and, seeing a better country, sets sail. Progress is the realization of Utopias. (Wilde, 1954, p.34)

Despite this, science-fiction is more often cast as a *dystopia*, or dire warning, than a utopia. One of the best known examples is Aldous Huxley's *Brave New World*, the opening pages of which appear in the Course Reader (Part 7, Section 7.8). There is also, however, a second crucial strand in science-fiction; one that has nothing to do with

allegory and contains no hidden message whether of gloom or uplift. Science-fiction is also a vehicle by which we can simply explore the possibilities of another and different world. 'What would happen to life if . . .?' This is often the central theme of the best science-fiction. It opens our eyes to fresh possibilities, however remote. A fine example of this style by a physicist, Desmond Bernal, also appears in the Course Reader (Part 7, Section 7.1). In an extract from his book, *The World, the Flesh and the Devil*, he argues that science can do better than mere biological evolution, by bio-engineering the future human — ultimately a disembodied brain interacting with the outside world via a multitude of mechanical sensors and robotic devices. Bernal's consideration of technical change is to some extent a feature of male science-fiction writers. In contrast, feminist writers (such as Marge Piercy) have tended to explore changes in human relationships as the most fundamental aspect in a utopian or dystopian future.

Both Huxley and Bernal speculated about science and society, health and disease in some far off time. Our concern in this chapter is more modest — a mere glance at some of the developments that might take place in health care over the next few decades. There are many aspects we could have chosen to consider — those we have selected partly reflect our own interests. To start, we consider the changing needs for care as a result of demographic changes, then discuss some ways in which patterns of care may alter, and finally we consider how the extent to which health services are accountable for their actions may increase.

Changing needs for health care

The nature of a health care system must depend on the amount of care of different kinds that is to be supplied, and that must in turn depend on the numbers of people needing care. How might these numbers change in the future, in the UK and the rest of the world? Let us begin by looking at the UK.

First, will the population increase or decrease? According to recent government population projections (OPCS, 1984), the population will rise slowly for the next forty years at least. In 1983, the estimated total population of the UK was 54.8 million; this is currently projected to increase by only about 4 per cent to 56.9 million by the year 2023. However, this overall change hides some important details that are likely to have a major impact on future needs for health care. The main one is that there will be far more elderly people, particularly elderly women, than there are today. This is especially true in the oldest age groups — for instance, the number of people aged ninety or over is projected to increase almost threefold, from 168 000 to 473 000, between 1983 and 2023.

But how accurate are these projections likely to be? As you have already seen, the future size of the elderly population can be fairly accurately forecast from knowledge of the existing number of young people. A few will die, but it is fairly easy to forecast how many. A few will emigrate and a few will immigrate to take their place, but these numbers are too small to make much difference to the total. Thus forecasts of the future size of cohorts of people who are already born tend to be accurate, though uncertainty about future age-specific mortality rates means that forecasts of the elderly population will be less accurate than forecasts of numbers of middle-aged people. (This is an aspect of 'Sod's law of service planning' — which states that the information you need most is exactly the information that is lacking or unreliable.)

In contrast, numbers of births are notoriously tricky to predict, and will remain so unless a breeding system like the one in *Brave New World* is introduced. Thus a projection of the total population forty years ahead is liable to be a long way out because it involves forty years' worth of birth rate predictions. And given the number of social and economic factors that affect the birth rate, it is hardly surprising that predictions of the rate tend to be highly inaccurate. Just how way out past projections have been can be seen in Figure 12.1. In 1965, it was predicted that the population of the UK would rise from 54 million to around 63 million by 1984 — in practice it only rose to about 56 million; for in 1965 it was predicted that in 1984 there would be over 1 200 000 births — in the event there were less than 750 000.

Future changes in Britain's population are, of course, tiny compared with what is expected to happen to the

Table 12.1 Percentage distribution of the world's population, 1980 and 2000

Region	1980	2000
Africa	10.6	13.9
Latin America	8.2	9.2
Northern America	5.6	4.9
East Asia	26.5	24.1
South Asia	31.7	33.9
Europe	10.9	8.4
Oceania	0.5	0.5
USSR	6.0	5.1

(Source: WHO, 1983, Table 21)

population of the whole world. The United Nations' demographers (WHO, 1983) predict that the world's total population will rise from an estimated 4 432 million in 1980 to 6 119 million in the year 2000 (though in the light of experiences in the UK discussed above, this prediction may also prove to be inaccurate). Table 12.1 shows how this population will be distributed among the regions of the world. As you might expect, the poorer regions of the world — Africa, Latin America and South Asia — are expected to have a larger share of the world's population in 2000 than they did in 1980. In 1980 the industrialised countries had a total population of 1 131 million, which is projected to increase by 12.4 per cent to 1 272 million by the year 2000. But the Third World, which already had the major share of the world's population — 3 300 million — in 1980, is projected to undergo a massive increase of 46.8 per cent to 4 847 million by 2000.

Not only is the total population of the world predicted to increase, but as in the UK, it is predicted that the proportion of elderly people will increase. This overall ageing of the population is much more marked in some regions than in others. The number of people aged seventy-five or over in the Third World is projected to double, more or less, between 1980 and 2000, rising from 37 million to 72 million. Meanwhile, the corresponding rise in industrialised countries is only (only!) about 40 per cent, from 46 million to 63 million. In other words, meeting the health care needs of an ageing population will be a relatively greater challenge for Third World than for industrialised countries. Given the difficulties the latter have faced, how will the elderly of the Third World fare?

Changing patterns of health care
If there are major changes in population structure, there are likely to be major alterations both in the pattern of disease, and in the demand for care. How can the world cope with a vast increase in population and disease? One possible answer lies in further scientific and technical developments

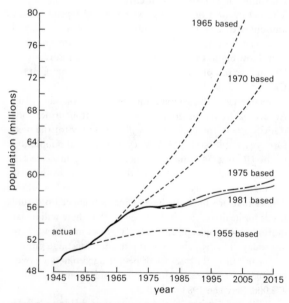

Figure 12.1 Actual and projected population of the UK. (Source: OPCS, 1984, Figure 4, p.30)

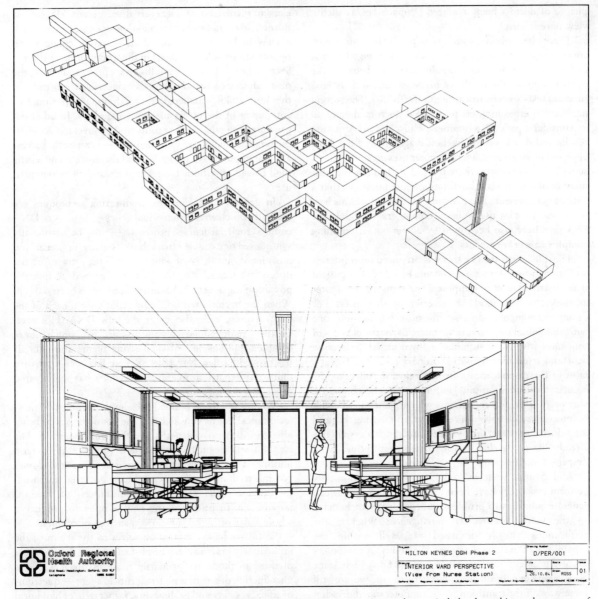

Figure 12.2 Milton Keynes District General Hospital opened in 1984. Computers were used extensively by the architects department of the Oxford Regional Health Authority during its design, producing ground plans, interior views and exterior perspectives such as these.

in natural science. Biology has made rapid strides in the last thirty years while, as you have already seen in Chapter 6, advances in physics and computing have provided medicine with scanners that can greatly increase the extent of biomedical exploration. There are many other examples, some of which are described in an article, 'High technology medicine' by Bruce Durie, which appears in the Course Reader (Part 7, Section 7.2). Here we will consider just two developments in greater detail — some of the impacts of

computers on health care and the potential role of genetic engineering.

Computers in health care

Since their introduction in the 1960s, *computers* have been applied to a diverse range of tasks: clinical diagnosis and decision-making, health service information systems, and even the design of hospitals (Figure 12.2). It is the first of these that has attracted most attention, as it conjures up the picture of doctors being replaced by machines. Is such a view pure fantasy?

There have been four principal ways in which computers have been applied to decision making. The first and most straightforward application has been in the interpretation of the results of investigations such as lung function tests and electrocardiograms (ECGs). The second has been to use computers to do what doctors already do — consider a patient's symptoms, signs, and investigation results and decide on the likeliest diagnosis and the most appropriate treatment. The computer uses *algorithms* — a series of simple instructions to lead it through the vast number of possible combinations and permutations that a patient may present. The main use of such algorithms has, so far, been for lay use on home computers, though in the USA they have also been used by doctors in determining complex cancer treatments.

The third use is the one that has produced most interest and speculation — *risk assessment*. Faced with a patient with a particular set of symptoms and signs, the computer assesses the likelihood of a series of diagnoses. For example, a computer can assess the probability of someone with abdominal pain having appendicitis, or the chances of someone who has suffered a myocardial infarction benefiting from admission to a coronary care unit. To date, most of these applications involve a doctor collecting the necessary information and putting it into the computer. However, in the future, patients who are not too ill could be interviewed directly by a computer, eliminating the need for a doctor at that stage of health care. Such a system has already been developed for patients suffering from dyspepsia (indigestion).

And finally, what of computers that can not only perform tasks they have been programmed to do but can generate solutions to problems independently of humans — the world of *artificial intelligence*? Whereas the applications already discussed are well within the capabilities of existing machines, the ability of computers to solve problems intelligently is still at a fairly early stage of development. In diagnosis and treatment, we are still some way off the transition from computer-*aided* decision making to computer decision making. Whether that point will ever be reached depends as much on what we see as the nature of health care and the role of doctors as it does on developments in computing science. After all, most people want something more than just an accurate diagnosis and an appropriate treatment when they seek care.

Genetic engineering

Compared with the impact that computers have had on health care, the techniques known collectively as *genetic engineering* promise to make an even greater impact. Some commentators have suggested that there is a genetic element involved in almost every disease state. Macfarlane Burnett, a world-famous immunologist, expresses just such a view in his article 'Biomedical research: changes and opportunities' which appears in the Course Reader (Part 2, Section 2.6). Whether or not his views prove to be true, the new industries based on genetic engineering are already, in the mid 1980s, challenging the dominant position of computing in the world of high technology. In addition, genetic engineering — the production of novel molecules or the refashioning of pre-existing ones — is attracting a vast amount of public attention. We will therefore spend a little time considering both the techniques and their potential uses.

In general terms, genetic engineering techniques are methods which enable individual genes — lengths of DNA coding for particular proteins — to be artificially synthesised or extracted from the cells of one organism and introduced into those of another, from the same or even a different species.* So far this has proved technically possible if the novel DNA is introduced into a bacterial cell. When the bacteria reproduce by cell division, each of the two offspring cells also carry the new DNA. However, because multicellular organisms are so much more complex, the business of engineering plants and animals has proved harder. Nevertheless there has been a massive industrial expansion in this area, which has made rapid progress.

What are the biomedical implications of these techniques? Let us consider first the possible uses of being able to insert novel lengths of DNA into bacteria. The bacteria will begin to make a new protein. As bacteria multiply very fast in suitable environments it becomes possible to think in terms of producing bacterial 'factories' to provide bulk supplies of substances of medical importance. In principle, the way is open to produce a whole range of useful substances, such as hormones.

So far we have confined ourselves to the realm of the immediately practicable. The obstacles to the development of these methods are primarily those involved with the introduction of any new pharmaceutical agent — questions of efficacy, safety and profitability, rather than of biological technique. The molecular products are all intended to be used in the same way as existing hormones, drugs and so forth. Although they are novel biological substances produced by new genetic techniques, they do not directly interact with an individual's genes but with their biological environment — such methods are sometimes referred to as *euphenics*.

However, could the techniques not be extended? Instead of inserting the DNA into bacteria, why not into animal,

---

*The roles of DNA and protein synthesis are discussed in *The Biology of Health and Disease*, Chapters 2–5, *ibid*.

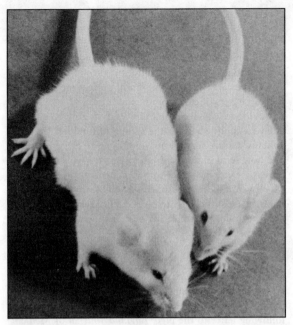

Figure 12.3 Littermate mice. The mouse on the left had DNA for rat growth hormone introduced into its genetic material.

plant or even human genes? Such a technique — just one example of a process called *eugenics* — is more complex but not impossible. Look for example at Figure 12.3, which shows littermate mice. The small one is the 'normal' control. Its littermate had had the gene for rat growth hormone inserted into it. If these supermice are mated their offspring also tend to express the inserted gene and therefore grow larger.

So what are the limits? Why not mice as big as humans? The answer lies in the complex processes involved in the growth of any multicellular organism. Increasing size is not just a problem of a single molecule speeding up growth but of overall *design*. A really giant mouse would need bones of quite different strength to avoid collapsing under its own weight, different circulatory and nervous systems, and it would have to behave in quite a different way too. In addition, all these changes require subtle combinations of many genes in complex interaction with each other and their environment during development. And finally, only a few per cent of the supermice would breed 'true' and produce supermice offspring. A multicellular organism's genotype is so complex, buffered and interactive that it tends to reject, during sexual reproduction and development, such foreign genes as may have been inserted into it.

Such problems are greatly multiplied if we consider the question of interfering with the human genome by *gene therapy* for eugenic purposes. Human eugenic proposals take two forms; in the first, *negative* eugenics, it is proposed to delete or replace deleterious or faulty genes; in the second, *positive* eugenics, it is proposed to insert advantageous ones.

There are a variety of diseases in which a single faulty gene is responsible, for example, P.K.U., Tay-Sachs disease, sickle cell disease and Huntington's disease. There are also conditions that arise from combinations of faulty genes and from chromosomal abnormalities, such as Down's syndrome. Estimates of the contribution of deleterious genes to human disease are hard to calculate. This is at least in part because it is very difficult to decide what is implied by the term 'deleterious'. For example, the sickle cell gene is deleterious in homozygous people but provides some protection against malaria in heterozygous people. Some molecular biologists argue that as much as half of the diseases and disabling conditions found in industrialised countries is the consequence of specified genetic predispositions. Others put the figure much lower. How much importance one attaches to the prospects for gene therapy obviously depends very much on whether one looks at the higher or lower end of this spectrum.

The methods currently available for the prevention of genetic disorders — genetic counselling, prenatal screening, selective abortion — were discussed in Chapter 8. The medical, social and ethical issues that such methods raise were also considered. As you may imagine, the problems posed by eugenics are even greater. First, as you have seen, only a small number of diseases are the consequence of *single* abnormal genes, and the problems of inserting multiple genes are formidable. Second, with most multiple-gene diseases there is only a possibility that the person with a particular combination of genes will show the deficit. Is it right to tinker with a person's genes to guard against a *possibility*, especially when interference could produce other and not easily predictable effects? Once again, the issue of 'the perfectibility of humans' is raised. Should the presence of a certain gene or genes be regarded as a deficit to be corrected, or should we instead accept the rich diversity of humankind that the mix of genes and environment produce? The example of growth hormone in mice comes to mind. There are certain human conditions where a genetic deficit in growth hormone results in very short people, for example, pituitary dwarfism. Presumably this condition might be rectified by insertion of the normal gene. But it is not merely pituitary dwarfism which could be corrected by additional growth hormone — very tall people could be produced for parents wanting their offspring to become basketball players. Should such positive eugenics be permitted? What priority, either within research or the NHS, should be given to such developments? And, if they do become permitted or even routine aspects of the future practice of medicine, do they take us along the path towards Bernal's utopia — or towards Huxley's Brave New World?

Systems of health care

If natural science seems likely to produce dramatic new types of technology, parallel changes may also reasonably be predicted on the social side of things. It is not just that *more* health care will be needed and that there will be new technologies to help in that care, but that the manner of delivering and controlling that care is likely also to undergo radical change.

Despite the vast resources invested both in the development of biomedicine and the provision of health services based on western medicine, there continues to be a considerable demand for *alternative systems of care*. Indeed, demand for the latter appears to have increased in Britain recently. An article in the Course Reader — 'Alternative medicine: prospects and speculations' by Ruth West (Part 7, Section 7.6), a supporter of alternative medicine, suggests some of the reasons why there has been renewed interest in some of the most ancient systems and speculates as to the future relationship between these systems and Western biomedicine. You should read this article now.

Whatever way the relationship between Western biomedicine and alternative systems develops, it seems likely that the latter will continue to play a part in health care in Western industrialised countries. One of the possible reasons for the support that these systems have attracted is people's desire for health care and carers to be more accountable for their activities to patients and the public (though it is by no means clear that alternative practitioners are any more accountable than their colleagues practising Western medicine).

Traditionally, doctors and health services have been subject to little or no *accountability* for their actions. Increasingly, this seems likely to change. Health professionals will be expected to account for their actions in three interrelated ways: to the public; to scientific evaluation; and to those who pay them. As you have seen in Chapters 3 and 4, the British public have little say in the choice of services provided and the particular way services are organised. Indeed, health authorities are increasingly accountable to central government, and virtually unaccountable to the local community they serve. Most of the local people on health authorities are selected directly or indirectly by the Secretary of State. Perhaps not surprisingly, the majority of these are white, middle-class, middle-aged or elderly men. Should this change? Two ways in which control of the NHS could be made more democratic are establishing directly elected health authorities or putting health services under the control of local authorities.

And just as the demand for public accountability is likely to grow, so too is that for scientific evaluation. Increasingly, only those investigations and therapies which have been scientifically evaluated will be acceptable. The effectiveness, efficiency and humanity of health care will have to be demonstrated before being implemented. And the methods of evaluation will grow more rigorous. While this will restrict the freedom of clinicians, it will increase the freedom of patients by freeing them from receiving ineffective care. In addition, it will protect the public and the purchasers of care from inefficient care.

An increase in accountability — to those who pay — is likely to apply whatever the system of funding. Decisions about which services are provided, who receives treatment, and how services and staff are organised will increasingly have to take the costs and the benefits into account. Moreover, if the total resources available for health care do not increase sufficiently to meet the increasing potential of new technology, then much more explicit, tragic choices will have to be made about who will and who will not receive care.

How will people react to such a state of affairs? Will people welcome the assistance of social science to help resolve the most pressing dilemmas, or might they provoke the kind of hostility expressed towards economics in the following letter to the *New England Journal of Medicine* (the leading American medical journal):

> Of late an increasing number of papers in this and other journals have been concerned with 'cost effectiveness' of diagnostic and therapeutic procedures. Inherent in these articles is the view that choices will be predicated not only on the basis of strictly clinical consideration, but also on the basis of economic considerations as they may affect the patient, the hospital and society. It is my consideration that such considerations are not germane to ethical medical practice, that they occupy space in journals that would be better occupied by substantive matters, and that they serve to orient physicians towards consideration of economics, which is not their legitimate problem. It is dangerous to introduce extraneous factors into medical decisions, since consideration of such factors may eventually lead to considerations of age, social usefulness, and other matters irrelevant to ethical practice. The example of medicine in Nazi Germany is too close to need further elucidation. (Loewy, 1980, p.697)

Every application of science can produce reactions of this kind: psychologists can be accused of manipulating minds, physicists of threatening us all with mass destruction. Just how alarmed should we be? Throughout this book discussion of science and scientific methods has been somewhat ambiguous. On the one hand, science offers new techniques and a cool approach to the many health issues that are sometimes muddied by the enthusiasm of evangelists. But on the other hand, we have emphasised that it cannot answer every question, for it itself is responsible for tragedies as well as blessings, while the pretence of science and 'scientific objectivity' is often used to mask specious and dangerous nonsense. For all these reasons it is worth reflecting on this subject just a little further and to do this we shall consider one of the most fashionable sciences of the moment — and one of the most developed of the social sciences — economics.

Dr Loewy's letter to the *New England Journal of Medicine* claims that the application of economics to medicine is new. In fact, there never was a time when medical practice was not influenced profoundly by economic considerations. None the less, there is genuine unease at the prospect of economists becoming ever more involved in health care decisions, roaming the wards, theatres and boardrooms with their 'tool-kits' of social scientific methods at the ready, claiming the ability to provide neutral, value-free advice and information (a claim echoed by other branches of science).

How plausible is this claim? Clearly some things are neutral. Measurement of money or volume can be conducted according to precisely specified standards. But as you have seen, theories about the social world — and those about the natural world too — require us to go beyond the facts, to make assumptions, such as those about human nature, or about evaluation, which can never be directly verified. Science too, therefore, for all its rigour, necessarily contains an element of ideology. As such it is always at least partly shaped by the values and prejudices of the age. The issue is particularly acute in the biological and social sciences, for their objects of study so clearly touch our own lives. Thus an economist, Joan Robinson, in reviewing the development of economics saw in it both a careful theoretical and empirical inquiry but also, and equally importantly, a method by which the prejudices and practices of successive ages might receive a dubious scientific blessing:

It was the task of the economist to overcome these sentiments and justify the ways of Mammon to man. No one likes to have a bad conscience. Pure cynicism is rather rare ... It is the business of the economist, not to tell us what to do, but to show why what we are doing anyway is in accord with proper principles. (Robinson, 1962, p.25)

In short, while science will undoubtedly continue to aid us in the future, it may also confidently be expected to serve as an ideological prop to many with special interests to advance.

One final point about science. Not only may it be mistaken because of ideological preconceptions or be used for harmful purposes, but also it may be wrong for wholly innocent reasons. The world simply is difficult to understand. This is why scientific knowledge undergoes continual change. It was once believed that scientific development occurs as the slow and patient accumulation of knowledge, brick upon brick. But more recently, sociologists and philosophers of science have seen it as in a perpetual state of revolution. Consider the following passage written by Paracelsus (1493–1541) one of the key figures in the development of scientific medicine, particularly in applying chemistry to medicine.

Nature works through other things, such as pictures, stones, herbs, or when she makes comets, similitudes, halos and other unnatural products of the heavens. (Cited in Hacking, 1983, p.70)

The passage sounds wholly bizarre. The problem is not one of whether Paracelsus was right or wrong but whether or not we can make any sense of what he is saying. Time has so changed things that what was clear and straightforward to Paracelsus and his contemporaries now seems wholly unintelligible to us. So it will undoubtedly be with some of the things that are central to our modern conceptions of health, disease and health care. Some aspects will remain recognisable even after the passage of many thousands of years, while others will appear not just wrong but unintelligible. What these will prove to be, only time will tell.

Some concluding thoughts

One thing, above all else, should be apparent to you about the dilemmas and prospects of caring for health — it is impossible to reach any simple, hard and fast conclusions. Dilemmas abound, and in turn, the very solutions proposed harbour their own intrinsic dilemmas. We therefore make no attempt to tie together the issues that have been raised nor to conclude any of the debates that have been aired. By their very nature, there are no easy answers. Instead, we end with three thoughts that should be considered when attempts are being made to resolve the dilemmas of caring for health.

The first is that whatever the dilemma, a multidisciplinary approach should be brought to bear in attempts to seek a solution. Each of the principal disciplines that have contributed to this book — biology, psychology, history, medicine, economics, sociology, social policy and statistics — have something to gain from working with the others. The same is true for research and for the development of health and social services. The days when biomedicine had a monopoly of interest in the subjects of health, disease and health care are long since over, but the days of a truly multidisciplinary approach have hardly begun.

Allied to the need for such an approach is the importance of adopting a comparative method. As you have seen, this can take several different forms — historical comparisons, comparisons between countries, and between social groups. There is, in addition, a comparative level that has received almost no attention in this book, that of comparison between species and the effect that diseases in other species have on the health of humans. The need for, and advantages of, such an approach may not be immediately apparent. What could we possibly learn from such comparisons? An example may serve as an answer.

Carlo Cipolla, an economic historian, was interested in the capital value that animals represented in non-industrial societies for such activities as transport, haulage, ploughing and wool. In seventeenth-century England, it was estimated that animals represented a sum equal to one quarter the value of all agricultural land. But as with humans, other animals are also subject to disease and the outbreak of epizootic diseases (epidemics in animals) in pre-industrial Europe could be as frequent as epidemics among humans, and as disastrous, for they knocked out a major part of society's acquired capital and reduced the prospects for economic growth:

> At times, these diseases assumed international political significance, as when in Pannonia, in 791, nine-tenths of Charlemagne's horses died and the Frankish King found himself in great military difficulties. More often, an epizooty was of purely local significance, but not infrequently it brought tragedy to entire regions. In 1275, 'A rich man of France brought into Northumberland a Spanish ewe, as big as a calfe of two yeares, which ewe being rotten infected so the country that it spread over all the realme: this plague of murrain continued for 28 years' ... When cattle died, the consequences for the economy of the time were comparable to the consequences of large fires which would destroy machines and power stations in a modern industrial economy. (Cipolla, 1976, p.99)

So, when considering the impact of disease upon humans, ideally we must also take into account its impact on the other species on which we depend. We might even take into account the fact that we ourselves might be a form of disease:

> Looked at from the point of view of other organisms, humankind therefore resembles an acute epidemic disease whose occasional lapses into less virulent forms of behaviour have never yet sufficed to permit any stable chronic relationship to develop. (McNeill, 1979, p.29)

What is the majesty of human progress from one point of view is merely a plague from another.

Finally, let us consider the importance we attach to the subjects of health and disease. There is a tendency for people committed or deeply involved in a particular area of research, work or study to think that that area is all important, that it takes precedence over all others. For example, throughout most of this book there is an assumption that *our* prime concern for health care is one that is shared by others. However, while most people attach a high value to good health and are concerned about the care they receive most do not view these issues as being of paramount importance in their lives. They (and we) attach as much importance to our relationships and our jobs, our homes and our families, our hopes and our fears.

The dangers of attaching too much importance to health and health care were recognised by Goethe (1749–1832), writing close to the beginning of the scientific revolution:

> ... I think it is actually true that humanity will win eventually. However, I am afraid at the same time the world will be a huge hospital and one will be the humane nurse of the other. (Goethe; cited in Fliedner, 1976)

Health is not the whole of life, merely the precondition. By itself it is a narrow subject. The best health science and the best health service, however specific its target, must also take the wider aspects of people's lives into account.

References and further reading

References

AARON, H. and SCHWARZ, W. (1984) *The Painful Prescription: Rationing Health Care*, Brookings Institution, Washington.

ADAMS, J. (1985) Medicine and the Media, *British Medical Journal*, 289, 1448.

ALLEN, D. (1981) An Analysis of the Factors Affecting the Development of the 1962 Hospital Plan for England and Wales, *Social Policy and Administration*, 15, 1, 3–18.

ALLDERIDGE, P. (1979) Hospitals, madhouses and asylums: cycles on the care of the insane, *British Journal of Psychiatry*, 134, 321–34.

ALLSOP, J. (1984) *Health Policy and the NHS*, Longmans, London.

BALL, K. P. (1979) *The heart patient I, Epidemiology*, Update Publications.

BAIN G. and PRICE, R. (1980) *Profiles of Union Growth: a Comparative Statistical Portrait of Eight Countries*, Blackwell, Oxford.

BARKER, D. and ROSE, G. (1984) *Epidemiology in Medical Practice*, Churchill Livingstone, third edn, London.

BERLIN, I., (1969) Two concepts of liberty, in *Four Essays on Liberty*, Oxford University Press, Oxford.

BEVAN, G., COPEMAN, H., PERRIN, J and ROSSER, R. (1980) *Health Care Priorities and Management*, Croom Helm.

BEVERIDGE, W. (1942) *Report on Social Insurance and Allied Services (The Beveridge Report)*, Command Paper 6404, HMSO, London.

BLAXTER, M. (1978) Power and inanity, in *Relationships between Doctors and Patients*, A Davis, (ed.) Saxon House.

BLAXTER, M. and PATTERSON, E. (1982) *Mothers and Daughters: a Three-generational Study of Health Attitudes and Behaviour*, Heinemann, London.

BLAXTER, M. (1983) Health services as a defence against the consequences of poverty in industrialised societies, *Social Science and Medicine*, 17, 16, 1139–48.

BLOOR, M. J., VENTERS, G. A. and SAMPHIER, M. L. (1978) Geographical Variation in the Incidence of Operations on the Tonsils and Adenoids: an Epidemiological and Sociological Investigation, Part I, *The Journal of Laryngology and Otology*, 52, 9, 772–80

BROTHERSTON, J. (1976) Inequality: is it inevitable?, in *Equalities and inequalities in health*, C. O. Carter and J. Peel (eds), Academic Press, London.

BROWN, M. and MADGE, N. (1982) *Despite the Welfare State*, Heinemann, London.

BURGHES, L. (1981) Unemployment and poverty, in *Unemployment: who Pays the Price?*, L. Burghes and R. Lister (eds), CPAG, London.

BURNINGHAM, S. (1984) Saved by a seatbelt, *Health and Social Services Journal*, 44, 532–3.

BUSH, M. (1984) Salt and hypertension (letter) *Lancet*, 2, 634.

BYRNE, P. S. and LONG, B. E. L. (1976) *Doctors Talking to Patients: a Study of the Verbal Behaviour of GPs Consulting in their Surgeries*, HMSO, London.

CARD, W. and MOONEY, G. (1977) What is the monetary value of a human life? *British Medical Journal*, 2, 1627–9.

CARTWRIGHT, A and O'BRIEN, M. (1976) Social class variations in health care and in the nature of GP consultations, *Sociological Review, Monograph 22*, University of Keele.

CARTWRIGHT, A and ANDERSON, R. (1981) *General Practice revisited — a Second Study of Patients and their Doctors*, Tavistock Publications, London.

CHAITMAN, B. R., *et al.* (1981) Effect of coronary bypass surgery on survival patterns, *American Journal of Cardiology*, 48, 765–77.

CHALMERS, I. (1983) Scientific inquiry and authoritarianism in perinatal care and education, *Birth*, 10, 3, 151–66.

CHARLTON, J. R. H., HARTLEY, R. M., SILVER, R. and HOLLAND, W. W. (1983) Geographical variation in mortality from conditions amenable to medical intervention in England and Wales, *Lancet*, 1, 691–6.

CIPFA (1985) *Health Care UK 1985: an Economic, Social, and Policy Audit*, CIPFA.

CIPOLLA, C. (1976) *Before the Industrial Revolution: European Society and Economy 1000–1700*, Methuen.

CIPOLLA, C. (1979) *Faith, Reason and the Plague*, Harvester Press, Brighton.

CLARK, J. M. (1981) Communication in Nursing, *Nursing Times*, January 1, 1981 12–18.

COHEN, D. and HENDERSON, J. (1983) A minister for prevention: an initiative in health policy, *HERU Discussion paper 2/83*, University of Aberdeen.

CONNOR, S. (1984) New Calls for Science Ministry, *New Scientist*, 20/27 December, 1984, 3–4.

CASS (1983) Coronary artery surgery study (CASS): a randomized trial of CABG. Survival data, *Circulation*, 68, 5, 939–50.

CORONARY DRUG PROJECT RESEARCH GROUP (1980) Influence of adherence to treatment and response of cholesterol on mortality in the coronary drug project, *New England Journal of Medicine*, 303, 1038–41.

CROSLAND, A. (1967) *The Future of Socialism* (abridged edn.) Jonathan Cape.

CROSSMAN, R. (1979) *The Diaries of a Cabinet Minister, Volume III*, Hamish Hamilton and Jonathan Cape.

DAVIS, K. and ROWLAND, D. (1983) Uninsured and undeserved: inequalities in health care in the United States, *Milbank Memorial Fund Quarterly*, 61, 2, 149–74.

DAVIS, M. S. (1966) Variations in patients' compliance with doctors' orders: analysis of congruence between survey responses and results of empirical investigations, *Journal of Medical Education* 41, 1037–48.

DEPARTMENT OF EMPLOYMENT (1983) *Employment Gazette*, 91, 5, 188–94, HMSO, London.

DEPARTMENT OF THE ENVIRONMENT (1983) Audit Inspectorate. *Social Services: Provision of Care to the Elderly*, HMSO, London.

DHSS (1976a) *Priorities for Health and Personal Social Services in England: a Consultative Document*, HMSO, London.

DHSS (1976b) *Prevention and Health: everybody's business*, HMSO, London.

DHSS (1977) *The Way Forward*, HMSO, London.

DHSS (1980) *Inequalities in Health*, Report of a research working group, DHSS, London.

DHSS (1981a) *Growing older*, Command Paper 8173, HMSO, London.

DHSS (1981b) *Care in the community*, HMSO, London.

DHSS (1982) *Health and Personal Social Service Statistics*, HMSO, London.

DHSS (1983a) *Health Care and its Costs*, DHSS, London.

DHSS (1983b) *Performance Indicators — Regional Summary for 1981*, DHSS.

DHSS (1984) *Annual Report*, HMSO, London.

DEUBNER, D. C., WILKINSON, W. E., HELMS, M. J., TYROLER, H. A. and HAMES, C. G. (1980) Logistic model estimation of death attributable to risk factors for cardiovascular disease in Evans County, Georgia, *American Journal of Epidemiology*, 112, 135–43.

DILNOT, A. W., KAY, J. A. and MORRIS, C. N. (1984) *The Reform of Social Security*, Institute for Fiscal Studies, OUP, Oxford.

DOLL, R. and PETO, R. (1976) Mortality in relation to smoking: 20 years' observation on male British doctors, *British Medical Journal*, 2, 1525–36.

DOWIE, R. (1980) The referral process and general medicine outpatient system. *First report: a statistical analysis, Health Services Research Unit, Report no. 41*, University of Kent.

DRAPER, P., GRIFFITHS, J., DENNIS, J. and POPAY, J. Three types of health education, *British Medical Journal*, 281, 493–5.

DRUCKER, P. F. (1979) *Management*, Pan.

ECKSTEIN, H. (1958) *The English Health Service*, Harvard University Press, Boston.

ECSS (1980) Prospective randomised study of coronary artery bypass surgery in stable angina pectoris, *Lancet*, 2, 491–6.

EGBERT, L. D., BATTIT, G. E., WELCH, C. E. and BARTLETT, M. K. (1964) Reduction of post-operative pain by encouragement and instruction of patients: a study of doctor–patient rapport, *New England Journal of Medicine* 270, 825–7.

EPSTEIN, F. (1984) Lessons from falling CHD mortality in the US, *Postgraduate Medical Journal*, 60, 15–19.

FARRANT, W. and RUSSELL, J. (1985) *'Beating heart disease': a case study in the production of Health Education Council publications*, Institute of Education, London.

FERRIS, P. (1967) *The Doctors*, Penguin, Harmondsworth.

FINLAYSON, C. (1983) Mental handicap in the family, in *Community Health*, J. Clark and J. Henderson (eds), Churchill Livingstone.

FINSBERG, G. (1982) *Prevention and Health Education*, Speech to Environmental Health Institution Congress, 22 September, DHSS, London.

FLIEDNER, T. (1976) *Priorities for the Uses of Resources in Medicine*, Fogarty International Centre Proceedings no. 40, Department of Health, Education and Welfare, Washington D.C.

FOOT, M. (1975) *Aneurin Bevan, 1945–1960*, Paladin.

FOSS, S. W. (1895) *Whiffs from Wild Meadows*, Lothrop, Lee and Shepard Co., Boston.

FOX, P. D. (1978) Managing health resources: English style, in *By Guess or By What? Information Without Design in the NHS*, G. McLachlan (ed.), Published for the Nuffield Provincial Hospitals Trust by Oxford University Press, Oxford.

FRIEDMAN, M. and FRIEDMAN, R. (1980) *Free to Choose: a Personal Statement*, Secker and Warburg.

FUCHS, V. (1972) The basic forces influencing costs of medical care, in *Essays in the Economics of Health and Medical Care*, V. Fuchs (ed.), Columbia University Press, New York.

GLENNERSTER, H., KORMAN, N. and MARSLEN-WILSON, F. (1983) Plans and practice: the participants' views, *Public Administration*, 61, 253–64.

GOFFMAN, E. (1968) *Asylums*, Penguin, Harmondsworth.

GOLDBERG, E. M. and HATCH, S. (1981) *A New Look at the Personal Social Services*, Policy Studies Institute, London.

GOUGH, I. (1979) *The Political Economy of the Welfare State*, Macmillan.

GRAHAM, H. (1956) *Surgeons All* (2nd edn) Rich and Cowan, London

GRAHAM, H. (1983) Health education, in *Women's problems in General Practice*, A. McPherson and A. Anderson (eds), Oxford University Press, Oxford.

GRAY, M. (1979) *Man against Disease*, Oxford University Press, Oxford.

GREEN, F., HADJIMATHEOU, G. and SMAIL, R. (1984) *Unequal Fringes*, Bedford Square Press.

GUEST, R. H. (1972) The role of the doctor in institutional management, in *Organizational Research on Health Institutions*, B. S. Georgopoulos (ed), Institute for Social Research, Michigan.

HACKING, I. (1983) *Representing and intervening: Introductory Topics in the Philosophy of Natural Science*, Cambridge University Press.

HAGGARD, H. W. *Devils, Drugs and Doctors*, Heinemann, London.

HALLETT, R. (1980) Why do we still dice with death?, *New Society*, 11 September 1980.

HANSARD, House of Commons, 24 November 1947.

HART, J. T. (1971) The inverse care law, *Lancet*, 1, 405–12.

HAUSER, M. M. (ed.) (1972) *The Economics of Medical Care*, Allen and Unwin, London.

HAYEK, F. V. (1944) *The Road to Serfdom*, Routledge and Kegan Paul.

HEALD, D. (1983) *Public Expenditure: its Defence and Reform*, Martin Robertson, Oxford.

HEALTH EDUCATION COUNCIL (HEC) (1981) Heart disease risks ignored, *Health Education News*, Sept./Oct.

HEALTH EDUCATION COUNCIL (1982) *Beating Heart Disease*, HEC, London.

HEALTH EDUCATION COUNCIL (1984) *Coronary Heart Disease Prevention. Plans for action*, Pitman, London.

HEATH, C. (1984) Participation in the medical consultation: the coordination of verbal and nonverbal behaviour between the doctor and patient, *Sociology of Health and Illness* 6, 3, 311–38.

HECLO, H. AND WILDAVSKY, A. (1974) *The Private Government of Public Money*, Macmillan.

HENDERSON, J. B. (1982) Measuring the benefits of screening for open neural tube defects, *Journal of Epidemiology and Community Health*, 36, 214–19.

HIMMELSTEIN, D. AND WOOLHANDLER, S. (1984) Pitfalls of private medicine: health care in the USA, *Lancet*, 2, 391–3.

HJERMANN, I., VELVE BYRE, K., HOLME, I. and LEVEN, P. (1981) Effect of diet and smoking intervention on the incidence of CHD, *Lancet*, 2, 1303–10.

HUGHES, E. (1958) *Men and their Work*, Free Press of Glencoe.

HUGHES, E. (1971) *The Sociological Eye*, Alldine-Atherton, Chicago.

HURST, J. (1979) Planning and hospitals costs, in *Economics and Health Planning*, K. Lee (ed.), Croom Helm.

JANIS, I. and FESHBACH, S. (1953) Effects of fear-arousing communications, *Journal of Abnormal and Social Psychology*, 48, 1, 78–92.

JEFFERYS, M. (1977) What are health services for: whom do they serve? *New Universities Quarterly*, 30, 2, 181–92.

JONES, K. (1972) *A History of the Mental Health Services*, Routledge and Kegan Paul.

KEYNES, J. M. (1922) General Introduction to Cambridge Economic Handbooks, Volume III, *Public Finance*, M. E. Robinson (ed.), Cambridge University Press.

KLEIN, R. (1983) *The Politics of the National Health Service*, Longman.

KOLATA, G. (1983) Some bypass surgery unnecessary, *Science*, 11 November 1983, 605.

LAMBERTS, H. (1980) Problem behaviour, in *Primary Care*, J. Fry (ed.), Heinemann.

LAND, H. and ROSE, H. (1985) Compulsory altruism for some or an altruistic society for all, in *In defence of Welfare*, P. Bean (ed.), Tavistock.

LANE, W. A. (ed.) (1934) *The Hygiene of Life*, British Books Ltd, London.

LE GRAND, J. (1978) The distribution of public expenditure: the case of health care, *Economica*, 45, 125–42.

LE GRAND, J. (1982) *The Strategy of Equality: Redistribution and the Social Services*, Allen and Unwin.

LEY, P. (1982) Satisfaction, compliance and communication, *British Journal of Clinical Psychology* 21, 241–54.

LILIENFELD, A. M. and KORDAN, B. (1966) A study of variability in the interpretation of chest X-rays in the detection of lung cancer, *Cancer Research*, 26, 2145.

LIPSEY, D. (1980) Random B-tests backed, *Sunday Times*, 8166, 28 December, 1980.

LOEWY, E. (1980) Letter, *New England Journal of Medicine*, 302, 697.

LONDON HEALTH PLANNING CONSORTIUM (1981) *Primary Health Care in Inner London*, Report of a study group, DHSS, London.

LRCP (1984) The Lipid Research Clinics coronary primary prevention trial results, *J.A.M.A.* 251, 351–64.

MCDONNELL, R. and MAYNARD, A. (1985) The costs of alcohol misuse, *British Journal of Addiction*, 80, 27–35.

MCKEOWN, T. (1976) An approach to screening policies, *Journal of Royal College of Physicians*, 10, **2**, 145–52.

MCNEILL, W. (1979) *Plagues and Peoples*, Penguin, Harmondsworth.

MCPHERSON, K., COULTER, A. and STRATTON, I. (1985) Increasing use of private practice by patients in Oxford requiring common elective surgical operations, *British Medical Journal*, **291**, 797–9.

MCQUILLAN, J. *Charity Statistics 1983/4*, Charities Aid Foundation, Tonbridge.

MADDISON, A. (1982) *Phases of Capitalist Development*, Oxford University Press.

MALINES, J. (1953) The fence or the ambulance, *Journal of the Soil Association*, 7, 24.

MAYNARD, A. and LUDBROOK, A (1980) Applying resource allocation formulae to constituent parts of the UK, *Lancet*, 1, 85–7.

MINISTRY OF HEALTH (1962) *A Hospital Plan for E and W*, Command Paper 1604, HMSO, London.

MINISTRY OF HEALTH (1963) *Health and Welfare. The Development of Community Care*, Command Paper 1973, HMSO, London.

MINISTRY OF HEALTH (1969) *Digest of Health Statistics for England and Wales*, HMSO, London.

MOONEY, G., RUSSELL, E. and WEIR, R. (1980) *Choices in Health Care*, Macmillan.

MORRIS, J. N. (1980) Inequalities in health, *British Medical Journal*, 281, 1003.

MORRIS, J. N., EVERITT, M. G., POLLARD, R., CHAVE, S. P. W. and SEMMENCE, A. M. (1980) Vigorous exercise in leisure-time: protection against CHD, *Lancet*, 2, 1207–10.

MURPHY, M. L. *et al.* (1977) Treatment of chronic stable angina: a preliminary report of survival data of the randomised Veterans' Administration cooperative study, *New England Journal of Medicine*, 297, 621–7.

NAHA (1979) Seat-belts — 'Challenge to MPs', *NAHA News*, Birmingham.

NIXON, P. (1984) The risk factors, *The Guardian*, 16 May 1984.

NORTON, A. AND ROGERS, S. (1981) The Health Service and Local Government Services: can they work together to meet the needs of the elderly and of other disadvantaged groups? Why is collaboration a problem?, in *Matters of Moment*. G. McLachlan (ed.), published for the Nuffield Provincial Hospitals Trust by Oxford University Press.

OAKLEY, C. (1984a) Coronary surgery for survival; paper given at Consensus Development conference on CABG, Kings Fund College.

OAKLEY, C. (1984b) Consensus development conference: CABG. (letter), *Lancet*, 289, 1690–1.

OFFICE OF HEALTH ECONOMICS (1981) *Alcohol — reducing the harm*, OHE, London.

OFFICE OF HEALTH ECONOMICS (1982) *Coronary heart disease. The scope for prevention*, OHE, London.

OFFICE OF HEALTH ECONOMICS (1985a) *Digest of Health Statistics 1985*, OHE, London.

OFFICE OF HEALTH ECONOMICS (1985b) *Pharmaceuticals in Seven Nations*, OHE, London.

OPCS (1984) *Population Projections: mid 1983-based*, OPCS Monitor, PP2 84/1, HMSO, London.

OLIVER, M. F. (1984) CHD — prevalence, clinical features, prognosis and medical management; paper given at Consensus Development conference on CABG, Kings Fund College.

PASTERNAK, B. (1958) *Dr Zhivago*, London, Collins.

PENDLETON, D. and BOCHNER, S (1980) The communication of medical information in GP consultations as a function of patients' social class, *Social Science and Medicine*, 14, a, 669–73.

POLITICAL AND ECONOMIC PLANNING (PEP) (1944) Medical care for citizens, *Planning*, 222.

POLLITT, C. (1985) Measuring performance: a new system for the NHS, *Policy and Politics*, 13, **1**, 1–15.

POSNETT, J. (1984) A profile of the charity sector, in *Charity Statistics 1983/4* J. McQuillan (ed.), Charities Aid Foundation, Tonbridge.

POWELL, J. E. (1976) *Medicine and Politics: 1975 and After*, Pitman Medical, London.

PUBLIC ACCOUNTS COMMITTEE (1981) *Seventeenth Report*, HC 225, HMSO.

PUBLIC MONEY (1984) Real resources and unreal assumptions: the case of the NHS, *Public Money* 4, 3, 58–62.

REVIEW PANEL ON CORONARY-PHONE BEHAVIOUR AND CHD (1981) Coronary-prone behaviour and CHD: a critical review, *Circulation*, 63, **6**, 1199–215.

RICHARDSON, J. J. and JORDAN, A. G. (1979) *Governing under Pressure: the Policy Process in a Post-Parliamentary Democracy*, Martin Robertson, Oxford.

RIMM, A. A. and BORTIN, M. (1978) Clinical trials as a religion, *Biomedicine Special Issue*, 28, 60–3.

ROBB, B. (ed.) (1967) *Sans Everything — A Case to Answer*, Nelson.

ROBINSON, J. (1962) *Economic Philosophy*, C. A. Watts.

ROSE, G. and MARMOT, M. (1981) Social class and CHD, *British Heart Journal*, 45, 13–19.

ROSENHAN, D. L. (1973) On being sane in insane places, *Science*, **179**, 250–8.

ROSSER, R. M. and WATTS, V. C. (1972) The measurement of hospital output, *International Journal of Epidemiology*, 1, **4**, 361–8.

ROTH, J. (1979) A Yank in the NHS, in *Medical Encounters*, A. Davis and G. Horobin (eds), Croom Helm, London.

ROYAL COLLEGE OF PHYSICIANS (1962) *Smoking and Health*, Pitman, London.

ROYAL COLLEGE OF PHYSICIANS (1983) *Health or Smoking*, Pitman, London.

ROYAL COMMISSION ON THE NHS (1978) *Patients' Attitudes to the Hospital Service*, Research Paper no. 5, HMSO, London.

ROYAL COMMISSION ON THE NHS (1979), Command Paper 7615, HMSO, London.

RUSSELL, M., WILSON, C., TAYLOR, C. and BAKER, C. D. (1979) Effect of GPs' advice against smoking, *British Medical Journal*, 2, 231–5.

ST GEORGE, D. (1981) Who pulls the strings at the HEC?, *World Medicine*, November 28, 1981, 51–4.

SALONEN, J. T., PUSKA, P., KOTTKE, T. E., TUOMILEHTO, J. and NISSINEN, A. (1983) Decline in mortality from CHD in Finland from 1969 to 1979, *British Medical Journal*, 286, 1857–60.

SHAPIRO, S. (1977) Evidence on screening for breast cancer from a randomised trial, *Cancer*, 39, 2772–82.

SHEFFIELD HEALTH COMMITTEE (1984) *Environmental Health: a Preventative Service*, Sheffield City Council.

SHEIHAM, A. (1983) Sugars and dental decay, *Lancet*, 1, 282–4.

SHULMAN, J. and RENTOUL, J. (1984) Profits of sickness, in *Who cares? The future of the NHS*, J. Rentoul (ed.), New Statesman, London.

SILVERMAN, D. (1984) Going private: ceremonial forms in a private oncology clinic, *Sociology*, 18, **2**, 191–204.

SIMPSON, D. (1984) Cigarette smoking, *Postgraduate Medical Journal*, 60, 20–5.

SIMON, J. (1980) *English Sanitary Institutions*, Cassell and Company.

SMAIL, R., GREEN, F. and HADJIMATHEOU (1984) *Unequal Fringes*, Low Pay Report no. 15, Low Pay Unit, London.

SMITH, A. (1984) Salt and hypertension (letter), *Lancet*, 2, 634.

SOCIAL SERVICES COMMITTEE (1982) *The Personal Social Services: Trends in Expenditure and Provision*, pp.168–89 of minutes of Social Services Committee, HMSO, London.

SOCIAL SERVICES COMMITTEE (1983) *Session 1982–83, Public expenditure on the Social Services*, HMSO, London.

SOCIAL SERVICES COMMITTEE (1985) *Community Care*, HMSO, London.

SPRING, J. A. and BUSS, D. H. (1977) Three centuries of alcohol in the British diet, *Nature*, 270, 567–72.

STACEY, M. (1983) A lay member's view of the GMC, *GMC Annual Report for 1982*, GMC.

STAMLER, J. and EPSTEIN, F. (1972) CHD: risk factors as guides to preventive action, *Preventive Medicine*, 1, 27.

STEEL, D. (1984) Managing Health Authorities: one member's view, *Public Money*, 4, **1**, 37–40.

STEWART, R. (1970) *The Reality of Organizations: a Guide for Managers*, Macmillan.

STIMSON, G. V. and WEBB, B. (1975) *Going to See the Doctor*, Routledge and Kegan Paul.

STIMSON, G. V. and OPPENHEIMER, E. (1982) *Heroin Addiction: Treatment and Control in Britain*, Tavistock, London.

STOCKING, B. (1985) *Initiative and Inertia*, Nuffield Provincial Hospitals Trust, London.

STORR, A. (1979) *The Art of Psychotherapy*, Secker and Warburg, London.

STRONG, P. M. (1979) *The Ceremonial Order of the Clinic*, Routledge and Kegan Paul.

TAYLOR, D. (1984) *Understanding the NHS in the 1980s*, Office of Health Economics, London.

TAYLOR, P. (1984) *Smoke Ring: the Politics of Tobacco*, Bodley Head, London.

TAYLOR, R. M. R., TING, A. and BRIGGS, J. D. (1985) Renal transplantation in the UK and Ireland — the centre effect, *Lancet*, 1, 798–803.

TIMES HEALTH SUPPLEMENT (1982) Abominable no-men (editorial), February 26 1982.

TITMUSS, R. (1976) The social division of welfare, in *Essays on the Welfare State* (3rd edn), Allen and Unwin.

TOWNSEND, P. (1962) *The Last Refuge*, Routledge and Kegan Paul, London.

TOWNSEND, P. (1979) *Poverty in the U.K.* Penguin, Harmondsworth.

TUC (1975) *Health and Safety at Work*, TUC, London.

TRENT, H. (1981) What the public wants, *Health and Social Services Journal,* June 5 1981, 665–8.

ULRICH, R. (1984) View through a window may influence recovery from surgery, *Science,* 224, 420–1.

US PUBLIC HEALTH SERVICE (1960) *Diabetes Program Guide,* Public Health Service Publication no. 506, US Dept. HEW, Washington.

WATKINS, B. (1975) *Documents on Health and Social Services: 1834 to the Present Day,* Methuen.

WALKER, A., WINYARD, S. and POND, C. (1983) Conservative economic policy: the social consequence, in *Thatcherism and the Poor,* D. Bull and P. Wilding (eds), CPAG, London.

WELLER, M.P.I. (1985) Friern hospital: where have all the patients gone?, *Lancet,* 1, 569–71.

WELLS, C. (1964) *Bones, Bodies and Disease: Evidence of Disease and Abnormality in Early Man,* Thames and Hudson.

WHEATLEY, D. (1984) Surgical prospects; paper given at Consensus Development conference on CABG, Kings Fund College.

WILDE, O. (1973) *De Profundis and Other Writings,* H. Pearson (ed.), Penguin, Harmondsworth.

WILLIAMS, A. (1974) The 'cost-benefit' approach, *British Medical Bulletin,* 30, **3**, 252–6.

WILLIAMS, A. (1985) Economics of coronary artery bypass grafting, *British Medical Journal,* **291**, 326–9.

WHO (1983) *World Health Statistics, 1983,* WHO, Geneva.

YATES, J. (1983) When will the players get involved?, *Health and Social Services Journal,* September 15, 1983, 1111–12.

Further reading

CIPFA (1985) *Health Care UK 1985: an Economic, Social and Policy Audit,* CIPFA.
Commencing in 1984, the Chartered Institute of Public Finance and Administration have published an annual review of the provision of formal health care in the UK. Although rather expensive to buy, these reviews provide a valuable up-to-date reference work for those interested in contemporary issues.

CORNWELL, J. (1984) *Hard-earned lives,* Tavistock Publications.
A revealing account of what 'ordinary people' living in East London think about health, disease and health care. It also illustrates one particular method of social research.

DAVIS, A. and HOROBIN, G. (1977) *Medical Encounters: the Experience of Illness and Treatment,* Croom Helm. A collection of essays written by sociologists who have themselves been patients, i.e. participant observers.

DILNOT, A. W., KAY, J. A. and MORRIS, C. N. (1984) *The Reform of Social Security,* Oxford University Press.
An account of the social security system, which explains the basis of the problems facing the welfare state in the 1980s and the measures that might be taken to reform the system.

FRIEDSON, E. (1970) *Profession of Medicine,* Dodd, Mead and Co.
The classic analysis of the modern medical profession.

GLOVER, J. (1977) *Causing Death and Saving Lives,* Penguin Books.
A philosopher considers the moral difficulties brought about by the advance of modern medicine, and sets these against the morality of life and death decisions in other areas of the social world — capital punishment, revolution, war and the relief of poverty.

GRAY, J. A. M. (1979) *Man against Disease: Preventive Medicine,* Oxford University Press.
Although in danger of becoming out of date, this remains one of the best accounts of disease prevention in all its ramifications. The chapters on ways and means and on obstacles to prevention are particularly good.

KLEIN, R. (1983) *The Politics of the NHS,* Longman.
An account of the political history of the NHS, written by a political scientist who is one of the leading British health policy analysts.

MOONEY, G., RUSSELL, E. and WEIR, R. (1980) *Choices for Health Care,* Macmillan.
A short review of the contribution that economics can make to planning and managing the NHS. It makes both the methods and some of the key issues in health economics accessible to the lay reader.

OHE (Office of Health Economics)
Publish several pamphlets and booklets each year on health care topics. In addition, they produce an annual *Compendium of Health Statistics* which gives detailed, up-to-date information on health services. OHE publications can be obtained from 12, Whitehall, London SW1A 2DY.

OPCS (Office of Population, Censuses and Surveys)
Publish many statistical works relevant to the study of health, disease and health care. Most publications are annual, though some are more frequent. In addition, OPCS also carry out and publish the findings of *ad hoc* surveys. Details of publications can be obtained from HMSO bookshops or bookshops which stock HMSO publications.

SALMON, J. W. (ed.) (1985) *Alternative Medicines: Popular and Policy Perspectives*, Tavistock Publications.

A collection of articles that examines the current interest in alternative medicines in the context of historical and contemporary developments in conventional medicine.

SILVERMAN, W. (1980) *Retrolental Fibroplasia: a Modern Parable*, Grune and Stratton.

A fascinating account of how the connection between blindness in infancy and the use of high concentrations of oxygen in the care of premature babies was unravelled. A revealing insight into the nature of scientific inquiry.

TAYLOR, P. (1984) *Smoke Ring: the Politics of Tobacco*, Bodley Head.

An investigative journalist describes the interests and powers that help maintain the strength of the tobacco industry both commercially and politically.

Answers to self-assessment questions

Chapter 1

1 Between 1948 and 1974 the NHS was organised in three parts (tripartite): general practitioner services (including dentists and ophthalmic services) were administered by Executive Councils; hospitals were the responsibility of Regional and Teaching Hospital Boards; and community and environmental health services were provided by the Local Health Authorities (see Figure 1.1). After 1974 the hospital and community services were integrated under the new Regional and Area Health Authorities. However, a form of tripartite structure persisted (see Figure 1.2).

2 The creation of a series of tiers of management in which the responsibility for providing services is delegated out from the centre to the periphery. In return, each tier is accountable for its performance to the tier immediately above it.

3 There were three key changes: the scrapping of one of the tiers of management (AHAs) in 1982; the replacement of the multidisciplinary teams with general managers; and the introduction of management units in an attempt to shift the administration of services closer to the staff providing them.

Chapter 2

1 The patients' *need* for treatment is clear from the fact that many died while waiting. The *demand* for transplant operations results from the availability of the operation — there was no demand before the 1980s because both lay people and GPs knew that the operation was not being supplied in the UK. The existence of a waiting list for the operation means that the level of supply is insufficient to meet the demand. As with nearly all hospital services in the NHS, supply is limited by the constraints on overall funding from the government.

2 With volume planning, the level of provision of services was guaranteed. If pay increases for hospital staff exceeded the amount allowed for them, then the government made up the shortfall to the health authorities. In contrast, under cash limits, any shortfall has to be found by the health authority. This may mean that services to patients have to be reduced to achieve the necessary savings.

At the time of writing (1985) cash limits have not been introduced for general practitioner services. The provision of these services has been demand-led. Whether or not this arrangement continues in the future is not clear.

3 Rationing is inevitable because the demand for health care is very great while the supply of care is limited. The existence of supplier-induced demand means that any increase in supply (such as the introduction of a new technique) will lead to an increase in demand.

Health care is rationed:

(a) In the NHS by restriction of the total amount of care available. This results in patients having to queue (on waiting lists), and doctors having to set their criteria for treatment in the light of realistic assessments of the availability of care. In some instances direct charges, such as for prescriptions, lead to some rationing.

(b) Rationing in a fee-for-service system is by price barriers — care is made available to those who can afford it, either by direct payment or more usually through insurance schemes.

(c) The form of rationing by HMOs lies somewhere between the other two systems. As with the NHS, cost-conscious doctors restrict the use made of services in the hope of avoiding unnecessary expenditure. However, as with fee-for-service systems, price barriers also exist. The higher the subscription to an HMO, the less the services will be rationed. Thus the poorest members of society will face greater rationing than the better off, though this difference would be considerably less than exists in fee-for-service systems.

4 (a) Until the 1970s English regions were allocated resources according to their existing level of hospital services. Thus, the more hospital facilities a region had, the more funding it received, and vice versa. In addition, the provision of general practitioner services favoured the more prosperous regions of the country.

(b) The per capita expenditure in Scotland is higher than in England because the demographic changes that have occurred since the Goschen formula was adopted have not been taken into account.

The main difficulty that has prevented a more rapid reduction in geographical inequalities within England has been the need to level down resources as a result of tight restrictions on total NHS spending since the late 1970s.

5   First, central government's priorities documents are only advisory — most decisions on how to spend resources are taken locally by the health authorities. Second, the priorities of central government may clash with those of staff groups in the NHS. And third, changes in services for groups such as the mentally handicapped have implications for other agencies such as local authorities. Without the agreement and cooperation of such agencies, change may be difficult or impossible to bring about.

Chapter 3

1   Compared with central or local government, DHAs are not very democratic. The members are selected, rather than elected, and the selection process is increasingly under the influence of the Secretary of State. DHAs are severely limited by central government in the decisions they can make about local services. For example, privatisation of services and reductions in the provision of care are measures that DHAs have little or no control over.

2   (a) Rational planning.
    (b) Central.
    (c) Consensus.

3   GPs are vital because it is they who control most referrals to the hospital - patients can only refer themselves directly to the Casualty Department. Thus GPs are a key factor in determining the overall level of work faced by hospitals. And social services and housing are vital because the extent to which some patients need hospital care is heavily dependent on the extent to which alternative forms of care are available in the community. For example, discharging elderly people from hospital depends upon their being alternative community services.

4   (a) 'A manager sets objectives' — planning in the NHS rarely meets the criteria of rational planning. Muddling through is the norm. Moreover, such is the power of doctors, that it is often they as much as the managers who shape the objectives.
    (b) 'A manager organizes' — Drucker's analysis assumes that managers have the power to control the division of labour between occupational groups. But within the NHS this is often not true. For example, the division of doctoring into different types of specialist and the relations between them (e.g. the demarcation agreement between the GPs and the consultants) is decided by the medical profession itself, not by health service managers. Professional bodies, such as Royal Colleges, may also dictate such aspects as the level of staffing that is needed. The same is true also of many occupations that are far less powerful than the doctors, e.g. the maintenance workers

may also have demarcation agreements. Finally, in all of the occupations, but particularly in the case of the doctors, it is very far from the case that it is the managers who analyse which activities are needed. The NHS up till now has been built primarily around the principle of clinical freedom - the right of individual doctors to decide as they think best for their patients.
    (c) 'The manager motivates and communicates' — for the professions in the NHS, the professional bodies such as the Royal Colleges are probably more important for motivation than the managers. Moreover, even amongst the non-professional staff, such as the kitchen-maids, management may not in fact do much in the way of motivation. The maids in Paterson's study clearly did not feel part of a team.
    (d) 'The manager establishes targets and yardsticks' — NHS managers have certainly attempted to do this. However, at present (1985), it is striking just how little basic information is routinely recorded on some major activities, e.g. out-patients. Moreover, even where information is available on the performance of individual doctors, little action is taken compared with, say, the USA. (Finally, insofar as individual appraisal of medical performance does occur, it is often conducted by doctors themselves — not by managers.)
    (e) 'A manager develops people' — there was little sign of this happening amongst Paterson's kitchen-maids. And, at the other end of the scale, most of the development of medical staff is conducted by the profession itself and its elaborate training system. The only staff-development conducted by management has been the attempt to train staff in greater awareness of management and its problems.

Chapter 4

1   As can be seen in Tables 4.1 and 4.2, there are three main areas of complaint: the physical environment of the surgery, waiting area or outpatient department; the length of time spent waiting; and aspects of communication with medical staff. In contrast, fewer people complain about the treatment they receive.

2   (a) Whereas some doctors and nurses often employ a quick-fire style which allows patients little chance to express or elaborate their point of view, the student nurse here explicitly encourages the patient to say more. Her repetition of the word 'sick' enables the patient to elaborate on his or her problems.
    (b) There are several possible answers. At one level, the problem is common to all personal service work. Staff often have many other tasks to do, many patients to see and little time in which to do this. What to them is work of a highly routine kind is to the patient a particular personal problem. This general tendency may be strengthened by the lack of

communications training received by most staff, by an imbalance of power between the two sides, and, in the case of doctors, by the differences in social class, ethnicity and gender.

3 (a) Drug addicts, like 'rubbish' in casualty, may break some of the main rules of the sick role. Some staff may view them, like drunks, as irresponsible — as suffering from self-induced ailments. Staff may also feel that, supposedly like tramps, these people put nothing in to society. However, the treatment that addicts receive is more hostile than that received by deviant patients in casualty. Heroin addicts are engaging in a far more stigmatised activity than that of either tramps or drunks. And while the clinic remains the sole legal source of methadone, its staff have a power over patients' addiction which is not true of that over drunks.

(b) Although some research literature pictures patients as 'unreliable' and there is evidence that, for whatever reason, up to 50 per cent of medications are not taken by patients, most doctors in fact assume that their patients do follow their advice. By contrast, the use of urine tests and good behaviour contracts suggest that staff in Drug Treatment Clinics are convinced that their patients are untrustworthy and that their compliance must be systematically investigated.

4 A private system of nursing care might ensure more personal service for some. There are, however, problems. Patients in all forms of fee-for-service system can be vulnerable to commercial exploitation, due to their lack of technical expertise. But those elderly patients with psychogeriatric conditions are doubly vulnerable, since they may also lack many everyday competences.

Chapter 5

1 (a) The prescriptive use of the term 'community care' refers to the way people with long-term health and social needs might be cared for: maintaining them in their own homes rather than caring for them in isolated institutions.

(b) Community care can be used to describe the services that are involved in caring for people in the community: domiciliary services such as home helps, the support of friends and relatives, day centres, and small homely residential hostels.

(c) The main factors that have promoted community care are the beliefs that it is better and that it is cheaper than institutional care. It is thought to be better because it avoids incarceration and institutionalisation of people, and cheaper because it shifts many of the costs of caring from the public to the private purse.

2 There have been three main reasons:

(a) The slow rate of establishment of alternative forms of care in the community, such as residential hostels. This,

in turn, reflects the financial and managerial difficulties that health and local authorities face in working together.

(b) Unlike mental illness, there are no prospects of medical treatments reducing the size of the population needing care (although it is hoped that preventive measures before and during pregnancy may reduce the number of mentally handicapped children — such measures are discussed further in Chapter 8).

(c) There is thought to have been relatively less family support for mentally handicapped people than for those who are mentally ill.

Chapter 6

1 From what is reported about the 'big banger', it seems likely that its development largely resulted from science-push. Product innovations of this kind tend to arise from scientists and engineers looking around for a use to which they can put their discoveries and new technology. However, the need for an alternative method of treatment to surgery may have contributed an element of market-pull also.

2 (a) The MRC is principally concerned with biomedical research, including that of pure science.

(b) The DHSS concentrates on health services research — the evaluation of the effectiveness, efficiency and humanity of health services.

(c) The pharmaceutical industry's main concern is profit, through the development of new drugs or new combinations of existing ones.

(d) The charities vary in their interests: some, such as the Cancer Research Campaign, concentrate on biomedical research, while others, such as the King Edward Hospital Fund, are interested in health services research.

3 (a) Factors that might assist its introduction would be similar to those that helped CT scanners: it has advantages over the existing treatment; the machine can be tested out by potential customers; it would involve only minor process changes in hospitals; it would be welcomed by the public and the mass media; and it would have the support of a powerful group of clinicians — the surgeons.

(b) The main obstacle it would meet would be its high capital and revenue costs.

Chapter 7

1 The major obstacle would be finding a suitable, objective measure of outcome. The measure would have to reflect the objectives of community care, such as reducing people's levels of dependency — factors that are extremely difficult to quantify. A second obstacle might be resistance from managers or staff involved in providing the service who might feel threatened by such a study of a form of care they were committed to implementing. They might object

on such grounds as the difficulty or impossibility of getting informed consent for an RCT from mentally handicapped people, and the spending of money on a study when the services themselves were short of funds.

2   (a) It may do, but without more information on the effects of such a change, it is not certain that reducing the length of time people stay in hospital is more efficient for the health service. It may be that patients sent home earlier would develop medical problems at home and have to be readmitted for further hospital care.

(b) The efficiency of such a change could be investigated by means of a cost-effectiveness study. The costs and benefits for two groups of patients — one group treated conventionally and the other group sent home three days earlier — would need to be compared.

(c) Using a cost-benefit study, in which are compared the benefits that would result from different uses of the available money. The major difficulty in a cost-benefit study is to find a way of comparing the benefits of diverse uses. For example, comparing the benefits of a residential home for the mentally ill with surgery for varicose veins. One recent attempt to resolve this dilemma is the use of QALYs.

3   The first possible explanation is that women in highter social classes have a greater medical need for hospital care than women in lower social classes. In fact, the opposite is true — virtually all measures of need demonstrate the highest levels in the lower social classes. The same is true of social needs such as poor housing and a lack of domestic help at home. In addition, women in social classes IV and V are likely to be younger and have more children to care for than women in higher social classes.

The difference in length of stay must therefore either reflect the hospital's policy of sending women in lower classes home earlier or the women themselves choosing to leave hospital earlier. The latter might be because they have to get home sooner to look after their other children (their husbands are less likely to be able to get paid leave to help at home) or because women in lower classes may not enjoy being in hospital as much as those from higher classes. This in turn may reflect the predominantly middle-class attitude of hospital staff.

4   Quantitative methods, such as further surveys, are unlikely to provide much more information as to the reason for this high level of dissatisfaction. On the other hand, qualitative methods might reveal why so many people express dissatisfaction. Through in-depth interviews you could find out more about why patients felt dissatisfied. However, it would only be possible to validate their claims by observing the encounters they have with staff.

5   Information on the overall level of prescribing of each GP is not sufficient in itself to know which are the 'good' and the 'bad' practitioners. It may be that the high prescribers are working harder and meeting the needs of all their patients. Alternatively, they may be over-prescribing and being wasteful. On the other hand, the low prescribers may be lazy and under-prescribing or alternatively they may be more discriminatory and offering non-medical treatments, such a counselling. This shows how monitoring only reveals the relative performance of staff or hospitals. The interpretation of such comparisons requires additional information and understanding of the nature of the activity being monitored.

Chapter 8

1   First, the nature of the test. Taking a child's blood pressure would be quite safe, but as you have seen, the repeatability of the test is poor as a person's blood pressure varies considerably over time and its measurement is subject to observer variation. The validity of the test (its sensitivity and specificity) would have to be investigated.

Second you would want to be sure that children with high blood pressure would benefit from being treated. Is there scientific evidence that early treatment of blood pressure actually reduces the risk of heart attacks later in life?

Third, what are going to be the costs of screening all schoolchildren? What is the prevalence of high blood pressure? What are the possible 'hidden' costs of labelling children as having a chronic condition and informing them of the risk they live with — particularly if it turns out there is nothing that can be done?

Finally, could there be some unexpected disadvantages for children found to have high blood pressure, such as disqualification from certain jobs?

Chapter 9

1   It would only be justified if it could be shown that smoking harmed people other than the smoker. This is now known to be so: passive smoking can harm the health of non-smokers. It could also be justified on the grounds that scarce health care resources used for smoking-related diseases were not available for the care of non-smokers when they are ill. However, such an attitude is in danger of victim-blaming — taken to extremes, those suffering from smoking-related diseases would not receive medical treatment.

2   There are four main 'answers' to consider. First, regulation of the price of alcohol by means of regressive taxes, such as excise duty. Second, a change in the legal availability of alcohol by altering licensing laws. There is still debate over what changes should be made to reduce the amount of alcohol-related disease. Third, greater control of

advertising might reduce levels of consumption and assist health education initiatives on the dangers of alcohol abuse. And fourth, action to limit the damage caused by alcohol abuse, such as tougher drink-drive legislation. Some of these measures would have less effect on the personal lives of high-income groups, such as doctors, than on low-income groups. (It is also worth noting that as an occupational group, doctors have one of the highest SMRs for cirrhosis of the liver.)

3 The first point to note is that for each of the four decisions it is unlikely that any of the other three were taken into account. Instead, two other factors were probably of importance — responsibility and explicit costs. If the government feels and is thought by the public to be responsible, then the government is more likely to act. This was true of the Ronan Point disaster (as the government of the day had publicly sponsored the new methods of building construction used in the tower block). Conversely, accidental self-poisoning by children was seen as an individual parental responsibility. Secondly, if the costs of a preventive strategy are explicit and fall on the government — such as the provision of child-proof drug containers — then the implicit value of life will tend to be low. The high implicit values arise as a result of strategies that appear to have no immediate explicit costs — such as a change in the building regulations.

4 The first is the psychological obstacle of persuading any particular individual that they *need* to reduce their consumption. Most people do not drink excessively, and of those who do, few believe that they themselves have a drink problem. The second obstacle is the counteracting influence of the drinks industry which by means of advertising encourages people to drink. The third obstacle is that drink has become progressively cheaper over the years as governments have failed to maintain the real price.

Chapter 10
1 Social insurance was a scheme in which people in employment paid a flat-rate weekly contribution and received in return a basic cash benefit when their earnings were interrupted or lost (e.g. through sickness or unemployment). National assistance was funded out of central taxation and provided cash benefits for those who had no other source of income and were not covered by the insurance scheme. Whereas social insurance was provided on a universal basis, entitlement to national assistance was on the basis of means-testing.

2 First, the Beveridge Plan was built on a model of a two-parent family with a male breadwinner and a dependent wife. Second, that the labour force was primarily made up of full-time male workers who would follow largely uninterrupted employment all their working lives. Third, they would earn enough to keep themselves and a dependent wife and child. And fourth, full employment would be maintained.

3 The radical right has argued that the post-war welfare system has seriously damaged national economic prosperity and threatened personal freedom. In their view, it is only through a free market that economic efficiency can be achieved, and that political freedom can only be guaranteed by a system of complete economic freedom.

The Marxist left argues that post-war economic policy has simply been postponing the working out of certain inherent contradictions in capitalism. While welfare spending contains some progresssive features that alleviate some aspects of social and economic deprivation, it also serves to maintain the capitalist system by ensuring a trained, healthy workforce is available. Thus while the positive aspects need expanding, the negative aspects call for radical revisions of the welfare system.

4 The *Black Report* recommendations both supported the welfare state and radical changes to social and economic structures, such as the redistribution of income and wealth. One explanation for this is that the working group believed that it was possible to bring about radical change gradually, rather than changing the complete system. Alternatively the group, while believing that radical change was needed, may have accepted the impossibility of achieving a national consensus for such change and therefore adopted a more pragmatic approach.

Chapter 11
1 There have been a number of reasons. First, RCTs of surgical operations are expensive to perform — the third CABG trial cost $24 million (in the 1970s). Second, the results of the three RCTs have been inconsistent — they have included different categories of patients; medical treatment for the control groups has varied; and surgical skills have varied.

2 Very few people have levels of cholesterol over 300 mg/ 100 ml. So even though the risk of death from CHD for these individuals might be markedly reduced, because they are few in number this would have little impact on the population mortality rate. The majority of people dying from CHD have blood cholesterol levels around the 'normal' level.

3 First, the control of medical research funds is largely in the hands of doctors and scientists who adhere to biomedical explanations of disease. Second, research into psycho-social factors presents greater difficulties: factors are harder to define and quantification is awkward. Third, biomedical explanations lend themselves to biomedical

responses, which often provide commercial and financial benefits to individual practitioners and industrial enterprises. Finally, psycho-social explanations may require changes in social and economic conditions and structures rather than measures aimed at changing the behaviour of individuals. The former tends to be resisted by those with an interest in the status quo.

Acknowledgements

Grateful acknowledgement is made to the following sources for material used in this book:

Text

'A worker's speech to a doctor' by Bertolt Brecht, trans. Frank Jellinick, Methuen, London, 1976; 'The fence or the ambulance' by Joseph Malines, in *Journal of the Soil Association*, vol. 7, no. 4, 1953; D. Steel, 'Managing Health Authorities: one member's view' in *Public Money*, June 1984, © 1984 *Public Money*, *Public Money* is available on subscription from the publishers, Chartered Institute of Public Finance and Accountancy, 3 Robert Street, London; D. Taylor, *Understanding the NHS in the 1980s'*, OHE, 1984.

Tables

Table 2.2 from K. Davis and D. Rowland, 'Uninsured and undeserved' in *Millbank Memorial Fund Quarterly*, vol. 61, no. 2, 1983; *Table 3.1* from M. J. Bloor, *et al.* 'Geographical variations on the incidence of operations on the tonsils and adenoids' in *Journal of Laryngology and Otology* vol. XCII, 1978; *Table 4.1* from A. Cartwright and R. Anderson, *General Practice Revisited*, Tavistock Publications, 1981; *Table 4.3* from J. Clark, in *Nursing Times*, 1 January, 1981; *Table 4.4* from P. Ley, 'Satisfaction, compliance and communication' in *British Journal of Clinical Psychology*, vol. 21, 1982; *Table 4.6* from D. L. Rosenhan, 'On being sane in insane places' in *Science*, vol. 179, 19 January, 1973, copyright © 1973 by AAAS; *Table 4.8* from D. A. Pendelton and S. Bochner, in *Social Science and Medicine*, vol. 14A, Pergamon Press, 1980; *Tables 5.1 and 5.4* from *Health Care UK 1985*, edited by Anthony Harrison and John Gretton, available from CIPFA, 3 Robert Street, London, price £24.50, all rights reserved by Policy Journals Ltd; *Tables 5.3 and 6.1* reproduced by permission of the Controller of HMSO; *Table 7.1* from R. Roser and V. Watts, 'The Measurement of hospital output' in *International Journal of Epidemiology*, vol. 11, no. 4, 1972; *Table 7.3* from J. Le Grand, 'The distribution of public expenditure' in *Economica*, vol. 45, 1978, Ticto Ltd; *Table 7.5* © MORI/*Sunday Times*, 28 December, 1980; *Table 9.3* from R. Hallett, 'Why do we still dice with death?' in *New Society*, 11 September, 1980; *Table 10.4* from D. Lipsey, 'Cost of tax relief schemes soars' in *The Sunday Times*, 27 January, 1985; *Table 10.7* from A. Maddison, *Phases of Capitalist Development*, Oxford University Press, 1982.

Figures

Figures 2.6, 2.18, 5.5, 5.7, 6.3 and 12.1 reproduced by permission of the Controller of HMSO; *Figure 2.12* Gina Glover/Photo Co-op; *Figure 2.20* from H. Trent, 'What the public wants', in *Health and Social Services Journal*, 1981; *Figure 3.2* Crown Copyright (COI); *Figure 3.5* courtesy of Royal College of Physicians; *Figure 3.6* from R. Dowie, *General Practitioners and Consultants: a study of outpatients referrals*, King's Fund/Oxford University Press, 1983; *Figure 3.8 Bradford Argus*; *Figure 4.1* from A. Davis, *Relationships between Doctors and Patients*, Gower, 1978; *Figure 4.2* from 'How much do you know?', *Self Health*, no. 2, 1984; *Figure 5.1* Aerofilms; *Figure 5.2* Vicky White/Photo Co-op; *Figure 5.4* Corry Bevington/Photo Co-op; *Figure 5.6* Gina Glover/Photo Co-op; *Figure 5.9* Vicky White/Photo Co-op; *Figure 5.10* Vicky White/Photo Co-op; *Figure 6.2 New Scientist*, December 1984; *Figure 6.5* from *Charity statistics 1983/4*, Charities Aid Foundation; *Figure 6.7* courtesy of I.G.E. Medical Systems Ltd; *Figure 6.9* Camera Press; *Figure 7.2* from A. A. Rimm and M. Bortin, 'Trialism' in *Biomedicine: Special Issue*, vol. 68, 1978, Masson S. A., Paris; *Figure 7.3* courtesy of A. Monk and Co. Ltd; *Figure 8.1* PACE; *Figure 9.1* courtesy of Sheffield Environmental Health Department/Central Policy Unit, 1984; *Figure 9.3* from P. Taylor, *Smoke Ring*, Bodley Head Ltd, 1984; *Figure 9.5* from C. Wells, *Bones, Body and Disease*, Thames and Hudson, 1964; *Figure 9.6* from J. A. Spring and D. H. Buss, 'Three centuries of alcohol in the British diet' in *Nature*, vol. 25, © Macmillan Journals, 1977; *Figure 9.7* from D. Taylor, *Alcohol*, Office of Health Economics, 1981; *Figure 9.8* HEC/*British Medical Journal*; *Figure 9.9* Royal College of Physicians, *Health and Smoking*, by permission of Pitman Publishing Ltd, London; *Figure 9.10* from D. Simpson, in *Postgraduate Medical Journal*, vol. 60, no. 699, 1984; *Figure 9.11* reproduced by kind permission of the Health Education Council, London; *Figure 10.1* Associated Newspapers Ltd; *Figure 10.2* courtesy of NUM; *Figure 10.3* from A. W. Dilnot, *et al.*, *The Reform of Social Security*, Oxford University Press, 1984; *Figure 10.4* Crispin Hughes/Photo Co-op; *Figure 11.9* from K. P. Ball, 'The Heart Patient' in *Update*, January 1979, Update Publications; *Figure 11.11* from G. Rose and M. Marmot, 'Social class and CHD' in *British Heart Journal*, vol. 45, 1981; *Figure 12.3* from *Nature*, vol. 300, no. 5893, 1982 © Macmillan Journals Ltd.

Index

Entries and page numbers in **bold type** refer to key words
which are printed in *italic* in the text.
NB: Sub-entries are in alphabetical order except
where page order is more significant.
NHS is used as an abbreviation for National Health Service.